D0022877

Strategic Human Resources Management in Health Services Organizations

Strategic Human Resources Management in Health Services Organizations

Third Edition

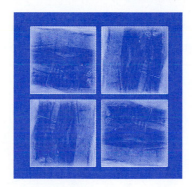

Edited by

S. Robert Hernandez, DrPH

Professor and Director
Doctoral Program in
Administration/Health Services
Department of Health Services Administration
University of Alabama at Birmingham
Birmingham, AL

Stephen J. O'Connor, PhD, FACHE

Professor and Director, MSHA Program
Department of Health Services Administration
University of Alabama at Birmingham
Birmingham, AL

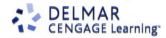

Australia • Brazil • Japan • Korea • Mexico • Singapore • Spain • United Kingdom • United States

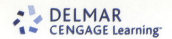
DELMAR
CENGAGE Learning

Strategic Human Resources Management in Health Services Organizations, Third Edition
S. Robert Hernandez, Stephen J. O'Connor

Vice President, Career and Professional Editorial: Dave Garza

Director of Learning Solutions: Matthew Kane

Senior Acquisitions Editor: Tari Broderick

Managing Editor: Marah Bellegarde

Product Manager: Natalie Pashoukos

Editorial Assistant: Anthony Souza

Vice President, Career and Professional Marketing: Jennifer McAvey

Marketing Director: Wendy Mapstone

Marketing Manager: Michelle McTighe

Marketing Coordinator: Scott Chrysler

Production Director: Carolyn Miller

Production Manager: Andrew Crouth

Senior Content Project Manager: James Zayicek

Project Manager: Pre-PressPMG

Senior Art Director: Jack Pendleton

© 2010, 1994 Delmar, Cengage Learning

ALL RIGHTS RESERVED. No part of this work covered by the copyright herein may be reproduced, transmitted, stored, or used in any form or by any means graphic, electronic, or mechanical, including but not limited to photocopying, recording, scanning, digitizing, taping, Web distribution, information networks, or information storage and retrieval systems, except as permitted under Section 107 or 108 of the 1976 United States Copyright Act, without the prior written permission of the publisher.

For product information and technology assistance, contact us at
Professional & Career Group Customer Support, 1-800-648-7450

For permission to use material from this text or product, submit all requests online at **cengage.com/permissions**. Further permissions questions can be emailed to **permissionrequest@cengage.com**.

Library of Congress Control Number: 2009927671

ISBN-13: 978-0-7668-3540-5

ISBN-10: 0-7668-3540-5

Delmar
5 Maxwell Drive
Clifton Park, NY 12065-2919
USA

Cengage Learning products are represented in Canada by Nelson Education, Ltd.

For your lifelong learning solutions, visit **delmar.cengage.com**

Visit our corporate website at **cengage.com**

Notice to the Reader
Publisher does not warrant or guarantee any of the products described herein or perform any independent analysis in connection with any of the product information contained herein. Publisher does not assume, and expressly disclaims, any obligation to obtain and include information other than that provided to it by the manufacturer. The reader is expressly warned to consider and adopt all safety precautions that might be indicated by the activities described herein and to avoid all potential hazards. By following the instructions contained herein, the reader willingly assumes all risks in connection with such instructions. The publisher makes no representations or warranties of any kind, including but not limited to, the warranties of fitness for particular purpose or merchantability, nor are any such representations implied with respect to the material set forth herein, and the publisher takes no responsibility with respect to such material. The publisher shall not be liable for any special, consequential, or exemplary damages resulting, in whole or part, from the readers' use of, or reliance upon, this material.

Printed in the United States of America
1 2 3 4 5 XX 11 10 09

CONTENTS

P A R T
ONE
Strategy and Organization Systems/1

P A R T
TWO
Organizing for Human Resources/61

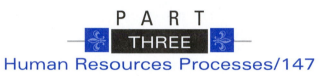

P A R T

THREE

Human Resources Processes/147

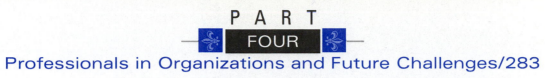

P A R T
FOUR
Professionals in Organizations and Future Challenges/283

ACKNOWLEDGMENTS

There are a number of individuals we wish to acknowledge and thank for their contributions to this book. Alice Johnson, a student in the Master of Science in Health Administration program at the University of Alabama at Birmingham provided significant and invaluable assistance to us on many aspects of this project. Gouri Gupte, Anantachai (Tony) Panjamapirom, David Au, and Katrina Graham, doctoral students in Health Services Administration at UAB provided superb research assistance. Our faculty colleagues and administrators at UAB continue to uphold a stimulating and encouraging work environment that is supportive of our work.

This book would have been impossible without significant editorial, production, and marketing support. Natalie Pashoukos of Cengage Learning worked closely with us throughout the entire process of developing the manuscript, keeping us on task, and ensuring our best work. Rathi Thirumalai of Pre-PressPMG worked personally with all of the authors through the final stages of production. Her attention to detail, patience, and agreeable demeanor was greatly appreciated. Tari Broderick, Senior Acquisitions Editor at Cengage Learning encouraged our ideas and was a positive resource for us as we entered the final phase of this project.

A special thanks to our wives, Joy and Vicki, for their support and encouragement of this book. Dr. O'Connor wishes to acknowledge his daughters, Lauren and Maggie, for the important place they fill in his life.

Finally, to our many remarkable colleagues who authored their respective chapters, our sincere appreciation for their time, effort, and professionalism. We will be eternally in their debt for their efforts.

PREFACE

The Third Edition of *Strategic Human Resources Management in Health Services Organizations* is designed for those interested in a broad understanding of the human resources management function in health care organizations, especially as it relates to organizational strategy, behavior, and design. The principal audiences for this book are graduate students in health services administration and management as well as health policy programs. It should also be of value to students in undergraduate and executive education courses as well as professional health services managers seeking the most current thinking and developments in the field.

WHY WE WROTE THIS TEXT

The human resources function in health care continues its evolution from the "Personnel Department"—traditionally an organizational backwater concerned with maintaining employee records and meeting payroll—to a modern, sophisticated activity that is centrally important to the strategic, operational, and clinical goals of any health care organization. Given the speed and intensity of change in the health care environment, it is more important than ever for health care human resources departments to become an integral part of the organization's strategy. Regrettably, many have not advanced as far from the traditional "Personnel Department" as we might think. This absence of strategic orientation can be attributed to continued growth in the number of labor laws and a traditional mindset that is more inwardly and operationally directed, resulting in a situation whereby many human resource functions remain chiefly concerned with staying within the laws and pursuing operational consistency of procedures and processes. The latter occurs despite a health care workforce that is becoming more diverse and multifaceted.

A contemporary approach to human resources is essential as health care is extremely labor-intensive and continues its emphasis on productivity, quality, and cost containment. A strong human resources function is necessary for building a staff that is adequate in number, sufficiently qualified, easy to recruit, motivate, retain, and appropriately balanced in terms of organizational needs. It is also essential for achieving strategic goals. The field of health care management requires an up-to-date human resources management book which advances our understanding of these important functions.

ORGANIZATION OF THE TEXT

The book is organized into four parts. Part One examines strategy and organization systems as it relates to human resources, including the legal and financial environment. Part Two focuses on organizing for human resources, emphasizing the health care workforce, human resource management competencies, culture, workforce diversity, and leadership development. Part Three deals with human resources processes including job analysis, recruitment and retention, selection and onboarding, training and development, performance appraisal, compensation, and labor relations. Part Four addresses physicians in health care organizations and future human resources challenges.

FEATURES

Each chapter begins with several principal learning objectives to be achieved. In addition, a new feature to this edition is the introduction of key terms within each chapter and a glossary at the end of the book which provides definitions for these terms. This feature will allow the reader to easily find definitions of concepts, principles, or terms with which they may not be familiar. Other features include end-of-chapter summaries, practical managerial guidelines, discussion questions, a chapter case and case discussion questions. Some chapters include additional case studies, learning vignettes, and illustrations.

NEW TO THIS EDITION

Seven chapters have been significantly revised and ten are completely new to this edition. New chapters addressing important trends in the field and new developments in human resources include the health care workforce, human resources management competencies, leadership development, succession planning and mentoring, job analysis, personnel selection and onboarding, training and development, compensation principles, and a focus on physicians.

SUPPLEMENTARY PACKAGE/ ANCILLARY MATERIALS

A supplementary teaching package is available that corresponds closely to each of the respective chapters, allowing for a comprehensive teaching experience. Resources include PowerPoint presentation slides, a test bank with answers, and an Instructor's Resource Guide.

CONTRIBUTORS

G. Ross Baker, PhD
Professor
Department of Health Policy, Management and
    Evaluation
Faculty of Medicine
University of Toronto
Toronto, Ontario, Canada

Lee W. Bewley, PhD, FACHE
Program Director and Assistant Professor
Graduate Program in Health and Business
    Administration
U.S. Army-Baylor University
Fort Sam Houston, Texas

Richard L. Clarke, DHA, FHFMA
President and CEO
Healthcare Financial Management Association
Westchester, Illinois

Stephen N. Collier, PhD
Professor and Director
Office of Health Professions Education and
    Workforce Development
School of Health Professions
University of Alabama at Birmingham
Birmingham, Alabama

Leonard H. Friedman, PhD, MPH
Professor and Director
Department of Health Services Management
    and Leadership
George Washington University
Washington, DC

Andrew N. Garman, PsyD, MS
Associate Chair
Health Systems Management Department
Rush University
Chicago, Illinois

Katrina Graham, MBA
Doctoral Candidate
PhD Program in Administration-Health
    Services
Department of Health Services
    Administration
University of Alabama at Birmingham
Birmingham, Alabama

S. Robert Hernandez, DrPH
Professor and Director
PhD Program in Administration-Health
    Services
Department of Health Services
    Administration
School of Health Professions
University of Alabama at Birmingham
Birmingham, Alabama

William F. Jessee, MD, FACMPE
President and CEO
Medical Group Management Association
Englewood, Colorado

Alesia Jones, CCP, MBA
Interim Chief Human Resources Officer
University of Alabama at Birmingham
Birmingham, Alabama

Naresh Khatri, PhD
Associate Professor
Department of Health Management and
    Informatics
School of Medicine
University of Missouri
Columbia, Missouri

Amy Yarbrough Landry, PhD
Assistant Professor
Department of Health Services Administration
School of Health Professions
University of Alabama at Birmingham
Birmingham, Alabama

Christy Harris Lemak, PhD
Associate Professor
Department of Health Management and Policy
School of Public Health
University of Michigan
Ann Arbor, Michigan

Louise Lemieux-Charles, PhD
Professor
Department of Health Policy, Management and
    Evaluation
Faculty of Medicine
University of Toronto
Toronto, Ontario, Canada

Cheryl Locke, BA
Vice President and Chief Human Resources
    Officer
Wake Forest University Baptist Medical Center
Winston-Salem, North Carolina

Stephen J. O'Connor, PhD, FACHE
Professor and Director
Master of Science in Health Administration
    Program
Department of Health Services Administration
School of Health Professions
University of Alabama at Birmingham
Birmingham, Alabama

Anantachai Panjamapirom, MS, MBA
Doctoral Candidate
PhD Program in Administration-Health
    Services
Department of Health Services Administration
University of Alabama at Birmingham
Birmingham, Alabama

Elena Platonova, PhD
Assistant Professor
Department of Public Health Sciences
College of Health and Human Services
University of North Carolina at Charlotte
Charlotte, North Carolina

E. José Proenca, PhD
Professor and Department Head
Department of Management, Health and
    Human Resources
School of Management
Widener University
Chester, Pennsylvania

Daniel P. Russell, MS
Senior Vice President and Regional Practice
    Leader
Aon Consulting
Atlanta, Georgia

Grant T. Savage, PhD
Chair and Health Management and Informatics
    Alumni Distinguished Professor
Department of Health Management and
    Informatics
School of Medicine
University of Missouri
Columbia, Missouri

Winsor Schmidt, JD, LLM
Professor and Chair
Department of Health Policy and
    Administration
Washington State University
Spokane, Washington

Connie Schott, MBA, SPHR
SchottWorks LLC
Human Resources Consulting and Coaching
Gainesville, Florida

Richard M. Shewchuk, PhD
Professor
Department of Health Services Administration
School of Health Professions
University of Alabama at Birmingham
Birmingham, Alabama

Windsor Westbrook Sherrill, PhD, MBA, MHA
Associate Professor
Department of Public Health Sciences
Clemson University
Clemson, South Carolina

J. Larry Tyler, FAAHC, FACHE, FHFMA, CMPE
CEO and Chairman
Tyler & Company
Atlanta, Georgia

Barbara A. Wech, PhD
Associate Professor
Department of Management, Information
   Systems, and Quantitative Methods
School of Business
University of Alabama at Birmingham
Birmingham, Alabama

REVIEWERS

Gregory O. Ginn, PhD
Associate Professor of Health Care
Administration and Policy
University of Nevada
Las Vegas, Nevada

Lloyd Greene, EdD
Senior Lecturer, School of Health
Administration
Texas State University
San Marcos, Texas

Judith Schiffert, EdD
Professor, Graduate Program in Health Services
Administration
D'Youville College
Williamsville, New York

Pamela Walsh, PhD, MPH
Assistant Professor, Health Administration
Eastern Michigan University
Ypsilanti, Michigan

ONE

Strategy and Organization Systems

CHAPTER 1

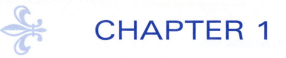

Integrating Strategic Management and Human Resources

S. Robert Hernandez, DrPH and Stephen J. O'Connor, PhD, FACHE

LEARNING OBJECTIVES

Upon completing this chapter, the reader will be able to:

1. Describe and discuss the changing health care environment and its impact on human resources.
2. Describe and discuss a model for the strategic management of human resources in health services organizations.
3. Describe and discuss the structural, behavioral, and human resource systems that impact health care organizational outcomes.

KEY TERMS

Contingency Theory

Job Analysis

Job Description

Mission

Performance Appraisal

Six Sigma

Strategic Human Resource Management

Strategic Planning

INTRODUCTION

Like most other service industries, the health care industry is very labor intensive. One reason for the reliance on an extensive workforce is that it is not possible to produce a "service" and store it for subsequent consumption. The production and consumption of the service occurs simultaneously. Thus, the interaction between consumers and health care professionals is an integral part of the provision of health services. Given the dependence on health care professionals for service delivery, the possibility of heterogeneity of service quality must be recognized, both within an employee as skills and competencies change over time and among employees as different individuals or representatives of different professions provide a service.

The intensive use of labor for service delivery and the possibility of variability in professional practice require that the attention of health care leaders be directed toward managing the performance of the professionals involved in service delivery. The effective management of people requires that health services executives understand the factors that influence the performance of individuals employed in their organizations. These factors include not only the traditional human resources management activities (i.e., recruitment and selection, training and development, appraisal, compensation, employee relations) but also environmental and other organizational factors that impinge on human resources activities.

The strategic management of human resources ensures that qualified, motivated personnel are available to staff the portfolio of business units that are operated by the organization. This book explains and illustrates the methods and practices that can be used to increase the probability that competent personnel will be available to provide the services delivered by the organization and that these personnel will perform necessary tasks appropriately. Implementing these methods and practices means that requirements for positions must be determined, qualified persons must be recruited and selected, employees must be trained and developed to meet future organizational needs, and adequate rewards must be provided to attract and retain top performers.

Of course, these functions are performed within the context of the overall activities of the organization. They are influenced or constrained by the environment, the **mission** and strategies that are being pursued, the structure of the organization, and the behavioral systems indigenous to the institution. To manage human resources strategically, health care executives must understand the relationships that exist among these important organizational components and the human resources functions so that appropriate methods can be selected to accomplish service delivery objectives desired by the organization.

The next section presents an overview of fundamental changes occurring in the health services environment that affect the numbers, types, and roles of health practitioners. This material is followed by a model of the relationships that exist among strategy, selected organizational design features, and human resources management activities.

Health Care Workforce

In the United States, employment in the health services industry has grown more rapidly than overall employment. In 1900, persons employed in health occupations accounted for 1.2% of the labor force. This proportion increased to 2.1% in 1940, 3.0% in 1960, and 7.6% in 1990 (Freudenheim, 1990; U.S. Department of Labor, Bureau of Labor Statistics, 1990). The health care workforce accounted for about 13.6 million jobs in 2006, making it the largest industry in the United States. Between 2006 and 2016, total employment in the health care industry will rise by 21.7% through the addition of 3 million new jobs. This level of employment growth will exceed that of any other industry sector (U.S. Department of Labor, Bureau of Health Statistics, 2007).

Changes in the types and characteristics of health professionals have been dramatic. Health professions requiring a college education or professional preparation accounted for approximately 200,000 persons in 1900 as compared to 4.9 million in 1990 (Ginzberg, 1990; U.S. Department of Health, Education, and Welfare, 1970). For instance, in 1900, three in five health professionals were physicians. By 1990, rapid growth in other occupations reduced the proportion of physicians to about one in eight professional health workers (Ginzberg, 1990). A further decline is expected as other disciplines experience more rapid rates of growth and as new categories of personnel emerge.

The most rapid growth in the supply of health professionals has occurred in the recently developed occupations of physician assistants, nurse practitioners, multiskilled health practitioners, laboratory technicians, occupational and physical therapists, medical records personnel, radiologic technologists, and so forth. More than two-thirds of all people employed in the health care industry in 1990 were employed as nontraditional allied health or support service personnel (U.S. Bureau of the Census, 1991).

The primary reasons for this growth in these nontraditional health occupations were the interrelated forces of technological change, specialization, and the emergence of the hospital as the central focus of the health care system. The technological revolution led to the increased concentration and specialization of numerous types of health personnel in acute care hospitals.

Table 1.1 provides an overview of the estimated supply of selected health care personnel from 1970 to 2000. Few industries have the diversity of personnel and the wide variation in educational preparation, technical skills, professional responsibilities, and professional values seen in health services. Preparation ranges from 6 to 8 weeks of on-the-job training for nursing assistants to more than 10 years of post baccalaureate education for some medical specialties. Health practitioners share a common duty to provide services to consumers, but diversity exists in the responsibilities of these groups.

The numbers of practitioners and their roles have evolved over time and are expected to undergo radical change because of three factors that have transformed the health services industry. These factors are scientific and technological change, patterns of utilization, and funding for health services.

Advances in scientific understanding and technology in health services have triggered significant change in the industry and in the responsibilities of practitioners. Individual roles have become more specialized, since one person or profession cannot possess all the knowledge in a specific area of medicine. This has caused not only specialization of medical practice but also the creation of new types of health practitioners with up-to-date and unique skills to staff new technologies.

The evolution of medical knowledge, concentration of technological capability in the hospital, and improved reimbursement have led to increases in the absolute number of employees in non-federal short-term general hospitals from 662,000 in 1950 (American Hospital Association, 1986) to over 4 million in 2005 (American Hospital Association, 2007). Recent changes in utilization of services have occurred because of a number of factors described elsewhere (Shi & Singh, 2007). Hospital admissions and patient days per 1000 population appear to have peaked in the 1970s, after years of increase. The absolute number of hospital admissions for non-federal short-term general hospitals have increased every year from 1994 to 2005 (American Hospital Association, 2007).

Certainly, more extensive discussions are available on the health services industry (Shi & Singh, 2007; Starr, 1982; Williams & Torrens, 2008), the health professions labor force (Barton, 1999; U.S. Department of Health and Human Services, 2007), and personnel planning (Bach & Sisson, 2001). This brief review suggests that the labor force expanded and became specialized during the past 50 years in response to increased utilization of services. A more in-depth discussion and overview of the health care workforce and future trends in the United States is presented in Chapter 4.

Environmental shifts that influence demand for services and trends in the health labor force must

Table 1.1. Estimated Supply of Selected Health Personnel and Practitioner-To-Population Ratios, Selected Years: 1970–2000.

Health Occupation	Estimated Active Supply				Percent Change	
	1970	1980	1990	2000	1970–2000	1995–2000
Number						
Physicians	323,800	453,100	601,700	782,200	141.6	14.7
Allopathic (MD)	311,200	435,500	572,700	737,500	137	14.2
Osteopathic (DO)	12,600	17,600	29,000	44,700	254.8	25.2
Dentists	96,000	121,900	147,500	168,000	75	9.6
Optometrists	18,400	21,900	26,000	32,200	75	11.4
Pharmacists	112,600	142,400	168,000	196,100	74.2	8.3
Veterinarians	25,900	36,500	48,700	60,100	132	9.5
Registered nurses	750,000	1,272,900	1,789,600	2,201,800	193.6	4.1
Practitioners per 100,000 Population						
Physicians	155.6	195.9	237	279.8	79.8	9.7
Allopathic (MD)	149.6	188.3	225.6	263.8	76.4	9.1
Osteopathic (DO)	6.1	7.6	11.4	16	164	19.7
Dentists	46.5	53.2	58.7	60.7	30.5	4.7
Optometrists	9	9.6	10.4	11.7	30	6.4
Pharmacists	55.2	62.7	67.3	71.3	29.2	3.5
Veterinarians	12.7	16.1	19.5	21.8	71.7	4.3
Registered nurses	367.7	560.2	717.4	807.4	119.6	0.3

SOURCE: U.S. Department of Health and Human Services (2007). National Center for Health Workforce Analysis: U.S. Health Workforce Personnel Factbook. Accessed December 21, 2007, from http://bhpr.hrsa.gov.

be considered during human resources planning. It cannot be assumed that skilled personnel will be freely available in the labor market when services are started or expanded; thus, adequate time for recruitment and training must be allowed. When services are downsized or terminated, use of tactics such as attrition or employee retraining may reduce the probability that layoffs and terminations will be required. Attention to external trends and proper planning provides for the maintenance of the organizational staff at near optimum levels of size, skills, and experience. It also reduces problems from personnel shortages or surpluses such as reductions in quality, inefficiencies, inability to deliver services, and practitioner dissatisfaction.

STRATEGIC MANAGEMENT OF HUMAN RESOURCES

Among the major environmental trends affecting health care institutions are the changing financing arrangements, the emergence of new competitors, changes in physician/health care organizational relationships, changes in workforce demographics, increases in the number of uninsured, technological changes, and capital shortages. The result has been increased competition, the need for higher levels of performance, and concern for institutional survival. Many health care organizations are providing services with fewer resources, changing their organizational structures and/or job designs, and developing leaner management structures with fewer levels and wider spans of control. Moreover, many are incorporating techniques such as **Six Sigma** efforts to significantly improve quality and change operational processes (Langabeer, 2009). Others are seeking positive, systemic, transformative change to become an employer of choice by seeking Nurse Magnet Status or the Malcolm Baldrige Award.

Strategic human resource management involves generating and implementing human resource policies and practices to supply the complement of employee skills, knowledge, and abilities required by an organization to attain its strategic aspirations.

A variety of major competitive strategies might be pursued to respond to a changing environment, including low-cost provision of traditional health services, offering superior patient service through high technical quality or attentive customer service, or specialization into a few key clinical areas. Hence, staffing profiles are increasingly characterized by a limited number of highly skilled and well-compensated professionals. At the same time, most health care organizations are experiencing shortages of nursing and various other types of health professional personnel.

Involving key personnel such as human resources managers in strategy formulation is crucial to the success of any strategic plan. For example, if the human resources executives are not actively involved, then the employee planning, recruitment, selection, development, appraisal, and compensation necessary for successful implementation are not likely to occur. Dessler (2008) has noted: "[T]op management needs the input of the human resource team in designing the strategy, since it is the team charged with hiring, training, and compensating the firm's employees" (p. 87). As such, "[h]uman resource professionals need to understand the basics of **strategic planning** and the basic business functions such as accounting,

finance, production, and sales, so they can take (as human resource advocates put it) their 'seat at the table' when top management is crafting the firm's strategic plan."

Such an approach to strategic human resources management activities includes human resource professionals in formulating the organization's strategy, determining the human resources requirements based on that strategy, comparing the current inventory of personnel to the future organizational requirements, developing plans and tactics to ensure that the necessary personnel are available, and implementing the appropriate practices to reinforce the strategy. Figure 1.1 provides some examples of possible linkages between strategic decisions and human resources management practices. There is fairly strong evidence that organizations utilizing more progressive (i.e., strategically linked) human resources approaches achieve significantly better financial results than comparable (but less progressive) organizations (Gomez-Mejia, 1988; Kravetz, 1988).

An organization that is managed strategically ensures that the functional and operational administrative systems are linked to the strategic and tactical decision-making activities of the organization. The planning, control, and management systems must be joined for the organization to be able to ensure that the plans developed by senior management are executed as intended.

As illustrated in Figure 1.2, organizations are complex entities that require constant interaction with the environment. If they are to remain viable, health services organizations must adapt their strategies to external changes. The internal components of the organization are then affected by these changes in that shifts in the organization's strategy potentially necessitate modifications in the internal structural systems, behavioral systems, and human resources process systems. There must be harmony, in turn, among these systems. The characteristics, performance levels, and the amount of coherence in operating practices among these systems influence the outcomes achieved in terms of organizational- and employee-level measures of performance.

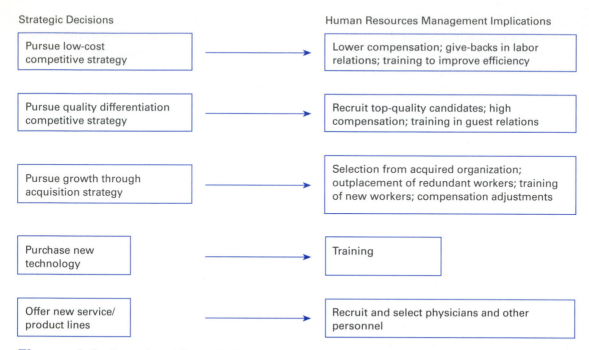

Strategic Decisions

Human Resources Management Implications

| Pursue low-cost competitive strategy | → | Lower compensation; give-backs in labor relations; training to improve efficiency |

| Pursue quality differentiation competitive strategy | → | Recruit top-quality candidates; high compensation; training in guest relations |

| Pursue growth through acquisition strategy | → | Selection from acquired organization; outplacement of redundant workers; training of new workers; compensation adjustments |

| Purchase new technology | → | Training |

| Offer new service/ product lines | → | Recruit and select physicians and other personnel |

Figure 1.1. **Examples of Strategic Decisions and Corresponding Human Resources Management Implications**

The strategic management of human resources involves attention to the effects of environmental and internal components on the human resources process system. Because of the critical role of health professionals in delivering services in this labor-intensive industry, a major concern of health services managers should be the development of personnel policies and practices that are closely related to, influenced by, and supportive of the strategic thrust of their organizations. In addition, managers must ensure that the human resources functions are linked to the other internal design features of the organization.

Organizations, either explicitly or implicitly, pursue a strategy in their operations. Deciding on a strategy means to determine the products or services that will be produced and the markets to which the chosen services will be offered. Once these selections have been made, the methods to be used to compete in the chosen market must be

identified. The methods adopted are based on internal resources available, or potentially available, for use by managers.

As illustrated in Figure 1.2, strategies should be based on consideration of environmental conditions and organizational capabilities. To be in a position to take advantage of opportunities that are anticipated to occur, as well as to parry potential threats from changed conditions or competitor initiatives, managers must have detailed knowledge of the current and future operating environment. Cognizance of internal strengths and weaknesses allows management to develop plans based on an accurate assessment of the firm's ability to perform in the marketplace at the desired level.

A more detailed discussion of the significance of the legal and economic environment is presented in Chapter 2. Chapter 3 focuses on a more detailed discussion of approaches for determining organization strategy.

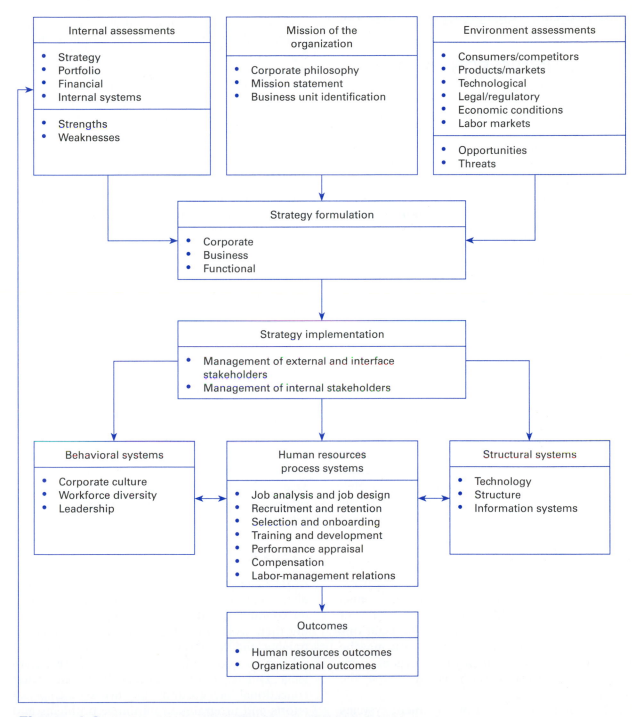

Figure 1.2. **Model of the Strategic Management of Human Resources**

ORGANIZING FOR HUMAN RESOURCES

The structure of an organization has a profound effect on the activities of employees. Structural concerns include deciding how task responsibilities will be allocated among employees and determining how coordination among the tasks will be achieved (Mintzberg, 1979), and these involve two features. One is the formal allocation of work roles to individuals; the second is the use of administrative mechanisms to control and integrate work activity.

Implementation of strategies occurs through specific programs or services by the assignment of work to individuals, the control of worker activities so that standards of performance are achieved, and the coordination of tasks among workers for efficient operation. Thus, organizational structure should be determined by the strategy being pursued by the organization, since different strategies require work routines, control methods, and coordination patterns of distinctive types.

The actual delivery of health services, the provision of most support functions, the development of plans, and the coordination and control of work occur through the behavior of people and the processes by which they interact. Thus, the ability to achieve an organizational strategy depends on the nexus between organizational management systems and the mission and objectives of the institution.

The actions and behaviors of individuals within the organization constitute a major focus of management systems. If management is sensitive to the personal and professional requisites of these individuals, their needs and expectations from participation in the organization may be translated into commitment to the organization and motivation to accomplish tasks desired by the institution.

Additional emphasis of management systems is on group attributes, the quality of leadership available for guiding the institution through major change, and the corporate culture (i.e., the characteristic day-to-day internal environment that is experienced and shared by those working within the organization). The approaches to leadership and organizational change must be handled properly and linked to the mission of the firm if human resources are to be directed strategically by management.

Corporate Culture

The system of informal customs and rules that transmit the behaviors expected of employees in most situations constitutes corporate culture. The quality of the relationship between the culture of an organization and its strategy has significant implications for the potential performance of that organization. Strong cultures do an excellent job of transmitting the values and beliefs of the organization to the individual. Thus, individuals are able to determine what they are to do in the vast number of situations for which no formal rules or guidelines exist.

Corporate culture should complement the human resources management process systems. The shared values and expectations that are reinforced by culture should blend with the systems that have been established for selecting organizational members, developing their skills, and rewarding desirable behavior. It is important that management assess cultural norms and plan interventions as required. Methods for managing the corporate culture are discussed in Chapter 6.

Workforce Diversity

As the demographic characteristics of the U.S. population are changing, health care organizations face the continuing challenge of managing and integrating their workforce. The recruitment, selection, training, and development of ethnic minorities and other nontraditional employees also pose a challenge. Differences in language, culture, values, and educational backgrounds may necessitate special efforts and programs to minimize problems and conflict. The management of a diverse workforce is discussed in Chapter 7.

Leadership Development, Succession Planning, and Mentoring

The importance of effective leadership in determining the overall mission and direction of an organization and guiding the institution through major change cannot be overstated. Whereas **contingency theory** posits that appropriate organizational strategy and design are determined by environmental conditions, senior management must be cognizant of those environmental conditions and determine the response the organization should initiate. In addition, the implementation of organizational transformation and change is the responsibility of senior executives.

To survive, organizations must constantly adapt. This is demonstrated by the radical changes that have been occurring in the health care sector. Managers must provide leadership and develop the leadership capabilities within the organization in order to make the transformations necessary in a changing environment. In Chapter 8, the approaches that are available for renewing the organization and for developing future leaders are discussed.

HUMAN RESOURCES PROCESSES

The processes used for human resources management may be viewed as a cycle of related activities. **Job analysis,** recruitment, retention, selection and onboarding, training and development, **performance appraisal,** compensation, and labor relations may be envisioned as a continuum of tasks and responsibilities that flow logically from one to another. These functions must be performed to ensure that the necessary human resources are available to support the strategic thrust of the organization.

Although each of these areas is important and must be performed competently for the organization

to function, the importance of the activity to sustaining excellence varies depending on the strategies chosen. Some strategic initiatives emphasize selection and onboarding activities, while others require health services managers to concentrate on refining the appraisal system. The relationships of selected strategic activities to human resources functions within the organization are discussed in Chapter 3. The association between other organizational activities and human resources functions, as well as the contribution of these functions to organizational performance, are discussed in the sections that follow.

Job Analysis

Job analysis is a systematic process of gathering information about jobs, which results in a **job description.** Job descriptions provide basic information necessary to implement all of the other human resources functions successfully. Chapter 9 discusses job analysis and job design in more detail.

Recruitment and Retention

Health services organizations must have a constant influx of candidates for potential employment. New employee positions are required as market areas are expanded or services are initiated. Recruitment occurs even in the face of limited growth or decline in service capacity, because individuals with specialized skills or training who leave the organization must be replaced and because services or technologies that have been revised or modified must be staffed.

The recruitment of personnel plays an important role in helping the organization to adapt and remain competitive. Employees who have recently finished professional training are the source of information on new methods and techniques in service delivery that allow the organization to remain competitive in its traditional services. In addition, it may be necessary to recruit outside the institution if personnel with the managerial or professional skills needed to implement new strategic thrusts are not available internally.

As discussed previously, the health services industry employs a wide variety of workers. Thus, the sources of applicants and types of method used to expand the applicant pool vary depending on the occupational classification being considered. A description of recruitment methods is provided in Chapter 10, together with a discussion of retention and turnover. Obviously, it is self-defeating to invest significant resources in a successful recruitment effort if such effort is offset by high turnover rates. Retention of high-performance employees is as essential as their original recruitment.

Selection and Onboarding

A responsibility highly correlated with recruitment is employee selection and onboarding. Once the applicant pool has been filled, methods must be in place to choose the persons who will be most qualified for each job. Successful implementation of organizational strategy requires that management have a thorough understanding of the jobs that must be performed and the qualifications of individuals to fill these jobs.

Selection of competent personnel for new or unique positions created by initiation of services may be problematic. For example, an institution initiating an innovative, nontraditional service may have difficulty identifying the activities that must be performed by individuals to be employed. In addition, it may have little experience in evaluating candidates for new positions.

A number of steps are critical in the selection and onboarding process. Job analysis must be conducted to determine the tasks to be performed and the qualifications required to perform them. Then, criteria for predicting employee effectiveness are required, with adequate attention given to validity and reliability of the selection instrument. These activities are examined in Chapter 11.

Training and Development

Investment in the existing human capital of a health services organization through a well-managed training and development activity offers potential for significantly enhancing the ability of the enterprise to achieve its objectives. Indeed, improvement in the skills and abilities of current employees will contribute to sustained levels of performance because the technological change occurring in the health services industry requires the constant updating of the knowledge base of health professionals. The increased competency of the health services organization staff will provide significant benefits to the enterprise no matter what strategy is being pursued.

The changing environment of the health services industry itself ensures that the training and development of current staff members will contribute to organizational performance. Institutions are required to develop innovative responses to the competitive reformations taking place today. The providers of health services within organizations must be informed of the factors causing these changes, as well as the roles they can potentially play in helping management cope with change. Information on competitive shifts and marketing alternatives conveyed to current employees and medical staff will help these professionals to understand the rationale for fundamental changes that are occurring. An improved understanding should make it easier to obtain their support and advice on implementation issues.

A third factor relating the strategic thrust of the enterprise to staff training and development is that the initiation of unique strategies and tactics may call for programs to be implemented by current employees who do not possess the necessary skills. For example, strategies to become a low-cost provider may dictate the use of internal management control methods that are foreign to supervisory staff. Management must ensure that plans for strategic initiatives include an inventory of the skills required for program implementation and must design necessary developmental activities. These and other issues in training and development are discussed in Chapter 12.

Performance Appraisal

Performance appraisal is the systematic evaluation of an employee's work behavior on criteria measuring important job-related activities.

To determine the extent to which work requirements and responsibilities are met, valid, reliable criteria must be developed for a job, and job behaviors must be measured.

Performance appraisal can serve multiple purposes for management. First, it can provide guidance for the selection of individuals for promotion. When advancement criteria have been determined, employees who meet or exceed those criteria can be identified as promotion opportunities arise. Second, it can be used as a method for determining increases in employee compensation. Levels of employee performance can be measured and comparisons can be made to improve the probability of equitable rewards being given for desired performance. Third, performance appraisal can serve as a tool for identifying areas in which personnel need training and development or additional counseling. Areas in which one or a number of employees exhibit consistently inadequate performance can be identified and remedial programs to improve performance developed.

If properly designed, an appraisal system complements the strategic planning of an organization because it translates the initiatives desired by the organization into specific behaviors required of individuals. Management must identify the key activities necessary for the achievement of the institutional mission and translate those activities into employee appraisal criteria. Performance appraisal methods are discussed in more detail in Chapter 13.

Compensation Management

The compensation system of an organization can influence the strategic direction of an organization and organizational effectiveness in a number of ways, as identified by Lawler (2003). First, a compensation system may foster the achievement of desired outcomes by motivating employees if an organization can link valued rewards to the performance of essential behaviors. Second, performance appraisal and compensation systems can contribute to the corporate culture that is perceived by organizational members as well as serve to reinforce the structural systems of the organization. Third,

terminating individuals on the basis of appraisal and compensation systems is associated with more positive performance appraisal outcomes.

The linking of compensation systems to the mission and strategies of the organization occurs through several vehicles. An assessment of the current compensation systems and their influence on behaviors should be an input to strategy development. Once a strategy has been generated, the firm must focus on the type of human resources needed and the behaviors required to make the plan effective. Then, compensation systems should be designed to reward the behaviors necessary for obtaining desired outcomes. The coupling of compensation to the behaviors required to support diverse strategic thrusts is a major component of strategic human resources management.

A difficulty health services managers face in developing compensation systems is the heterogeneity of personnel employed within an institution. This heterogeneity suggests that unique methods for compensating different types of employees may need to be developed. Variability also must be faced by larger health services delivery systems across facility sites or, as the merger of larger systems occurs, across systems in compensation programs. Such diversity means that managers must be sensitive to the need for blending these potentially different approaches for employee remuneration into a logical framework that is supportive of the mission of the organization. The methods for development of compensation packages for rewarding the diverse activities of health services organizations are discussed in Chapter 14.

Labor Relations

Senior managers seek to retain flexibility in selecting among alternatives when determining organizational strategy. Preservation of administrative flexibility is critical for long-term adaptability and survival for health services organizations, especially in today's volatile environment. Thus, development of a positive relationship between management and employees by practicing "preventive health" in labor-management relations is important for strategic management of human resources. This is because if groups of employees feel that management is not interested in their welfare, they may elect to have a union represent and bargain for them.

Nonunion status allows management greater flexibility in exercising its prerogatives. Loss of flexibility accompanies union status when provisions of the labor-management contract serve as a barrier to the implementation of programs or options that are being considered by management.

For example, a hospital may have agreed with a union that workers whose jobs are terminated will be shifted to other comparable positions or that present workers will be hired first if new jobs are created within their job classification. If such a facility desires to cease offering obstetric services while initiating new inpatient services for psychiatric patients, there may be an impasse. It will be almost impossible to shift personnel from obstetrics to psychiatry without significant retraining, and the obvious alternative (i.e., for the hospital to hire new personnel for psychiatric services) may be blocked, at least temporarily, by the terms of the union agreement. Thus, the change in services desired by the hospital cannot be implemented without major costs and delays.

Health services organizations that already have unions should consider the future strategic thrusts they wish to follow when they negotiate new collective bargaining agreements. Otherwise, an agreement may serve as an internal constraint that inhibits the performance of the organization. If the institution decides to follow a low-cost strategy in the marketplace, the management team must be tough negotiators, granting few wage demands, holding the line on numbers of workers, and stressing productivity standards in an attempt to restrain costs.

Conversely, the negotiations of an organization wishing to compete on the basis of service quality should reflect that desire. Management should bargain to gain concessions that focus on quality of care, such as use of employee assessment criteria that stress job performance and quality of care. Bonuses may be paid to employees for quality

enhancement activities. The organization may emphasize funding for training and development for job improvement rather than providing larger pay increases. Less stress may be placed on reducing staffing ratios or controlling overtime pay.

These factors suggest the importance of integrating strategic considerations into the handling of labor relations and negotiating collective bargaining agreements. Discussion of approaches to labor relations, including methods to create a positive human relations climate in order to reduce the probability of unionization, is provided in Chapter 15.

Future Human Resources Challenges

As previously mentioned, the mission and objectives of the organization will be reflected in the outcomes that are stressed by management and in the strategies, general tactics, and human resources practices that are chosen. Management makes strategic decisions that, combined with the level of fit achieved among the internal organizational systems, determine the outcomes the institution can achieve. For example, almost all health services organizations need to earn some profit for continued viability. However, some organizations refrain from initiating new ventures that might be highly profitable if the ventures would not fit the overall mission of the organization for providing quality services needed by a defined population group.

Conversely, an organization may start some services that are acknowledged to be break-even propositions at best, because the services are viewed as critical to the mission of the institution and the needs of the target market. The concerns of such an organization would be reflected not only in the choice of services offered but also in the human resources approaches used and the outcome measures viewed as important. This organization would likely place more emphasis on assessment criteria for employee performance and nursing unit operations that stress the provision of quality care and less emphasis on criteria concerned with efficient use of supplies and the maintenance of staffing ratios. This selection of priorities does not mean that efficiency of operations is ignored, but that greater weight is placed on the former criteria. The outcome measures used to judge the institution should reflect those priorities.

Another institution may place greater emphasis on economic return, profitability, and efficiency of operations. While quality of care also is important, the driving force for becoming a low-cost provider causes management to make decisions that reflect that resolve. Maintenance or reduction of staffing levels is stressed. Prohibition of overtime is strictly enforced. Recruitment and selection criteria stress identification and selection of employees who will meet minimum criteria and expectations and, possibly, will accept lower pay levels.

In an organization striving to be efficient, less energy may be spent on "social maintenance" activities designed for employee needs and to keep them from leaving or unionizing. It can be anticipated that the outcomes in this situation will reflect, at least in the short run, higher economic return and lower measures of quality of work life. Chapter 18 examines present and future human resource challenges that must be met in order to achieve positive outcomes.

strong influence on human resources systems. The behavioral systems of the organization (i.e., commitment and motivation, culture, leadership) also influence the personnel functions performed by the organization.

The outcomes achieved by the organization are influenced by numerous factors. The mission determines the direction that is being taken by the organization and what it desires to achieve. The amount of integration of mission, structural systems, behavioral systems and human resources systems defines the level of achievement that is possible. The remainder of the text addresses these issues in detail.

DISCUSSION QUESTIONS

1. Describe the changes that have taken place in the distribution of health care personnel among various occupational categories. What changes do you anticipate in this distribution during the next decade? Why?
2. What are the organizational advantages of integrating strategic management and human resources management? What are the steps involved in such an integration?

SUMMARY

The intensive reliance on professionals for service delivery requires health services executives to focus attention on the strategic management of human resources in the delivery of services and to understand the factors that influence the performance of persons employed in their organizations. To assist managers in understanding these relationships, this chapter presented a model of the association that exists among strategy, selected organizational design features, and human resources management activities.

Since different strategies require work routines, control methods, and coordination patterns of distinctive types, the structure of a health services organization is determined by the strategy being pursued. Components of an organization's structure have a

CASE

Affiliated HealthSystems, a regional, nonprofit hospital system, was founded in 1986 by the merger of three large, urban hospitals. These institutions were tertiary care facilities that had a combined capacity of 2000 inpatient acute care beds. During the next 7 years, Affiliated HealthSystems purchased 12 hospitals located in rural communities or small towns that were within 150 miles of the three original institutions. In addition, five management contracts were initiated between Affiliated and smaller facilities. These 17 institutions were added by Affiliated in hope of increasing, or at least retaining, referrals for the three urban hospitals.

From 1995 to 1998, Affiliated began to diversify and offer a broader array of programs and services to its urban marketplace. A health maintenance organization and a preferred provider organization were initiated successfully. Special services for target markets, such as the elderly and women, were offered with positive results.

In contrast, the rural hospitals are not doing so well; for example, occupancy levels are down, the cash flow at some institutions is poor, and it is difficult to recruit competent physicians and other professional staff. The system is not certain that its urban centers are receiving the volume and type of referrals that it desires. As a result, Affiliated is considering the development of outcome measures that would allow it to monitor the performance of its rural hospitals as well as its new urban community initiatives.

CASE DISCUSSION QUESTIONS

1. Describe the steps you would take to identify the measures that should be included in the performance measurement system.
2. List suggested measures you believe are important items to include in this analysis. Discuss your rationale for including each item.

REFERENCES

American Hospital Association. (1986). *Hospital Statistics.* Chicago: Author.

American Hospital Association. (1991). *Hospital Statistics.* Chicago: Author.

Bach, S., & Sisson, K. (2001). *Personnel Management: A Comprehensive Guide to Theory and Practice.* Boston: Blackwell Publishing.

Donabedian, A. (1980). *Explorations in Quality Assessment and Monitoring, Vol. 1: The Definition of Quality and Approaches to its Assessment.* Ann Arbor, MI: Health Administration Press.

Freudenheim, M. (1990, March 5). Job growth in health care areas. *New York Times,* p. 1.

Galbraith, J., & Nathanson, D. (1978). *Strategy Implementation: The Role of Structure and Process.* St. Paul: West Publishing.

Ginzberg, E. (1990). Health personnel: The challenge ahead. *Frontiers of Health Services Management,* 7(1), 3–22.

Gomez-Mejia, L.R. (1988). The role of human resources strategy in export performance. *Strategic Management Journal, 9,* 493–505.

Kravetz, D.J. (1988). *The Human Resources Revolution: Implementing Progressive Management Practices for Bottom Line Success.* San Francisco: Jossey-Bass.

Lawler, E.E. (1973). *Motivation in Work Organizations.* Pacific Grove, CA: Brooks/Cole.

Lawler, E.E. (2003). Reward practices and performance management systems. *Organizational Dynamics, 32*(4), 396–404.

Mintzberg, H. (1979). *The Structuring of Organizations.* Englewood Cliffs, NJ: Prentice-Hall.

Starr, P. (1982). *The Social Transformation of American Medicine.* New York: Basic Books.

U.S. Bureau of the Census. (1991). *Statistical Abstract of the United States.* Washington, DC: Government Printing Office.

U.S. Department of Health and Human Services. (1986). *Fifth Report to the President and Congress on the Status of Health Personnel in the United States.* (DHHS Publication No. HRS-P-OD-86-1.) Hyattsville, MD: Author.

U.S. Department of Health and Human Services. (1991). *United States Health and Prevention Profile 1991,* (DHHS Publication No. PHS 92-1232). Hyattsville, MD: Author.

U.S. Department of Health, Education, and Welfare. (1970). *Health Manpower Sourcebook.* Washington, DC: Government Printing Office.

U.S. Department of Labor, Bureaus of Labor Statistics. (1990). *Employment and Earnings.* Washington, DC: Government Printing Office.

Williams, S.J., & Torrens, P.R. (2008). *Introduction to Health Services* (8th ed.). Albany, NY: Delmar.

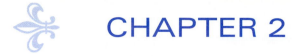

CHAPTER 2

The Legal and Financial Environment

Winsor Schmidt, JD, LLM and Richard L. Clarke, DHA, FHFMA

LEARNING OBJECTIVES

Upon completing this chapter, the reader will be able to:

1. Describe and discuss a definition of law and its implications for human resources management.

2. Recognize, describe, discuss, and apply the employment-at-will doctrine and its three exceptions.

3. Explain the purposes and major requirements of the *Fair Labor Standards Act* and the *National Labor Relations Act*, including their historical context of a relatively unregulated legal environment before 1964.

4. Recognize, describe, discuss, and apply the major federal statutes establishing the extent of equal opportunity in employment, including not only Title VII of the *Civil Rights Act of 1964* (42 U.S.C. sections 2000e-2000e-17) but also the *Age Discrimination in Employment Act* [29 U.S.C. sections 621-634, 663(a)], the *Americans with Disabilities Act of 1990* (29 U.S.C. section 706), the *Rehabilitation Act of 1973* (29 U.S.C. section 701), and the *Equal Pay Act of 1963* (29 U.S.C. section 201).

5. Describe the importance of labor costs to overall financial performance.

6. Identify the key drivers of financial performance in health care organizations.

7. Understand the role of management and governance in dealing with these drivers.

8. Synthesize the roles and issues described to strategies necessary for human resource management given the legal and financial frameworks.

KEY TERMS

Age Discrimination in Employment Act (ADEA)

Americans with Disabilities Act (ADA)

Civil Rights Act of 1964

Cost Shifting

Employment-At-Will Doctrine

Equal Pay Act of 1963 (EPA)

Fair Labor Standards Act (FLSA)

Health Insurance Portability and Accountability Act of 1996 (HIPAA)

Law

National Labor Relations Act of 1935 (NLRA)

Occupational Safety and Health Act of 1970 (OHSA)

Pay-for-Performance (P4P) Systems

Public Policy Exception

Rehabilitation Act of 1973

Role of Management

Sarbanes-Oxley Act

Sexual Harassment

INTRODUCTION

Law is the rules of the "game" for the business of human resources management in health services organizations. Finance is about ensuring resources are available so that the organization can fulfill its mission and achieve its vision.

More formally, law is "a body of rules of action or conduct prescribed by controlling authority, and having binding legal force" (Black, 1979, p. 795). Mr. Justice Oliver Wendell Holmes wrote to Sir Frederick Pollack: "I can imagine a book on the law, getting rid of all talk of duties and rights [and] beginning with the definition of law . . . as a statement of the circumstances in which the public force will be brought to bear upon a [person] through the Courts" (Howe, 1941). Law is a formal identification of the boundary for risking and experiencing formal accountability and finality of judgment.

Although it is tempting to dispense with all talk of rights and duties, as well as all talk of money, this chapter addresses two fundamental facets of the human resources manager's surroundings: law and finance. Dunlop (1958) recognized the legal and financial frameworks as major milieus for human resources management.

Dunlop (1958) appreciated the power context of law. While law is perceived as constraining, a more constructive view sees law as empowering. Law provides an answer to a fundamental human resources management question: by what authority do I act? If the authority to act is not identified, then a conservative approach may be to not act. An unnecessarily risk-taking approach confuses enforcement with law. Identification of the authority to act in law provides the power to act.

In *The Federalist No. 51*, James Madison wisely observed: "If men were angels, no government would be necessary. . . . [T]he great difficulty lies in this: you must first enable the government to control the governed, and in the next place oblige it to control itself." If people were angels, no law would be necessary. Rule of law is a distinction of American and Western industrialized systems. Law enables nonviolent control of those who govern and manage, as well as control of government itself.

The purpose of this chapter is not to provide legal advice. The most recent judicial decisions and agency regulations, and a comprehensive treatise on health care human resources law, are beyond the scope of this chapter. Individuals needing legal assistance should seek advice from a qualified attorney licensed to practice in their state. Just as preventive health care is more cost effective than acute care, so preventive legal service is more cost effective than litigation service. Legal problems are easier to prevent than fix.

A purpose of this chapter is to assist acquisition of the ability to recognize, describe, discuss, and apply the significant and major issues in the legal and financial environment for health care human resources management. Legal issue identification should facilitate timely consultation of an attorney. The first part of this chapter addresses the legal environment for health care human resource management and the second part of this chapter focuses on the financial environment.

LEGAL ENVIRONMENT

Employment-At-Will

Managers who work without an employment contract, as well as physicians, nurses, and others working without an employment contract in private health services organizations, are generally subject to the **employment-at-will doctrine.** The employment-at-will doctrine also generally applies to employees working under a contract that does not have either a particular term of employment or require cause for termination. The employment-at-will doctrine means that termination of the employment relationship can occur without cause at the choice or will of either the employee or the employer, subject only to such restrictions as anti-discrimination statutes (Furrow, et al., 2000).

The St. Francis Regional Medical Center in Kansas suffered a damage award of $552,756 for breach of contract where the hospital's contract provided that the medical director was to be "mutually acceptable" to both the hospital and the current radiologist of the hospital. The phrase "mutually acceptable" did not mean employment-at-will [*Dutta v. St. Francis Regional Medical Center*, 850 P.2d 928 (Kan.App.1993), affirmed 867 P.2d. 1057 (Kan.1994)].

As with much of the law, the extent of application of the employment-at-will doctrine varies significantly among the states, ranging from states like New York that are more employer-oriented to states like California that are "much more forward thinking and in harmony with the constitutional rights of the employee" (Pozgar, 2007, p. 424).

There are three recognized exceptions to the employment-at-will doctrine. Most states accept implied contract as an exception to the at-will doctrine. A personnel manual or employee handbook can create a contractual right to continued employment. For example, an Illinois court held that in terminating a nurse, the St. Mary of Nazareth Hospital Center must conform to its employee manual [*Duldulao v. St. Mary of Nazareth Hospital Center*, 505 N.E.2d 314 (Ill.1987)]. An employer can avoid creating a contract with a personnel manual or employee handbook by including a prominent, clear, and unambiguous disclaimer saying the manual or handbook is not a contract and that employees are subject to termination at will [e.g., *Hrehorovich v. Harbor Hospital Center*, 614 A.2d 1021 (Md.App.1992)]. Also, while medical staff bylaws are a contract for purposes of the procedures to limit or revoke medical staff privileges, the bylaws are not an implied contract preventing termination of an at-will employee (Furrow, et al., 2000).

A second exception to the employment-at-will doctrine is the **public policy exception.** An employee has a legal claim for wrongful discharge if the employee is terminated for activity that is protected by a specific state law, for example, a health care worker who reports abuse of a nursing home patient under an abuse-reporting statute [*McQuary v. Bel Air Convalescent Home, Inc.*, 684 P.2d 21 (Or. App.1984)]. The worker is authorized, even mandated, to report such abuse. Health care professionals terminated for criticizing or trying to improve patient care quality do not qualify for the public policy exception (Furrow, et al., 2000).

There is a minority view endorsing a broader scope for the public policy exception. A Wisconsin court allowed a wrongful discharge claim for $39,344 in lost wages against Beloit Memorial Hospital for the termination of a nurse who refused to "float" to another hospital unit because she would have performed services for which she was not qualified [*Winkelman v. Beloit Memorial Hospital*, 483 N.W.2d 211 (Wis.1992)]. A federal district court in Ohio allowed a wrongful discharge claim by a physician against the Bryan Medical Group where he was allegedly terminated for his deposition testimony in a malpractice case [*Hicks v. Bryan Medical Group*, 287 F.Supp.2d 795 (N.D. Ohio 2003)].

Several commentators ask rhetorically whether physicians and nurses who are employees-at-will should receive more extensive legal protection for conduct and complaints concerning patient care quality or illegal financial arrangements than other employees (Furrow, et al., 2008). They note that while many states and the federal government have "whistle-blower" statutes that protect public employees who report misconduct, the statutes are usually narrow and strictly interpreted by the courts. However, several courts have allowed wrongful discharge claims when a nurse was terminated for suggesting that a family obtain a patient's medical record, and when another nurse advised a family to replace a patient's doctor [*Kirk v. Mercy Hospital Tri-County*, 851 S.W.2d 617 (Mo.App.1993); *Deerman v. Beverly California Corp.*, 518 S.E.2d 804 (N.C.App.1999)]. The National Labor Relations Act may protect activities and statements about the quality of patient care. At-will employees in public hospitals may have First Amendment protection when terminated for statements about patient care quality or in opposition to policies [*Waters v. Churchill*, 511 U.S. 661 (1994); *Ulrich v. City and County of San Francisco*, 308 F.3d 968 (9th Cir. 2002)].

A dilemma theoretically arises between encouragement of physicians to whistle-blow on incompetent colleagues and the need for collaborative work. Some health care management commentary worries that the potential mutual suspicion and internal strife from whistle-blowing are unlikely to inspire "the transformational models of leadership and cohesive teamwork necessary to high quality care" (Morton-Cooper & Barnford, 1997, p. 236). On the other hand, failure to self-regulate stimulates a demand for external regulation. Transformational models of leadership presumably include transformation in compliance with law.

A third exception to the employment-at-will doctrine is the implied duty of fair dealing and good faith. Bozeman Deaconess Hospital was liable for wrongful discharge in failing to investigate the charges before terminating the employee [*Crenshaw v. Bozeman Deaconess Hospital*, 693 P.2d 487 (Mont.1984)]. However, this exception is not extended to health care workers like physicians as a special group because of the equal bargaining position between the hospital and a well-educated doctor (Furrow, et al., 2000).

The employment-at-will doctrine reflects a relatively unregulated legal environment for managers and employees. With the exception of wage-and-hour laws (i.e., Fair Labor Standards Act) and labor relations laws (i.e., National Labor Relations Act), managers before the "pivotal year" of 1964 had broad discretion in their treatment of employees (Fallon & McConnell, 2007, p. 41). The **Civil Rights Act of 1964** was the beginning of a more heavily regulated legal environment for human resources management in health services organizations.

Fair Labor Standards Act

The **Fair Labor Standards Act (FLSA;** 29 U.S.C. sections 201-219) was passed in 1938 in response to the high unemployment rate of the Great Depression. The FLSA sets minimum wages, time-and-a-half guaranteed overtime, maximum overtime pay, and prohibition of employing minors. The FLSA covers nonprofit and for-profit hospital employees (Miller, 2006). The Wage and Hour Division of the U.S. Department of Labor administers the FLSA, including workplace inspections and the conducting of audits. There are significant financial incentives for private federal litigation by employees and their attorneys (Pozgar, 2007).

Bona fide executive, administrative, and professional employees who are salaried are exempt from the wage and hour rules. While administrators and physicians are clearly exempt, the courts are split about other employee classifications. A staff nurse at Rush-Presbyterian-St. Luke's Medical Center in Chicago was not found not exempt as a professional from FLSA and therefore entitled to overtime [*Klein v. Rush-Presbyterian-St. Luke's Medical Center*, 990 F.2d 279 (7th Cir. 1993)]. However, another court listed nursing as an example of an exempt professional [*Reich v. Newspapers of New England, Inc.*, 44 F.3d 1060 (1st Cir. 1995)]. Department of Labor regulations [69 Fed. Reg. 222122 (April 23, 2004)] should be consulted (Miller, 2006).

If work is longer than 40 hours in seven days, the FLSA requires most employers to pay overtime rates. However, section 7(j) of the FLSA allows hospitals to contract with employees for an alternative work period of 14 consecutive days. Under the "8/80" system, a hospital employee is not eligible for overtime as long as the employee works no more than eight hours in any one day, and no more than 80 hours in 14 consecutive days (Miller, 2006).

The courts disagree about paying employees in on-call status and about paying employees in on-call status at a different rate (Miller, 2006). One court held that a hospital's security staff is not entitled to lunch break compensation though on call. Another court held that hospital employees should receive compensation for lunch breaks if on call. A third court allowed Mercy Hospital in Pennsylvania to pay nurses and operating room technicians who were on-premises-on-call one and one-half times minimum wage, instead of one and one-half times their hourly wage, for the time period in which they did no other work [*Townsend v. Mercy Hospital*, 689 F. Supp. 503 (W.D. Pa. 1988) affirmed 862 F.2d 1009 (3d Cir. 1988)].

National Labor Relations Act

Congress passed the **National Labor Relations Act of 1935 (NLRA**; 29 U.S.C. sections 141-187) to govern management–labor relationships of businesses engaged in interstate commerce. The NLRA defines unfair labor practices for employees and employers, authorizes the National Labor Relations Board (NLRB) to conduct secret elections for employees to determine any representation by a labor organization, and authorizes the NLRB to investigate and conduct hearings for complaints about unfair labor practices. Amendments to the NLRA include the *Taft-Hartley amendments of 1947* and the *Labor-Management Reporting and Disclosure Act of 1959*.

The NLRA did not explicitly exempt health care employees, but Taft-Hartley specifically excluded private, nonprofit hospitals and health care organizations in its definition of employer. While the NLRB asserted jurisdiction over for-profit hospitals and nursing homes, it took the *1974 Health Care Amendments* to authorize the NLRB to cover private nonprofit health care organizations (Furrow, et al., 2000; Pozgar, 2007). The NLRA does not cover government hospitals except for those where a private contractor exercises daily control [cf., *Pikeville United Methodist Hospital v. United Steelworkers of America*, 109 F.3d 1146 (6th Cir. 1997)].

The NLRA has several provisions that are unique to health care organizations. So that health care organizations have sufficient advance notice of a strike, the 1974 Amendments require a 10-day strike and picket notice to the health care organization and to the Federal Mediation and Conciliation Service (Furrow, et al., 2000). The definition of bargaining units is a hotly contested issue for health care organizations and employees. Management usually prefers larger units of employees with conflicting, heterogeneous interests. Unions usually prefer smaller units with homogenous interests. In 1989, the NLRB issued a rule recognizing eight possible bargaining units in acute-care hospitals: registered nurses; physicians; professionals except for registered nurses and physicians; technical employees; skilled maintenance employees; business office clerical employees; guards; and other nonprofessional employees (29 C.F.R. section 103.30). Units must have at least six employees for certification. The U.S. Supreme Court upheld the rule against a challenge by the American Hospital Association [*American Hospital Association v. NLRB*, 499 U.S. 606 (1991)]. The frequency of union elections and the union success rate increased after the eight-unit rule (Hirsch & Schumacher, 1998).

Commentators report a surge in health care unionization, including physicians and nurses, at the beginning of the 21st century (Furrow, et al., 2008). Following recognition of the close association between nurse staffing ratios and quality of care (Government Accountability Office, 2002), and recommendations to increase quality of care by increasing nurse staffing levels in hospitals and nursing homes (Institute of Medicine, 2003), nurse unions in California achieved legislation instituting minimum nurse-to-patient ratios for specific hospital services.

Another NLRA provision unique to health care organizations relates to solicitation about union matters and distribution of union materials. Health care organizations can limit solicitation and distribution to nonpatient care areas [*NLRB v. Baptist Hospital*, 422 U.S. 773 (1979)].

Supervisors are not protected by the NLRA. The Supreme Court held that registered nurses at Kentucky River Community Care, a residential mental health care facility, could be supervisors to the extent that they exercise independent judgment in responsibly directing other employees in the employer's interest [*NLRB v. Kentucky River Community Care*, 532 U.S. 706 (2001)]. However, the NLRB continues to find that registered nurses in nursing homes, and licensed practical nurses serving as charge nurses in nursing homes, are not supervisors [Miller, 2006; *Golden Crest Healthcare Center*, 348 NLRB No. 39 (2006); *Oakwood*

Healthcare, Inc., 348 NLRB No. 37 (2006)]. The federal circuit courts are split regarding charge nurses (Furrow, et al., 2008; Miller, 2006).

Equal Opportunity Employment Statutes

The "pivotal year" of 1964 (Fallon & McConnell, 2007, p. 41) began the paradigm shift in the legal environment for human resources management. The major federal statutes establishing the extent of equal opportunity in employment include not only Title VII of the *Civil Rights Act of 1964* (42 U.S.C. sections 2000e-2000e-17) but also the *Age Discrimination in Employment Act* [ADEA, 29 U.S.C. sections 621–634, 663(a)], the *Americans with Disabilities Act of 1990* (ADA, 29 U.S.C. section 706), the *Rehabilitation Act of 1973* (29 U.S.C. section 701), and the *Equal Pay Act of 1963* (29 U.S.C. section 201).

Title VII of the *Civil Rights Act of 1964* prohibits employment treatment in hiring, dismissal, promotion, discipline, terms and conditions of employment, and job advertising that is disparate based on race, color, religion, sex, national origin, or pregnancy (*Pregnancy Discrimination Act of 1978*). Employees must exhaust administrative remedies by filing a complaint or charge with the Equal Employment Opportunity Commission (EEOC) before they can file a lawsuit. There are criminal penalties for false claims (Miller, 2007). Legal theories for finding employment discrimination include disparate treatment, disparate impact, and carryover from past discrimination (Miller, 2007). Disparate treatment is inconsistent application of employment practices or work rules with discriminatory intent. For example, there was no discrimination where an African American registered nurse terminated for mixing up telemetry strips did not show that there was more favorable treatment of white nurses [*Beene v. St. Vincent Mercy Medical Center*, 111 F.Supp.2d 931 (D. Ohio 2000)]. Disparate impact is an adverse impact on a minority caused by an employment practice that does not have a job-related justification. More than statistics are required to establish

disparate impact [*Watson v. Ft. Worth Bank & Trust*, 487 U.S. 977 (1988)]. Claims of illegal discrimination in staff privileges and contracting decisions have been infrequent, but may increase because civil rights claims are now exempt from the immunity available to peer review decisions in the *Health Care Quality Improvement Act* (Furrow, et al., 2000). Many states also have anti-discrimination statutes.

Sex discrimination under Title VII includes not only unjustified preference of one gender for certain jobs, but also **sexual harassment** [*Meritor Savings Bank v. Vinson*, 477 U.S. 57 (1986). Sexual harassment is defined by Section 703 of Title VII and the EEOC as "unwelcome sexual advances, requests for sexual favors, and other verbal or physical conduct of a sexual nature when this conduct: explicitly or implicitly affects an individual's employment; unreasonably interferes with an individual's work performance; or creates an intimidating, hostile, or offensive work environment" (Pozgar, 2007, p. 418). Sexual harassment includes a quid pro quo form where work conditions are altered for refusal to submit to sexual demands. Supervisors perpetrating quid pro quo sexual harassment subject their employers to general liability (Miller, 2006). Sexual harassment also includes a hostile environment form of unreasonable work interference or an intimidating or hostile environment. Supervisors do not subject their employers to strict liability for hostile environment sexual harassment unless they have actual knowledge of the misconduct (Miller, 2006). Perception of abusiveness constitutes a hostile work environment; proof of injury or serious effect on employee psychological well-being is not necessary [*Harris v. Forklift Systems, Inc.*, 510 U.S. 17 (1993)].

The **Age Discrimination in Employment Act (ADEA)** prohibits discriminatory treatment of individuals 40 years of age or older for employment-related purposes, including mandatory retirement (Miller, 2007). Employment purposes include hiring, job retention, compensation, discharge, and other privileges, conditions, and terms of employment. The purpose of the ADEA is employment of older persons based on the ability of an individual to fulfill job requirements without regard to age limitations or stereotypes related to age. Georgia Osteopathic Hospital was found responsible for age discrimination when its medical director terminated a 56-year-old secretary for a 34-year-old secretary and told the 34-year-old that she was hired for her appearance [*O'Donnell v. Georgia Osteopathic Hospital, Inc.,* 748 F.2d 1543 (11th Cir. 1984)]. A CEO's statements about the need for "new blood" and a 62-year-old day-shift nurse supervisor's "advanced age" caused another court to find that a jury could decide whether this created intolerable working conditions that forced the nurse supervisor to resign in violation of the ADEA [*Shaw v. HCA Health Services,* 79 F.3d 99 (8th Cir. 1996)].

The **Americans with Disabilities Act (ADA)** "is the most important civil rights act ever passed by Congress to deal with the problems of discrimination against persons with disabilities" (Perlin, 2000, p. 145). Congress recognized that 43 million Americans have one or more mental or physical disabilities. Title 1 of the ADA prohibits employers with more than 15 employees from discriminating "against a qualified individual with a disability because of the disability in regard to job application procedures, the hiring, job assignment, advancement, or discharge of employees, employee compensation of fringe benefits, job training, and other terms, conditions, and privileges of employment" [42 U.S.C. section 12112(a)]. Disability is broadly defined and includes having "a physical or mental impairment that substantially limits one or more of the major life activities of such individual, a record of such impairment, or being regarded as having such an impairment" [42 U.S.C. section 12102(2)]. A qualified individual with a disability is "an individual with a disability who meets the skill, experience, education, and other job-related requirements of a position held or desired, and who, with or without reasonable accommodation, can perform the essential functions of the position" [42 U.S.C. section 12111(8)]. One court upheld a jury verdict of $325,000 against Charleston Area Medical Center in West Virginia where an employee was not accommodated for asthma aggravated by

job exposure to chemicals and was terminated (Pozgar, 2007).

Many of the terms in the ADA are the subject of extensive litigation to clarify the meaning. Judicial decisions address such issues as whether correctable conditions are disabilities (generally no); the scope of "major life activities" involved (a symptomatic HIV-positive person is covered but a nurse with a lifting limitation is not considered disabled); whether an employer may prohibit alcohol and illegal drug use and require compliance with the *Drug Free Workplace Act of 1988* (generally yes); whether the essential functions of a job can be performed by the employee with an accommodation (an RN with rheumatoid arthritis had no claim because she could not perform essential functions even with accommodation); direct threats to public health (not qualified under the act) and safety issues (HIV-positive persons are legally considered a direct threat in some hospital positions despite low risk of transmission compared with, e.g, hepatitis C) (Furrow, et al., 2008); the hiring process (job criteria and tests must be job related); reasonable accommodation for the employee without undue hardship to the employer; and insurance benefits (e.g., caps on coverage for HIV-positive employees do not violate the ADA) (Miller, 2006).

The **Rehabilitation Act of 1973** forbids discrimination in employment of the handicapped, including advertising, recruitment, processing of applications, promotions, pay rates, fringe benefits, and work assignments. There is overlap with the ADA, and judicial decisions under the Rehabilitation Act are considered in interpreting the ADA. Section 504 applies to employers receiving federal financial assistance; for example, health care organizations participating in such federal programs as Medicare and Medicaid. Section 504 states: "[n]o . . . qualified handicapped individual in the United States . . . shall solely by reason of his handicap, be excluded from participation in, be denied the benefits of, or be subjected to discrimination under any program receiving federal financial assistance." The organization is prohibited from discriminating against any qualified handicapped persons who can perform a job's essential functions with reasonable accommodation [*Tuck v. HCA Health Services*, 7 F.3d 465 (6th Cir. 1993)]. A discharged teacher with a tuberculosis history was entitled to reasonable accommodation [*School Board of Nassau County v. Arline*, 480 U.S. 273 (1987)]. A dentist's patient infected with HIV was found handicapped and protected [*Bragdon v. Abbott*, 524 U.S. 624 (1998)]. Other conditions ruled as protected handicaps include: a nursing home director of nursing with multiple sclerosis; a person with obstructive lung disease needing a smoke-free environment; and a recovering addict in a nursing position who had narcotics administration authority restricted (Miller, 2006).

The **Equal Pay Act of 1963 (EPA)** prohibits discrimination in pay for women and men performing substantially equal work in similar situations. The EPA requires equal pay for equal work. Pay differences are allowed if they result from earnings measured by the quality or quantity of production or a formal seniority system. One court found violations of both the EPA and Title VII by Nucare, Inc. in Minnesota for payment of higher wages to male orderlies than a female nurse's aide for similar work [*Odomes v. Nucare, Inc.*, 428 N.W.2d 574 (Minn. Ct. App. 1988)]. Some states have comparable worth legislation requiring comparable or equal pay for jobs of similar responsibility, effort, and skills performed in comparable working conditions (Greenlaw & Kohl, 1995).

Another important federal law is the **Occupational Safety and Health Act of 1970 (OSHA)** (29 U.S.C. sections 651-678). OSHA establishes standards for occupational health and safety. OSHA has taken initiatives for the protection of health care employees from blood-borne diseases and, "latex allergies, needle-stick injuries, tuberculosis, and waste anesthetic gasses," as well as general initiatives and citations regarding employee vaccinations, ergonomics, and workplace violence (Miller, 2006, p. 186).

Limitations

There are legal issues that are beyond the limited scope of this chapter on the legal and financial framework for human resources management in health services organizations. Legal issues regarding the employment relationship from the more comprehensive subject of health care law include, but are not limited to, such concerns as selection of employees; health screening; training and supervision; staffing and staffing ratios; constitutional searches and seizures in the workplace; discipline and dismissal; drug and other substance testing; genetic screening and testing; other behavioral screening; polygraph tests; communications about former staff [e.g., libel or slander *per se* (on its face) issues requiring no proof of damages, such as accusations of criminality, accusations of having a loathsome disease, words affecting a person's business or profession, calling a woman unchaste]; Federal Wage Garnishment Law; *Employee Retirement Income Security Act of 1974* (ERISA); **Health Insurance Portability and Accountability Act of 1996 (HIPAA)**; *Family and Medical Leave Act of 1993;* state laws (e.g., anti-injunction acts, union security contracts and right-to-work laws, worker's compensation, unemployment compensation); independent contractors (e.g., taxes, benefits, discrimination, labor law, whistle-blowers, confidentiality of medical records, liability); volunteers; and students (Furrow, et al., 2000, 2008; Miller, 2007; Pozgar, 2006).

FINANCIAL ENVIRONMENT

At almost 13 million individuals, health care workers represent some 10% of the nonfarm workforce. In addition, firms that provide support to health care provider organizations (medical supply and device manufacturers, pharmaceutical companies, insurance companies, consultants, and so on) employ many thousands more. Clearly, these workers represent an important component of the overall economy of the United States. They also represent an important asset, as well as cost, to health care organizations (Bureau of Labor Statistics, 2007).

Table 2.1. **Employment and Total Compensation as a percent of Operating Expenses.**

Employer Category	Total Employment	Percentage of Operating Expenses
Community hospitals	4,490,800[1]	51.5[2]
Physician practices	2,204,300[1]	32.6[3]
Skilled nursing/nursing care facilities	1,603,900[1]	62.8[4]

[1] Data from March, 2007. (Bureau of Labor Statistics, 2007)
[2] Data from 2006. American Hospital Association Survey. (AHA, 2007)
[3] Data from 2005. Non-physician staff costs, multi-specialty clinic. Medical Group Management Association. (MGMA, 2006)
[4] Data from 2004. Federal Register, Aug. 3, 2007. Department of Health and Human Services/Centers for Medicare and Medicaid Services. (Federal Register, 2007)

For provider organizations, total compensation paid to these workers represents a sizable portion of overall expenses. Table 2.1 lists the percentage of total expenses from compensation by major employer categories.

The cost of labor impacts the overall financial performance of health care organizations. As a result, these organizations must manage within the resources available to them. The focus of the remainder of this chapter is on the broad-based financial issues that affect health care provider organizations and their need to appropriately manage human resource costs.

Finance and labor issues often are top priority for health care leaders. In a recent poll of chief executive officers, the American College of Healthcare Executives (ACHE) found that 72% identified financial issues as their greatest concern, and the area related to financial issues most cited by these executives was the increasing cost for staff, supplies, and so on (ACHE, 2006). Likewise, members of governing boards expressed concern about the financial vitality of health care organizations, including controlling costs (Kaufman, 2007).

In examining financial issues, the Healthcare Financial Management Association identified four areas of concern to health care financial leaders. Those areas are revenue cycle improvements, consumer-focused practices, Medicare payment trends, and business issues. Within business issues, managing labor cost was a key focus (HFMA, 2007).

Key Finance Drivers

The ability of a health care organization to continue to employ health care workers and thus to provide medical services depends on several factors that impinge on financial performance. According to Moody's Investors Service, the key factors that impact financial performance are:

- Payment rates from public and private payers
- Competition (especially between facilities and physicians) and volume shifts
- National and state economies
- Capital spending
- Management and governance (Moody's, 2007)

Following is an examination of these issues that provides a context for the strategic management of human resources within the financial environment in which health care organizations must operate.

Payment Issues

Annually, the Office of the Actuary of the Centers for Medicare & Medicaid Services projects figures for total health expenditures. A major category, "expenditures for personal health services," represents payments to providers for services to individuals. In 2007, those expenditures were projected to exceed $1.8 trillion. The lion's share of that amount is payments to hospital and medical professionals ($697.5 billion for hospitals and $703.9 billion for physicians, dentists, and other professionals). Nursing home care payments were projected at approximately $190 billion, with the remainder,

$293.9 billion, going to retail sales of medical products. Of those amounts, approximately 12% are out-of-pocket expenditures from patients, 33.9% are from private health insurance, 46.8% are from public sources (mainly Medicare and Medicaid), and the remainder are from other private sources, including foundations (CMS/OOA, 2007).

Payments from sources other than patient payments (third-party payments) represent a major portion of the revenue stream for most health care provider organizations. Government payments in the form of Medicare and Medicaid, as well as payments from private sources including employer-provided health insurance, drive much of this revenue. As such, the dynamics that impact these payments determine the extent to which providers can maintain or expand services and their labor force. Table 2.2 below lists the rate of change in payments for major public and private payers.

Tax support for public programs such as Medicare and Medicaid and employer payments for employee health insurance are growing faster then the underlying growth in tax revenues and/or profits. As such, major payers continually implement strategies to reduce the rate of increase in their outlays. Strategies used by government typically involve setting prices for services (for example, DRGs for inpatient hospitalization, or RBRVS for physicians) and controlling the rate of increase of these prices. Volume (services delivered and number of individuals covered) and acuity (intensity of services) increases continue to drive overall expenditures. Government payments, however, have not generally kept pace with the cost of care and inflation.

Actions by governments to hold payment increases at cost or below often result in a phenomenon known as "cost shifting" in which providers of care cause "systematically higher prices (above cost) paid by one payer group to offset lower prices (below cost) paid by another" (Dobson, DaVanzo, & Sen, 2006. See also Lee, et al., 2003). Figure 2.1 demonstrates this "cost shift hydraulic."

As a result of the cost shift, input prices (cost wages, supplies, etc.), and other factors, employer premium increases continue to outpace their ability to sustain coverage for employees (Angrisano, et al., 2007). Employers, seeking to better manage their rate of premium increases have shifted an increasing burden to employees in the form of higher deductibles and copayments. Increased employee payments as well as pressure to hold rate of premium increases are part of the overall slowing of payment increases experienced by providers of care described by Moody's.

Price transparency is an additional impact of this movement. The relationship of prices for health services to the cost of providing care often is difficult to explain. As a result, meeting market demands for clarity and pressure from employers to reduce cost requires a reexamination of pricing strategies—often resulting in reduced prices (Clarke, 2007). Additionally, increased deductibles and copayments may cause employees to reduce the volume of services consumed (Buntin, et al., 2006). The net effect of these actions is to reduce the pricing flexibility of providers and limit their ability to pass on cost increases. These dynamics cause providers to examine alternative revenue sources and cost-saving strategies.

Table 2.2. **Annual Percentage Change, Estimated and Projected: 2002–2007.**

Payer	2002e	2003e	2004e	2005e	2006p	2007p
Medicare	7.3	6.7	10.3	9.3	22.1	6.5
Medicaid	10.5	9.1	7.5	7.2	0.1	7.3
Private Health Ins	10.5	9.6	7.9	6.6	4.8	6.7

SOURCE: CMS/OOS 2007. Annual percentage change are estimates or projections by CMS/OOS; e = estimated; p = projected.

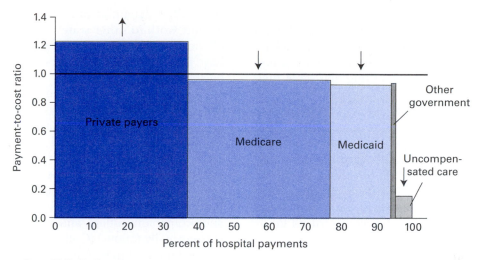

Figure 2.1. Cost Shift Hydraulic

SOURCE: Lewin Group analysis of data presented in Lewin Group, *Trendwatch Chartbook 2005: Trends Affecting Hospitals and Health Systems* (Washington: American Hospital Association, May 2005). Dobson, et al., 2006.

CREDIT: Copyrighted and published by Project HOPE/*Health Affairs* as Dobson, et al., "The Cost-Shift Payment 'Hydraulic': Foundation, History, and Implications," *Health Affairs*, 25(1): 22–23, January/February 2006. The published article is archived and available online at www.healthaffairs.org.

NOTE: The bold ruling line at 1.0 represents costs and payments in balance.

Finally, payment systems are moving toward better recognition of payment for quality, or **pay-for-performance (P4P) systems.** These systems reward providers (beginning with hospital payments and moving to physician payments) for reporting, then performing against, certain quality performance standards. Medicare, several state's Medicaid programs, and many private payers have programs that identify quality measurement sets and measure providers against them (Nichols & O'Malley, 2006; Wilensky, 2007).

Competition and Volume Shifts

Payment policy often drives a variety of decisions made by those impacted by the policy. As government and private payers reduce payment for certain types of services, hospital leaders, physicians, other medical professionals, and investors make up the difference through alternative revenue strategies. For example, to augment income, many physicians continue to expand ancillary services offered in their offices, investing in ambulatory surgery and diagnostics centers and even specialty inpatient facilities in competition with hospitals. Conversely, hospitals employ or contract with physician groups to ensure certain levels of coverage and referrals from those services. In some cases, these actions are conservative and maintain revenue. In other cases, the goal is to create new revenue streams.

Continuous care retirement communities with assisted-living and skilled nursing units compete with traditional nursing home facilities. Investors, including venture capitalists, seek to make investments where payment and/or cost savings opportunities exist. For the most part, these competitive actions are a direct result of payment policies (Ginsburg & Grossman, 2005).

This level of competition causes a shift of volume and revenue from traditional sites of care to new venues. The American Hospital Association reported that the number of hospital-owned outpatient surgery facilities declined from almost 95% of total facilities in 1981 to less than 50% by 2005, while freestanding facilities grew from less than 5% of the total to 38% during that same time period (AHA, 2006).

The combination of changes in payment policy and the resulting impact on revenue and volume drives investment decisions. Based on these trends within their markets, health care leaders must decide which services should be added, modified, reduced, or eliminated. These decisions impact the overall financial performance of the organization as well as the number and make up of its labor force.

National and State Economies

Payment for health care services is dependent on the ability of individuals and sponsors (primarily government and employers) to generate resources to pay for these services. For example, during times of economic growth, tax revenues increase, thereby providing a more stable revenue base for publicly funded programs such as Medicare and Medicaid. Although government often is a frugal purchaser (as demonstrated by Figure 2.1), aggressive budget cutting occurs only when tax revenues get tight. During the 2000s, the growth of the national economy, as measured by changes in gross domestic product, grew at an average rate of 2.6%. Current receipts by the federal government grew from $2.9 trillion in 2002 to $3.6 trillion in 2006 (Bureau of Economic Analysis, 2007). This level of growth reduced pressure of national policy makers to make drastic changes in payments. Beginning in 2008, however, economic growth slowed significantly producing an economic recession that continued into 2009.

The same is true for most state economies. There is, however, much more variability at the state level. States such as Michigan have experienced significant employment declines in manufacturing sectors; states such as Arizona have experienced significant employment growth, especially in the services sectors. At the state level, global competitive dynamics can drive private employers to shift work to other states or to move offshore. Obviously, those states with stagnant economies have more budget challenges than others where businesses are growing.

Clearly, the same is true for businesses in these states. Where the economy is growing, business revenue growth and profitability enables businesses to invest in technology and expand their labor force, adding to overall economic growth. Provision of health insurance to these workers is often a result of this growth. Conversely, during periods of economic stagnation or decline, business revenue and profitability suffers, and cuts in labor and benefits normally follows (Collins, et al., 2004).

The impact on health care providers is threefold. First, from the standpoint of Medicare, payment trends have been fairly stable, given the relatively stable economy. This will change when the national economy slows or moves toward stagnation or recession. Additionally, federal budget deficits are mounting, and once again (as in 1997 with the *Balanced Budget Act*), Congress and the administration may have to act to make significant reductions in the rate of payment increases.

The second impact is on state programs for the poor and long-term care. Medicaid, the largest of these programs, often is the largest single line item on the state's budget. As expenditures rise, and if tax revenues slow or fall, state government must take drastic action. Generally, their actions impact nursing homes more than hospitals or physicians because significant portions of most state Medicaid programs are designed to subsidize the poor elderly in nursing homes. Some hospitals, especially "safety net" hospitals (those who primarily treat the poor) also rely on Medicaid for substantial payments. These providers are especially hard hit when state economies slow or stagnate.

The third impact is on employer-provided health insurance. In states where employers are struggling, health insurance premiums are a primary target. These companies seek to limit their risk of premium increase by designing plans that shift increased risk to employees (as described earlier in the chapter). Or, they may reduce their workforce through layoffs, to reduce their payroll and benefit expenses. In some cases, employers may drop health insurance all together. These last two options increase the number of uninsured persons, which puts additional financial burdens on both state and local governments and the providers of care (Collins, et al., 2004).

Capital Spending

Capital spending represents expenditures for durable items such as medical equipment, information technology, bricks and mortar, and so on. Advances in medical technology, medical procedures, and pharmaceuticals pressure health care providers increasingly to invest in capital equipment and facilities. Additionally, many nursing homes and hospitals were built in the 1950s and are in need of replacement or major renovation to meet current building and safety codes. According to the HFMA, hospitals plan to increase capital expenditures by about 14% annually for the next five years. Significant spending is expected for digital imaging storage and retrieval, information systems, and capacity increases for emergency and surgery departments (HFMA, 2003).

Capital spending places financial performance demands on providers. Resources for capital spending come primarily from internal funds and secondarily from debt. Investor-owned organizations also use equity financing in the form of stock and joint ventures. Investor-owned and nonprofit organizations must generate enough positive cash flow (cash inflows in excess of cash outflows) to fund needed capital expenditures and reserves for future expenditures. Lenders (banks and bondholders) require a level of financial performance that ensures that the interest and principle on their loans will be paid in a timely manner. Likewise, investors expect performance that rewards them for the financial risk of their equity investment.

Capital spending also adds to the expense of operating the equipment or facility. Depreciation, maintenance, interest costs, and labor often are part of the additional expenses incurred by an organization as a result of capital spending.

Interestingly, there is a delicate balance between spending on capital assets and financial performance. Underspending on capital can lead to a "using up" of capital assets, resulting in additional costs (maintenance and inefficiencies) and loss of revenue (loss of referrals, slower throughput, or perceived lower quality). Overspending on capital increases the fixed expenses mentioned above that must be covered by operating cash flow. Health care leaders must determine the optimal level of spending given the condition of current capital assets, market forces, and available financial resources.

Management and Governance

Management and governance (board of directors or trustees) have a significant impact on the financial performance of health care organizations. Management is responsible for the development and execution of strategic direction. Governance is responsible for policies that drive strategy development and management oversight to ensure that those policies are maintained. Lenders and investors rely on both management and governance to ensure that proper systems of internal control are in place to protect their investments (loans or stock) and to report fairly on the financial performance of the organization. Governance also has a special responsibility to the community to ensure that organizational policies and strategies are in the interests of the community served.

Reporting and accounting scandals during the late 1990s and early 2000s increased the focus of legislators and regulators on the appropriateness of financial reporting and internal controls of publicly owned companies. The law known as **Sarbanes-Oxley** increased significantly the accountably of management and governance in ensuring proper accounting, financial reporting, and internal control (see Securities Lawyers Deskbook: http://www.law.uc.edu for more information on this law). Publicly owned companies have invested heavily to develop systems to increase this accountability and to obtain the assurance of external auditing firms related to these systems (Howell, de Mesa Graziano, & Sinnett, 2005). In addition, health care provider organizations, especially tax-exempt, nonprofit organizations, are under scrutiny to ensure that the public benefit they provide is worth the public cost of the tax exemption they enjoy. Issues such as billing practices and services provided to poor and uninsured individuals, as well as compensation levels for top executives, are issues being examined at both federal and state levels. Governance, especially, has an obligation to ensure that the organization is meeting and properly reporting on the community benefits provided (see HFMA "Valuation and Presentation of Charity Care and Bad Debt" available at http://www.hfma.org).

From an operational level, management has a responsibility to ensure that a culture of caring and a concern for quality is an integral part of operations. A working relationship between physicians, nurses, and other professionals that is respectful and has a spirit of teamwork is a key component of this effort. Inattention to the needs of employees, poor employee interaction and teamwork, and inadequate or dysfunctional IT systems foster employee dissatisfaction and turnover. Management's responsibility to ensure a positive work environment directly impacts the financial performance of the organization. The cost of turnover (recruitment costs, training costs, productivity issues, etc.) and the impact of employee dissatisfaction on work performance and quality is well documented (see Institute of Medicine, 2001).

The issues identified in this section of Chapter 2 drive financial performance. Key factors include payment for services, competition for volume of services, underlying economic conditions, and expenditures for the provision of services (both operating expenses and capital purchases). Management and governance must be focused on all of these issues. As noted above, however, management of labor costs is a key component of financial performance. Labor shortages, especially for nurses, technicians, and physicians in some specialties, drive labor costs. According to research performed by May, Bazzoli, and Gerland (2006), short-term strategies used to combat shortages include use of temporary staff, foreign workers, and increases in pay and benefits. Long-term strategies related to education include professional development, orientation, partnering with schools, and faculty support. As indicated above, improvement in the work environment is a key **role of management.**

Strategies related to improved work environment often focus on improvements in productivity. But, unlike cost-cutting efforts that reduce the workforce without reorganizing job processes, the current focus is on ensuring that the right tools (technology, workflow, training) are in place so that time is not wasted on nonproductive rework, paperwork, or processes that do not add value (HFMA, 2007).

Management of health care organizations in an environment of constrained revenue (e.g., price inflexibility and increased competition) requires effective management of human resources and labor costs. Effective management of labor costs involves creating a positive work environment, including tools for improved productivity and long-term strategies that ensure increased employee satisfaction. Without this focus, the health care organization will not be able to deal effectively with the challenges to financial performance described above.

SUMMARY

Law specifies the rules of the "game," for the business of human resources management in health services organizations. Finance assures that resources are available for the organization to fulfill its mission and achieve its vision. This chapter addressed two fundamental facets of the human resources manager's surroundings: law and finance. The major milieus for human resources management are the legal and financial frameworks (Dunlop, 1958).

Legal Environment

A constructive perspective sees law as empowering rather than constraining. Law addresses a fundamental human resources management question: by what authority do I act? An unnecessarily risk-taking approach confuses enforcement with law. Identification of the authority to act in law provides the power to act, a context appreciated by Dunlop (1958).

A purpose of this chapter is to teach the ability to recognize, describe, discuss, and apply the most significant issues in the legal and financial environment for health care human resources management. Legal issue identification should include timely consultation of an attorney.

The employment-at-will doctrine results in a relatively unregulated legal environment for managers and employees. With the exception of wage-and-hour laws (e.g., *Fair Labor Standards Act*) and labor relations laws (e.g., *National Labor Relations Act*), managers before the "pivotal year" of 1964 had broad discretion in their treatment of employees (Fallon & McConnell, 2007, p. 41).

The *Civil Rights Act of 1964* was the beginning of a more heavily regulated legal environment for human resources management in health services organizations, consisting of the major federal statutes establishing the extent of equal opportunity in employment, including not only Title VII of the *Civil Rights Act of 1964* (42 U.S.C. sections 2000e-2000e-17) but also the *Age Discrimination in Employment Act* [29 U.S.C. sections 621-634, 663(a)], the *Americans with Disabilities Act of 1990* (29 U.S.C. section 706), the *Rehabilitation Act of 1973* (29 U.S.C. section 701), and the *Equal Pay Act of 1963* (29 U.S.C. section 201).

Legal issues regarding the employment relationship from the more comprehensive subject of health care law include, but are not limited to, such concerns as selection of employees; health screening; training and supervision; staffing and staffing ratios; constitutional searches and seizures in the workplace; discipline and dismissal; drug and other substance testing; genetic screening and testing; other behavioral screening; polygraph tests; communications about former staff; *Federal Wage Garnishment Law; Employee Retirement Income Security Act of 1974* (ERISA); *Health Insurance Portability and Accountability Act of 1996* (HIPAA); *Family and Medical Leave Act of 1993;* state laws (e.g., anti-injunction acts, union security contracts and right-to-work laws, worker's compensation, unemployment compensation); independent contractors (e.g., taxes, benefits, discrimination, labor law, whistle-blowers, confidentiality of medical records, liability); volunteers; and students (Furrow, et al., 2000, 2008; Miller, 2007; Pozgar, 2006).

Financial Environment

Ensuring resources are available to enable the health care organization to fulfill its mission is a key role of governance and management. The financial environment in which the organization operates often determines the strategic and tactical approaches that must be used by management, within the policy established by governance and the legal "rules of the game." Strategic human resource management is a critical component of overall organizational management because people provide the services and support necessary to fulfill the organization's mission. And, labor cost is the largest single component of a health care provider's overall cost structure.

The factors that drive organizational financial performance are payment rates, competition and volume shifts, national and state economies, capital spending, and the actions of management and governance in relation to these factors. These factors also are very interrelated.

For example, payment rates from governmental sponsors (Federal and state governments) often are determined by the level of tax receipts and number of enrollees in their programs which are dependent in large part on national and state economies. Competition among providers of health services impact the volume of services provided and payment levels received by various competitors. Capital spending is dependent on the adequacy of payment levels and the volume of services provided. All of these factors must be considered by management when developing strategies and tactics.

Strategic management of human resources recognizes the role of management and governance in creating a positive work environment that is empowered by the spirit and letter of the law as well as the need to fulfill mission within a financial framework.

DISCUSSION QUESTIONS

1. What is the purpose of law for human resources management in health services organizations?
2. Describe and discuss differences in the legal environment for human resources management before 1964 and after 1964, and the implications of the differences.
3. Describe and discuss the three most important legal issues in human resources management. What will you do as a manager about the three issues' respective importance?
4. What factors effect the level of payment from both public (Medicare and Medicaid) and private payers?
5. Management must seek a balance in the level of spending for capital items (equipment and facilities). What are the issues that impact this balance and why is a balance important?
6. What are the respective roles of management and governance in the effective financial management of the organization?

REFERENCES

American College of Healthcare Executives. (2006). *Top Issues Confronting Hospitals: 2006.* American College of Healthcare Executives survey. Accessed http://www.ache.org.

American Hospital Association. (2006). *Trend Watch: Trends Affecting Hospitals and Health Systems.* American Hospital Association and The Lewin Group. Special Report. March.

American Hospital Association. (2007). *AHA Hospital Statistics.* Health Forum an American Hospital Association Company.

Angrisano, C., Farrell, D., Kocher, B., Laboissiere, M., & Parker, S. (2007). *Accounting for the Cost of Health Care in the United States.* McKinsey & Company: McKinsey Global Institute. Special report. January.

Black, H. (1979). *Black's Law Dictionary* (5th ed.). St. Paul: West Publishing Company.

Buntin, M., Damberg, C., Haviland, A., Kapur, K., Lurie, N., McDevitt, R., & Marquis, M.S. (2006). Consumer-Directed Health Care: Early Evidence About Effects on Cost and Quality. *Health Affairs.* W516. October 24.

Bureau of Economic Analysis. (2007). U.S. Department of Commerce. Accessed from http://www.bea.gov.

Bureau of Labor Statistics. (2007). *Employees on Non-Farm Payrolls by Industry.* Accessed August 17, 2007, from http://www.bls.gov.

Clarke, L. (2007). Price Transparency: Building Community Trust. *Frontiers of Health Services Management.* American College of Healthcare Executives. 23:3. Spring.

CMS/OOA. (2007). *National Health Expenditure Projections 2006-2016.* Centers for Medicare and Medicaid Services/Office of the Actuary. Accessed from http://www.cms.hhs.gov.

Collins, S., Davis, K., Doty, M., & Ho, A. (2004). *Wages, Health Benefits, and Workers' Health.* Commonwealth Fund Issue Brief. Accessed October, 2004, from http://www.cmwf.org.

Dobson, A., DaVanzo, J., & Sen, N. (2006). The Cost-Shift Payment 'Hydraulic': Foundation, History, and Implications. *Health Affairs.* January/February, 25(1), 23.

Dunlop, J. (1958). *Industrial Relations Systems.* Carbondale, IL: Southern Illinois University Press, reprint, 1970.

Fallon, L., & McConnell, C. (2007). *Human Resource Management in Health Care: Principles and Practice.* Sudbury, MA: Jones and Bartlett Publishers.

Federal Register. (2007). Department of Health and Human Services. Part IV. Friday, August 3, 2007.

Furrow, B., Greaney, T., Johnson, S., Jost, T. & Schwartz, R. (2000). *Health Law* (2nd ed.). St. Paul: West Group.

Furrow, B., Greaney, T., Johnson, S., Jost, T. & Schwartz, R. (2008). *Health Law: Cases, Materials, and Problems* (6th ed.). St. Paul: West.

Ginsburg, P., & Grossman, J. (2005). "When the Price Isn't Right: How Inadvertent Payment Incentives Drive Medical Cost." *Health Affairs.* Aug. 9. W5-376.

Government Accountability Office. (2002). *Nursing Homes: Quality of Care More Related to Staffing than Spending.* Government Accountability Office report. June.

Greenlaw, P., & Kohl, J. (1995). The Equal Pay Act: Responsibilities and rights. *Employee Rights and Responsibilities Journal, 8*(4), 295–307.

HFMA. (2003). Financing the Future Report 1: How are Hospitals Financing the Future? Access to Capital in Health Care Today. Healthcare Financial Management Association report.

Hirsch, B., & Schumacher, E. (1998). Union wages, rents and skills in health care labor markets. *Journal of Labor Research, 19*(Winter), 125–147.

Howe, M. (Ed.) (1941). *The Correspondence of Mr. Justice Holmes and Sir Frederick Pollock 1874–1932.* Cambridge, MA: Harvard University Press, April 21, 1932.

Howell, R.A., de Mesa Graziano, C., & Sinnett, W. (2005). *Sarbanes-Oxley Section 404 Implementation— Practices of Leading Companies.* Financial Executives Research Foundation report.

Institute of Medicine. (2001). *Crossing the Quality Chasm: A New Health System for the 21st Century.* Institute of Medicine report. March.

Institute of Medicine. (2003). *Keeping Patients Safe: Transforming the Work Environment of Nurses.* Institute of Medicine report. November.

Kaufman, K. (2007). *Current Healthcare Trends and Their Strategic Implications—Critcal Financial Issues for Hospital Leadership.* BoardRoom Press. The Governance Institute. 18:4. August.

Lee, J., Berenson, R., Mayers, R., & Gauthier, A. (2003). Medicare Payment Policy: Does Cost Shifting Matter? *Health Affairs.* W3-480. October 8.

May, J., Bazzoli, G., & Gerland, A. 2006. Hospitals' Responses to Nurse Staffing Shortages. *Health Affairs.* W316. June 26.

Medical Group Management Association. (2006). *Cost Survey for Multi-specialty Practices.* 2006 Report.

Miller, R. (2006). *Problems in Health Care Law* (9th ed.). Sudbury, MA: Jones and Bartlett Publishers.

Moody's. (2007). *Not-for-Profit Healthcare Sector: 2007 Industry Outlook.* Moody's Investors Service. January.

Morton-Cooper, A., & Barnford, M. (Eds.) (1997). *Excellence in Health Care Management.* Cambridge, MA: Blackwell Publishing.

Nichols, & O'Malley, A. (2006). Hospital Payment Systems: Will Payers Like the Future Better Than The Past? *Health Affairs, 25*(1). January/February.

Perlin, M. (2000). *Mental Disability Law: Civil and Criminal* (2nd ed.; vol. 3). Newark: Matthew Bender & Company.

Pozgar, G. (2007). *Legal Aspects of Health Care Administration* (10th ed.). Sudbury, MA: Jones and Bartlett Publishers.

Wilensky, G. (2007). Pay for Performance and Physicians—An Open Question. *Healthcare Financial Management, 6*(12). February.

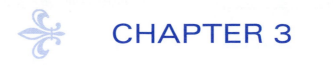

CHAPTER 3

Formulating Organizational Strategy

S. Robert Hernandez, DrPH and Elena Platonova, PhD

LEARNING OBJECTIVES

Upon completing this chapter, the reader will be able to:

1. Describe the evolution of planning systems used by American industry.
2. List and discuss the four corporate-level strategies available to health services managers.
3. List and discuss the business-level strategies available for health services organizations to gain strategic advantage over competitors.
4. Participate in formulation of an organization's strategy using the process illustrated in the text.
5. Describe the critical human resources issues facing strategists in each stage of the product/market life cycle.

KEY TERMS

Boston Consulting Group (BCG) Business Grid

Competitive Analysis

Cost Leadership Strategies

Differentiation Strategy

Distinct Competence

Financial Planning

Focus Strategy

Industry Analysis

Long-Range Planning

Mission Statement

Positioning

Product Life-Cycle Portfolio Matrix

Strategic Business Units

Strategic Management

Strategic Thinking

INTRODUCTION

A critical function of health care management is development of a plan for the future actions to be taken by the organization. Senior managers must identify the major tasks to be accomplished by their firm, assign responsibility for performance of those tasks, and monitor organizational actions to ensure that the tasks are executed satisfactorily. An adequate planning system allows a health care organization to achieve organizational objectives by identifying and being responsive to environmental change through deployment of internal resources in an efficient and effective manner.

The planning system or systems that are used by an organization vary based on the sophistication of management, rates of environmental change, and level of competition experienced within a geographic region or service sector. A planning system also must match the corporate culture of the firm as well as the complexity of the business in which the organization is competing. Major planning approaches available to health care managers are reviewed in the following section. Next, selected organizational strategies that might be used by health care institutions are presented. A guide for formulating the organization's strategy is then suggested. Selected relationships that should exist between possible business strategies and human resources functions are described at the conclusion of this chapter.

PLANNING METHODS

The methods used for the formulation of strategies and plans by organizations in the health services industry have evolved rather dramatically over the years. The major types of planning approaches that have been used are **financial planning** (1950s and earlier), **long-range planning** (1960s), strategic planning (1970s), and **strategic management** (since the 1980s). Financial planning mostly focused on budgets for a given time period, usually annually (Pettigrew, Thomas, & Whittington, 2002). Long-range planning is concerned with the projection of organizational goals, objectives, programs, and budgets during an extended period. This approach requires forecasting of environmental trends based on historical data. Strategic planning involves an organization's choices of mission, objectives, strategy, policies, programs, goals, and major resources allocations. This method is intended to define the strategy for the firm so that internal resources and skills are matched to the opportunities and risks created within the environment. Finally, strategic management is concerned with integration among administrative systems, organizational structure, and organizational culture for both strategic and operational decision making. This approach views strategic planning as one element of administrative functioning that must be blended with other management processes for an organization to function efficiently.

Each of these methods represents a fundamentally different approach for planning and organizing the activities of a health services organization. The evolution of each of these planning approaches in the health services industry is reviewed and implications for use of these techniques in strategy development are discussed.

Budgeting

Budgets are organizations' *financial* plans and are generally expressed in monetary terms. Thus, budgets are practical expressions of organizational financial goals. Budgeting was one of the first planning methods that emerged more than 60 years ago and, typically, early planning was mostly financial planning. Budgets were usually projections from the past into the future made by financial managers (Pettigrew, et al., 2002).

Budgeting continues to be an integral part of organizational long- and short-term planning. Its major function is to assist management in successfully implementing organizational strategies as well as planning, coordination, and control of operational activities of the organization (Henderson, 2003b; Rickards, 2006). Budgets provide essential information for managerial decision making and organizational control, for negotiating and monitoring managed care contracts as well as for helping management in overall financial planning (Fabrizio & Hertz, 2005; Henderson, 2003a; McVay & Cooke, 2006). Budgetary targets are typically set for a year and serve the basis of planning and control of organizational performance. Budgeting continues to be one of the most important tools of control in organizations (Rickards, 2006), and it is vital for reporting money received and spent, guaranteeing that organizations' financial guidelines are complied with, ensuring that financial resources are not wasted, and assisting managers to manage and develop services (Henderson, 2003b).

Budgeting has value for institutional planning because the process requires that the hospital direct its attention toward the future and plan for it. Thus, it *raises the priority of planning* within an organization. Additionally, budgeting *provides a structure* for the planning activity. It requires identification of projected revenues, expenses, capital needs, and cash flows for organizational units. Performance can be meaningfully planned, evaluated, and controlled by the responsibility centers identified

through the budgeting activity. Budgeting also ensures that the management team and physician leaders are *well-informed about the financial health* of the organization. Operationally, *budgets provide a benchmark* for the organization to regularly evaluate financial results, to assess the variances from the benchmarks, and to make appropriate operational changes as necessary. Further, the budget serves as a *motivator for employees* to strive for approved financial goals and as a *guide* for budgeted expenditures (Fabrizio & Hertz, 2005).

A typical process used in the decision-making process for budget development is illustrated in Figure 3.1. This simplified version of the process suggests that the facility board establish financial goals for the organization and give final approval to the budget. Senior management develops operational objectives and policies, establishes priorities for program development, plans for budget development including financial assumptions, and conducts the final administrative review after budgets have been developed. Line management must convert policy and operating objectives into programs by specifying resources required to accomplish approved projects.

If maximum benefit is to be obtained from this approach to planning, management must be sensitive to the importance of planning rather than

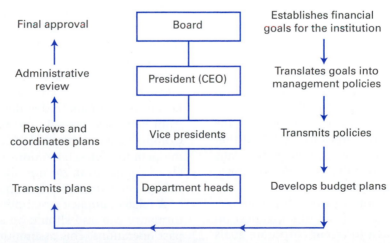

Figure 3.1. **Budget Preparation**

financial issues driving the budget process. The budget will have little value if it becomes a paper-shuffling exercise driven by finance rather than a comprehensive institutional plan driving projected revenues and expenses.

Budgeting will be inappropriately developed as a planning tool if the process does little more than use historical data for budget projections with only incremental change anticipated over past operations. One approach to overcome these incremental increases is to use the zero-based method that provides accurate and justifiable budget estimates. This approach uses historical data as a reference point but develops future projections from scratch using multiple sources of information (Fabrizio & Hertz, 2005). While traditional budgeting processes require only that a manager justify the increases planned over previous years, zero-based budgeting requires each department to defend its entire budget request each year. As a result, zero-based budgeting has been labelled as time consuming and inefficient (McVay & Cooke, 2006).

Another concern that arises if management uses budgeting as the only planning process for a health care facility is that the focus is only on organizational functional areas and on cost reduction and short-term profits rather than on the lasting, value-oriented execution of the strategy. It is important that management prevent preoccupation with short-term return on investment at the expense of the organization's long-term growth.

Long-Range Planning

Substantial improvement in planning future operations for a firm was made with the introduction of long-range planning. The use of this method followed the rapid growth of the U.S. economy in the post-World War II era. Corporations found that 1-year budget projections were inadequate means for identifying future operating plans for organizations in the rapidly expanding economy.

Long-range planning requires that management focus the energies of the organization on an integrated approach to attain corporate goals and objectives and be focused essentially on the planning of each of the functions—marketing, production, finance, human resources—necessary to reach long-term objectives. In the past, staffs were often employed and trained to develop long-range plans at the corporate level and for each function (Pettigrew, et al., 2002). Descriptions of long-range planning techniques were relatively widespread in the hospital and health services literature by the mid-1970s. Perlin (1976) presented a model outline for a hospital long-range plan that included several steps. The characteristics of the population residing in the facility's service area with projections of future demographic changes would be identified in one step. A planner then would forecast future community needs based on anticipated population changes and health delivery techniques, inventory current health resources and services, and conclude with future gaps or excesses in services based on a comparison of the preceding two factors. Historical utilization of an institution's programs and services would be chronicled. Then, based on the organization's mission and the gaps previously identified, the facility's plan to carry out future service programs would be developed. A long-range plan would conclude with an implementation plan that placed programs and services in short-range and long-range priorities and described physical plant requirements for plan accomplishment, manpower required, and financial resources needed. A typical flow of steps in long-range planning is illustrated in Figure 3.2.

This method represents a major improvement over the use of budgeting as a planning tool because it increases managerial awareness of and responsibility for planning. However, several limitations potentially detract from its use for charting future directions for an organization. One weakness is the assumption that the future is predictable from historical growth and utilization patterns. Complex environments that feature rapid change in operating rules, conditions of demand, and levels of competition do not allow the future to be extrapolated accurately from past operations.

A related, implicit assumption is that future performance can and should be an improvement on past operations. This assumption can lead managers to think they can control the future and achieve

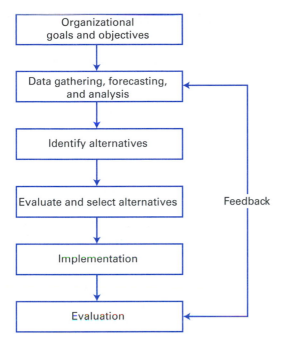

Figure 3.2. Long-Range Planning

sustained growth when, in fact, external forces beyond management's control may influence the organization's operations. Overly optimistic objectives can be identified because of this belief.

Another problem with long-range planning is that it frequently is developed by support staff or external consulting firms using exhaustive arrays of operating and environmental data, but without adequate involvement of either senior or line management. Meager participation by senior managers results in a plan that does not provide strategic direction for a firm because the plan may not address major issues critical for the organization's survival. This document becomes a dust gatherer that sits on a shelf and is reviewed annually, at best.

Strategic Thinking and Strategic Planning

Strategic planning in American industry is a reaction to changes in the nature of competition and increasing uncertainty in a firm's operating environment. Organizations had to confront environmental

fluctuations that had not been projected by their long-range planning systems, and discontinuities caused significant problems for the firms (Ansoff, 1977). Generally, strategic planning focuses on the examination of past trends and extrapolating future trends based on the past trends (Bonn, 2001; Heracleous, 1998). Strategic planning is about analysis and deals with articulation, elaboration, and formalization of existing strategies. Hence, it usually follows a predetermined strategy and helps senior management to allocate resources and to implement the strategy (Mintzberg, 1994).

Strategic planning has over time evolved into **strategic thinking.** The major characteristics of this shift is demonstrated by the decentralization of planning departments to business units, the change in planning responsibility from staff planners to line managers, more attention to market assessment, and more sophisticated quantitative techniques (Heracleous, 1998). Though strategic thinking is thought of as an evolution from strategic planning, strategic planning is also a process that takes place *after* strategic thinking (Bonn, 2001). Strategic thinking involves synthesis, which encourages intuitive, innovative, and creative thinking at all levels of the organization (Bonn, 2001; Mintzberg, 1994).

The ability to think strategically is crucial to stay competitive in an increasingly turbulent and global environment, and it is another dimension of the process of strategy making (Graetz, 2002). Strategic thinking is a method of thinking that has specific attributes, which include a holistic approach to the organization and the environment. A strategist must understand the vertical linkages within the system from multiple perspectives (Liedtka, 1998). Other important individual attributes pertain to creativity and a vision for the organization. However, it is the organization that creates the environment in which individual strategic thinking occurs. Hence, organizations must create structures, processes, and systems that facilitate a continuous strategic dialogue among the top management teams and which would benefit from the creativity of every individual employee

(Bonn, 2001). Strategic planning and strategic thinking are interrelated and are equally important for effective strategic management. Creative, ground-breaking strategies emerge from strategic thinking, but they still have to be operationalized through analytical thought (strategic planning); planning is important but cannot produce unique strategies that will challenge industrial boundaries and redefine industries (Heracleous, 1998).

Strategic planning focuses on the market environment facing a firm, including future actions by competitors and consumers. A major contribution of strategic planning is the use of market segmentation and portfolio analysis that allow management to assess the relative attractiveness and competitive strength of the business units of the organization. Typically, this approach to planning contains four steps (Ansoff & McDonnell, 1990). First, management conducts an *analysis of the anticipated results* of the firm's operations through projection of operating trends as well as identification of environmental threats and opportunities. These data provide levels of performance likely to be attained if management initiates no change in strategy. Then, **competitive analysis** identifies performance improvement that is possible from changes in the competitive strategies employed in current business units of the firm. Next, *portfolio analysis* allows management to establish priorities for the business units by comparing the anticipated future performance of all business areas. Because all subunits will not be anticipated to enjoy equal success, priorities for allocation of resources to business units can occur based on this analysis. Finally, *diversification analysis* provides management with an opportunity to identify new business opportunities if deficiencies exist in the current portfolio of services. The improvement in health services organization performance is possible following each of these analyses with related management actions that are suggested as appropriate. Incremental performance increases are possible, from improving competitive strategies in current businesses, more efficiently allocating resources among current portfolio of businesses, and diversifying into new areas.

Strategic Management

Strategic management is the most recent approach to planning that traditionally focused on business concepts that affect organizational performance (Hoskisson, et al., 1999). Strategic management is concerned with major intended and emergent strategies developed and executed by general managers and involves utilization of resources to enhance organizations' performances in their external environments (Nag, Hambrick, & Chen, 2007; Pettigrew, et al., 2002). It includes both strategic planning and implementation, and the measure of its success is the development of competitive advantage in each major line in the organization (Pettigrew, et al., 2002). In recent years, strategic management has become associated with flexibility and prompt responses to frequent discontinuous changes in the external environment. As a result, strategic management is viewed more as a basis for learning and adaptation than a permanent plan for the organization (Camillus, 1997).

Strategic management is also concerned with linking strategic planning activities with other internal management systems, the structure of the organization, and the culture of the firm. This means that management must work to see that the outcomes of strategic planning become an administrative reality. The next section of this chapter identifies the relationships and techniques for achieving the organizational strategies that are desired through strategic management of human resources within a health care organization. The remainder of this chapter is devoted to strategic planning and management processes that provide direction for the organization.

ORGANIZATIONAL STRATEGY

Many individuals do not distinguish between organizational strategy, operating tactics, and functional operating policy. The focus of strategic planning activities should be on *strategic* issues and *strategy* development, rather than operating tactics. Thus, a clear delineation of what constitutes strategy is critical. Because a complex health services orga-nization contains many operational units and can offer a vast array of products and services to a com-munity, a second area that requires clarification is how to identify the major subunits of an organi-zation. These subunits, called **strategic business units,** are the starting points for development of organizational strategy. A discussion of what con-stitutes strategy and how strategic business units are to be identified is provided here.

Types of Strategies

Although numerous management theorists and au-thors have definitions of what constitutes strategy,[1] Drucker (1974) captured the topic best when he stated that thinking about the mission and strat-egy of an organization involves answering the fol-lowing questions: *What is our business and what should it be?* These questions translate into *identifi-cation of the business areas in which the organiza-tion will compete.*

Health services organizations must determine what services they will provide to which market areas. Their current portfolio of services and/or business areas must be reviewed and a decision reached on what will be done with each of the ser-vices/businesses. This analysis is a corporate-level strategic decision that focuses on which areas will be *built, held, harvested, or divested.* Unique op-erating decisions concerning levels of investment, allocation of resources, functional policies, and related concerns are associated with each of these four strategic options that may be applied to a business unit operated by a firm.

Build

The decision by a health services organization to build a service/business area means that the insti-tution plans to invest heavily in the service in an attempt to increase its market share of consumers receiving the service. This approach may be taken even if it means that the institution forgoes some short-term profits to build market share. A system of emergicare centers may decide to implement a build strategy by retaining operating profits for develop-ment of new service delivery sites. Alternatively, the system may decide to implement its strategy by raising capital for growth by offering convertible debentures to a limited number of investors.

Hold

A decision to hold suggests that the institution has an objective to maintain its current market share. This strategy usually is associated with services or businesses that are expected to generate large cash flows that are to be diverted to other investment op-portunities. Increased levels of investment are made only to the extent that there are increases in patient demand. Many hospitals providing inpatient acute care have implicitly adopted this strategy.

Harvest

Organizations that attempt a harvesting strategy desire to increase short-term cash flows emanating from a service regardless of the consequences for that service. This strategy may be implemented by reduc-ing staffing levels, cutting maintenance, or allowing technical obsolescence or related tactics that decrease operating costs while maintaining prices. The long-term outcome will be that the service/business will be terminated or sold. A multi-institutional system may employ this strategy with a group of hospitals it owns in an attempt to reap short-term profits before disposing of the holdings to another system.

Divest

The decision to divest means that the organization will abandon the market. Resources that would have been consumed in service delivery will be di-verted to other parts of the organization. Divesting is illustrated by a multi-institutional system selling a hospital in a geographic area that it no longer

---

[1]For examples of strategy definitions, see Thompson, Strickland, and Gamble (2008); Swayne, Duncan, and Ginter (2006); Hofer and Schendel (1978); and Steiner (1979).

wants to serve, or it could entail termination of a major service (e.g., obstetrics) by a community general hospital.

A second, related, question that must be answered for strategy formulation is to determine *how the organization will compete in the delivery of the services to the markets that have been identified.* Managers must decide what general approach they will use to provide services to the areas they have identified. The answer to this question concerns what *competitive advantage* the organization will attempt to achieve. Three basic strategies that have been found to lead to sustained competitive advantage are overall **cost leadership, differentiation,** and **focus** (Hall, 1980; Porter, 1980, 1985).

Cost Leadership

Achieving overall cost leadership is an attempt by a health care provider to become the low-cost producer for an area. If a firm is able to provide services at a lower *cost* than its competitors and yet obtain reimbursement at *prices* that are comparable, it will receive above-average returns.

Although use of economies of scale through being the market share leader for a product is a common means of becoming the cost leader for industrial sector firms, numerous approaches may be used in the health services industry. Some investor-owned hospitals attempt to achieve cost leadership through management systems geared to control resource consumption (e.g., close monitoring of full-time equivalents per occupied bed). Health maintenance organizations attempt cost leadership through controlling utilization, especially hospital admissions. The methods for achieving cost leadership in health services depend on the type of organization providing the service, the consumers of the service, payer mix served by the institution, forms of reimbursement, and related other factors.

Differentiation

An organization seeking to achieve differentiation desires to be perceived by consumers as offering a service that is unique in important dimensions. This uniqueness is usually associated with a premium price that can be charged for the service.

Achieving differentiation may be associated with *technical quality* of the medical care that is being delivered. The medical staff, the level of technical sophistication of equipment provided, and related matters may be viewed by the community as being superior to competitors. Differentiation also may be associated with offering *patient amenities* that are valued (e.g., valet parking in crowded inner-city hospital locations; immediate access to medical personnel in emergency rooms; a reputation for having a responsive, caring nursing staff for inpatient acute care).

Focus

Organizations choosing to focus are those that target a narrow scope of competition within their community. The institution decides on a market segment or group to which it will provide a service or range of services. After choosing the target market, the institution may then have a *cost focus* or a *differentiation focus.*

One example of a focus strategy is initiation of pediatric emergency services by a community general hospital. Although there is increasing competition in many communities for the emergent patient, identifying pediatric patients as the market to be served may give a hospital a competitive advantage in a saturated urgent-care market. Targeted marketing strategies, special billing practices, separate entrances, unique employee uniforms, and related operating tactics support this strategy of focusing on the pediatric patient in need of urgent care and then differentiating the service from other emergency services available within the community.

Identifying Strategic Business Units

Most health care organizations are composed of logically grouped business units that are responsible for specific sets of activities and products. Some of these units compete in well-defined markets and have distinct competitors. These units are strategic and long-term-oriented parts of the organization that are used to establish long-term competitive advantage in their markets. Thus, they are focused on markets with greater strategic potential

(Samli & Shaw, 2002). These units are generally referred to as strategic business units (SBUs). One of the primary values of identifying SBUs is that the institution can discriminate among the divergent markets that it serves, develop logical strategies that will be successful in these unique markets, and assign responsibility for implementing the plan.

The composition of an SBU depends on the level of organization that is being examined. At the corporate level for HCA or Tenet, SBUs may be identified by groupings such as psychiatric hospital division, inpatient acute care hospital division, or outpatient diagnostic center division. Conversely, a multispecialty medical group may define its SBUs based on clinical services such as pediatrics, obstetrics, and general surgery.

For acute care hospitals, data may be collected and operational management decisions reached on the basis of diagnosis-related groupings (DRGs). However, it is *not* practical to plan using DRGs as the units for which strategies are developed because it would be almost impossible for a community hospital to develop unique market approaches for more than 400 business units. It is possible that clinical service groupings are appropriate units for SBU analysis by these hospitals.

Although there are a number of ways that one might identify SBUs, an ideal SBU might have the following characteristics (Kotler & Keller, 2006):

- It is a single business or collection of related businesses.
- It has a distinct mission.

- It has its own competitors.
- It has a responsible manager.
- It consists of one or more program units and financial units.
- It can benefit from strategic planning.
- It can be planned independently of the other businesses.

As previously stated, it is important that units designated as SBUs develop plans for the markets that they serve. In addition, these SBUs should receive resources to implement the plan and be held accountable for the plan's success or failure. Some health organizations do not delegate these latter functions to the managers at the operating unit level, requiring senior management oversight of these responsibilities. The separation of these activities currently appears to be working well. In any case, SBU plan development, resource allocation, and accountability for performance must be done in conjunction with an overall strategy for approaching the marketplace that is developed by corporate planning.

FORMULATING ORGANIZATIONAL STRATEGY

A model process used to generate strategy for a health care organization is illustrated in Figure 3.3. Planning begins with a **mission statement** that

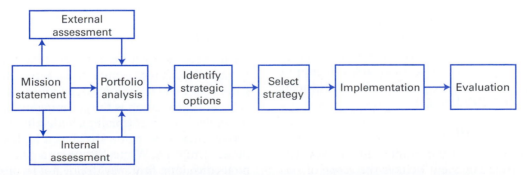

Figure 3.3. The Strategy Development Process in Health Services Organizations

has been articulated with sufficient detail to guide organizational decision making; external and internal analyses are then conducted; the portfolio is reviewed; strategies are identified and selected; implementation is accomplished; and evaluation begins. The material provided in this section, while not presented at the level of detail required to guide the production of a strategic plan, allows the reader to understand the flow of data and the rationale that supports corporate strategy development. This understanding is beneficial for comprehending the relationship between strategy and human resources functions. Detailed discussions of strategic planning approaches are offered by Bryson (2004), Swayne, et al. (2006), Hofer and Schendel (1978), Nutt (1984), and Thompson, et al. (2008).

Mission of the Organization

The first step in development of strategies is to identify the general direction in which the organization is headed. It is the responsibility of senior management to provide the institution with the goals and operating philosophy that will be a guide to direct the future of the firm. The communication of corporate purpose, scope of operations, self-concept, and image to important stakeholders occurs through a mission statement.

The principal value of a mission statement as a tool of strategic management is derived from its specification of the ultimate aims of the firm. It thus provides managers with a unity of direction that transcends individual, parochial, and transitory needs. It promotes a sense of shared expectations among all levels and generations of employees. It consolidates values over time and across individuals and interest groups. It projects a sense of worth and intent that can be identified and assimilated by company outsiders, that is, customers, suppliers, competitors, local committees, and the general public (Pearce, 1982, p. 24).

Product Definition

The identification of the product line of services means that management defines the *scope* of services that the organization will offer by determining the breadth of the line that will be provided. Will a complete range of patient needs be met or will the organization target a specific service? A multispecialty group may decide to change its product definition by broadening its services with the addition of a new specialty (e.g., neurology) that had not been offered previously. This decision allows the group to capture revenues that may have been lost to the group when patient referrals were made to other neurologists who were not members of the group.

Defining how an organization wishes its services to be perceived by consumers in relation to competitors providing the service is known as **positioning.** One example is positioning on the basis of a price–quality spectrum. An organization may attempt to be perceived as providing comparable services at a lower cost than its competitors. Emergicenters attempt to convince consumers that the centers can provide minor emergency service comparable to a hospital emergency room more rapidly and at a lower cost.

Products and services benefit from a positioning strategy that is clearly articulated to the target market for that service. Six potential approaches for a positioning strategy are listed as follows (Wind, 1982, pp. 79–81):

- Positioning on specific product features
- Positioning on benefits, problem solutions, or needs
- Positioning for specific usage occasions
- Positioning for user category
- Positioning against another product
- Product class dissociation

Market Definition

Defining the market for a business requires identifying the consumer groups to be served by the organization. The most logical delimiter for a health services organization is the *geographic boundary* of its service area. A hospital may identify its primary service area as a region that has a high relevance index (Griffith & White, 2006), or a generalist hospital consulting firm may decide not to offer its services beyond Midwestern states.

A market also may be defined by the *consumers that desire the product.* The consulting firm that is restricting its services to the Midwest also may identify its clients as senior managers of hospitals that are operating between 100 and 300 beds. This group may value the general management consulting package that is being provided more than other executives in more complex facilities.

The process of defining markets allows management to decide the *market segments* that will be served. Segmentation of a market is the process of breaking the total market into elements that share common properties. Organizations are able to develop appropriate services and provide those services more efficiently for groups that have common needs that have been identified through segmentation.

Distinct Competence

The **distinct competence** of an organization refers to an advantage that the institution holds over its competitors. The advantage may emanate from the competitive advantages of cost leadership, differentiation, or focus that were previously discussed. Alternatively, an organization may possess an asset that provides it with an advantage over competitors. A hospital may have a reputation for an outstanding nursing staff that is well-respected within the community. A nursing home may have evolved into an organization offering a complete array of vertically integrated services for the elderly. A hospital system may have facility sites that are conveniently located near transportation arteries. Articulating the distinct competence for the organization helps management to design strategies that reinforce strengths.

External Assessment

An external analysis focuses on elements that are relevant for organizational performance but are outside the institution's boundaries. The purpose of this assessment is to determine the major opportunities that might be available to the firm and potential threats that might prevent the organization from achieving desired outcomes. This analysis often consists of identifying and analyzing patient groups or consumers, competitors, industry conditions, and general environmental factors.

Consumer Groups

The first issue in external analysis is to identify the markets currently being served by the institution, to select markets that potentially could be served, and to determine how to segment these markets. As noted, the process of segmentation groups consumers into clusters that share common characteristics. The demand for services by consumers should be relatively homogeneous within the group and heterogeneous to demand by other groups. Analyzing consumer groups assists management in identifying increases or decreases in demand that might be associated with changing needs or requirements by the groups that are studied. This knowledge assists in making investment decisions across alternative product/market opportunities.

Competitor Analysis

The result of competitor analysis is identification of the threats or opportunities that will occur from the probable moves and reactions of competitors. This information is obtained by building a competitor's response profile (Wilson & Gilligan, 2005), which includes their future goals, current strategy, assumptions about market conditions, and current strengths and weaknesses.

This profile should include an estimation of the competitor's financial goals as well as a determination of its interest in long-term versus short-term performance. The extent to which the competitor will stress quality versus cost in the provision of services is important to note. Recording the values and beliefs of the competitor's senior managers will provide insight into the reason that specific services and programs are initiated. Knowledge of the structure of the competitor's organization provides information about who key decision makers are, the methods they use to handle the medical staff, and their ability to respond rapidly to its competition's initiatives.

The competitor's assumptions about its own operation and the health services industry also should be a component of the profile. How has it assessed its organization? What does it believe are its strengths and weaknesses? How will its perceptions influence likely thrusts? What does it view as future utilization patterns for the health services industry? What are the *actual* strengths and weaknesses of the competition?

The above information can be used to determine how the competitor will respond to new services that you may decide to offer or to your decision to terminate some of your current services. It also can be used to anticipate strategic thrusts it may be planning.

Analyzing competitors also improves understanding of consumer responses to product offerings. Cognition of the strategies, operating practices, and successes and failures of competing organizations helps management to know the attributes that appeal to various market segments. For example, close monitoring of an innovative service provided by a major competitor will allow management to decide which benefits and features will be included in their own version of the service.

Additionally, this analysis validates consumer analysis and provides clues as to potential market opportunities that may become available (Wilson & Gilligan, 2005). It is possible that identification of the product/markets served by competitors will result in recognition of an area unserved by other institutions.

Industry and Environmental Analysis

A third major component of external assessment is concerned with analyzing trends in the industry as well as overall environmental conditions. **Industry analysis** is intended to identify the competitive factors that lead to success in a given product/market and to determine the relative attractiveness of an industry/market for the firm. The forces that drive competition (Porter, 1980) and the manner in which firms are organized for delivery of services are areas to examine. An additional need is for projections of demand and number of competitors currently providing services or anticipated to begin

service delivery for the market. This information allows identification of the stage of the life cycle for the industry.

The environment provides the context in which industry operating rules and practices exist. *Environmental analysis* is concerned with identifying trends and major events that potentially have an effect on an industry and, ultimately, the strategy of an organization. Just as the environment is one step removed from and above an industry, so is environmental analysis related to, but broader than, industry analysis. Components of environmental analysis may be divided into five dimensions (Aaker, 1984), as follows:

1. Technology: new technologies and the life cycle of current technology;
2. Government: legislative and regulatory actions, tax policies, and values held toward the health industry;
3. Economics: interest rates, economic health of local firms, and general economic conditions;
4. Culture: lifestyle trends that affect consumption of health and related services; and
5. Demographics: trends in age, income, education, and geographic location.

A major component of industry and environmental analysis for health services organizations must include projections of the future availability of selected types of health professionals. For many types of professionals, state licensure boards provide counts of individuals practicing in an area. Of course, individuals may retain their licenses without intending to practice, so these figures are misleading. Historical labor force participation rates are helpful in determining the size of the current manpower pool.

Identifying the numbers of individuals in professional training is necessary to determine the potential size of the pool from which new employees may be recruited. Historical data on the success rate of the organization in attracting new recruits to work in the institution will provide at least a crude measure of the inflow of future workers that might be anticipated.

Internal Assessment

An internal assessment is intended to provide a detailed understanding of attributes of the organization that are of strategic importance. The outcome of this assessment should be a listing of the firm's strengths that might be used for competitive advantage. In addition, problems or weaknesses that might hinder performance must be recognized.

An inventory of current internal capabilities resources, operating characteristics, and actions provides the basis for this assessment. Webber and Peters (1983) suggest that the following areas be examined:

- Management and governance
- Functional programs and services
- Human resources
- Medical staff
- Financial resources and results
- Physical facilities
- Basic values and culture of the organization
- Interrelationships of the above

Although a description of each of these areas is beyond the scope of this chapter, some discussion of the human resources and medical staff inventory is required. Management must maintain separate databases on personnel and medical staff that can be used both for the day-to-day operation of the institution as well as for strategic planning. For strategic purposes, these databases include demographic information, career information, a skills profile, productivity measures, and utilization statistics. These data provide management with the basis for understanding the characteristics of its personnel and medical staff. This information can be used for determining how well the organization is currently functioning as well as for identifying the organization's future internal capabilities for implementation of programs and services that might be planned.

After current capabilities, resources, operating characteristics, and actions of the health care organization are inventoried, these attributes can be compared to performance levels that are standards in the industry or that are desired by management. The result of this assessment is a list of attributes viewed as institutional strengths and a list of organizational weaknesses. These attributes, when combined with the previously developed external opportunities and threats, provide data to be used in assessing the institution's portfolio of goods and services.

Portfolio Assessment

The analysis of the portfolio of SBUs operated by the firm examines the service mix of an organization to determine if the overall array of business units is appropriately balanced. This analysis typically requires that the SBUs of the organization be placed on a matrix that contains two parameters. One parameter describes characteristics (e.g., desirability) of the market or industry in which the SBU is competing, and the other illustrates the strength of the business unit in that unique market. Several techniques are used to conduct portfolio analysis, including the market growth rate-relative market share analysis known as the **Boston Consulting Group (BCG) Business Grid** and the industry maturity-competitive approach analysis known as the **Product Life-Cycle Portfolio Matrix.**

BCG Business Grid

This method of examining the holdings of an organization is based on pioneering work that was conducted by the Boston Consulting Group in the early 1960s. This easily understood analysis focuses on the growth rate for the market of a business and the relative market share that the business commands. As illustrated in Figure 3.4, the annual market growth rate for a business is shown on the vertical axis, and the relative market share of the SBU to its largest competitor is shown on the horizontal axis.

The market growth rate illustrated in Figure 3.4 ranges from 0 to 20%, although values above or below those numbers are possible. Because a growth rate above 10% is considered high, the vertical axis is divided into high and low growth markets

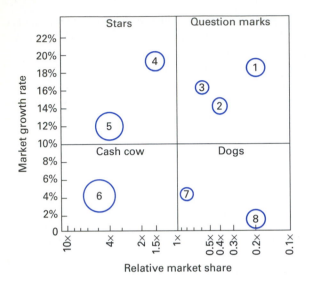

Figure 3.4. **The Boston Consulting Group's Growth-Share Matrix**

SOURCE: Reprinted from *Long Range Planning*, February 1977, Heldey, B., Strategy and the business portfolio, vol. 10, p. 12, Copyright 1977, with kind permission from Pergamon Press, Ltd., Headington Hill Hall, Oxford 0X3 0BW, UK.

at 10%.[2] The relative market share, shown in log scale with equal distances representing the same percentage increase, has the midpoint of the horizontal axis as 1. This occurs when the organization's share exactly equals its largest competitor. A value of 2 on the scale occurs when the firm's SBU has twice the sales as the next strongest firm and a market share that is half that of the strongest competitor is represented by the .5 value. The matrix is divided into four quadrants by these midpoints. The relative share and growth rate of these markets suggests management decisions for the SBUs operating in these four markets.

The lower left quadrant contains the *cash cows*. These SBUs operate in low-growth markets with relatively large market share. The strong market position suggests that they should be able to generate

positive cash flow because they have potential for economies of scale and higher profit margins. Investment needs should not be great because they are situated in a mature market with a low-growth rate. Funds from these businesses are used to support SBUs in other, high-growth, markets.

The upper left quadrant contains the *stars* that are high-growth, high-share SBUs. They require funds to support growth in demand for services, but they also are in a position to perform well financially because of their strong competitive position as market leaders. Stars usually do not generate surplus cash because this high-growth market attracts new firms, and the organization must reinvest to maintain share. These SBUs may be cash users if competitors begin major efforts to gain relative market share that must be countered.

The upper right quadrant contains *question marks,* also known as wildcats, that have relatively low market share in fast-growth markets. These SBUs need to fund growth, but are not able to obtain funding internally because they are not far enough down the experience curve. These businesses are in the worst position because of their growth needs and low market shares. They should be grown to become stars or should be divested.

The lower right quadrant contains the *dogs,* which are not profitable because of their weak competitive position in a low-growth market. Because growth in this market is low, increases in market share are costly. These businesses should be phased out when possible.

After the SBUs have been plotted on the matrix, the organization must determine how balanced the portfolio appears. Too many question marks or dogs or an inappropriate mixture of exclusively stars or cash cows cause management to attempt to change its investment mix.

Although this approach has merits, several factors detract from use of this analytical tool in the health care industry without modification. One issue is that growth rate is not an adequate criterion

---

[2]The cut off for high versus low growth rates is normally selected as the average growth for that industry, assuming that all SBUs are competing in the same industry (Hax & Majluf, 1984).

for determining the desirability of a market for investment decisions. Health care providers have multiple stake-holders with numerous, often conflicting, goals and objectives for the organization. The allocation of capital based on market growth alone is not a responsible approach to this complex situation.

Additionally, the success of market share leadership associated with cost reductions is meaningful only in volume businesses. Health care providers that concentrate on small segments of the market can focus on a defensible niche that is not easily penetrated by market leaders. Thus, market share leadership is not always an adequate criterion for determining the strength of a business.

Product Life-Cycle Matrix

The life-cycle approach is based on an analogy to the biological cycle that living matter experiences through stages of embryonic development, growth, maturity, and decline. Products and services (Kotler & Keller, 2006), organizations (Daft, 2007), and industries (Porter, 1980) are believed to follow a similar pattern from their inception to their decline. Each stage in the life of a service, business unit, or industry is characterized by changes in demand for the service, number of competitors, profitability, cash flow, and other features of market conditions. A generic life-cycle model is illustrated in Figure 3.5.

Although Figure 3.5 represents an expected, or "normal," life cycle, the curve does not always have the same shape as that illustrated. Some services

may have an introductory phase followed by rapid growth and then experience sharp, immediate decline. Other services may have long periods of maturity and never enter decline; still others may enter decline and then observe a revival in demand.

The general market conditions associated with each phase of the life cycle have been identified by Porter (1980) for industry evolution and by Kotler and Keller (2006) for product evolution. The first phase, or *introductory* stage, occurs when the service has just been introduced and there is limited consumer knowledge of the service, with resulting low utilization and revenue levels. Managerial time must be devoted to developing markets for the services because organization capacity is underused. Uncertainty exists among providers as to the technology that will be most effective, because no common standards have evolved. Because product quality may be erratic, control should be exerted over service delivery, possibly through narrowing the scope of service so that operations are better managed. Image and credibility with the financial community may be critical because of the funding required to support the growth and the uncertainty associated with new services.

During the second phase, the *growth* stage, consumer knowledge of the service increases and demand rises. Technical quality improves considerably. Reliability and differentiation become more critical because consumer expectations increase. Organizations experience increased use of existing capacity, and profits grow as costs are spread over larger volume. More providers enter the market and offer a broader scope of services that further expand the market. The potential exists for segmented services because of diverse consumer demand. Because the opportunities for shifts in relative market share are greatest during this stage, major efforts may be directed toward market penetration.

At *maturity,* Kotler and Keller (2006) identifies three substages that exist. They describe the three as follows:

> In the first phase, growth maturity, the sales growth rate starts to decline because of distribution saturation. There are no new

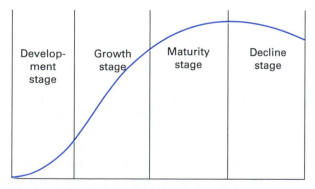

Figure 3.5. A Life-Cycle Model

distribution channels to fill, although some laggard buyers still enter the market. In the second phase, stable maturity, sales become level on a per capita basis because of market saturation. Most potential consumers have tried the product, and future sales are governed by population growth and replacement demand. In the third phase, decaying maturity, the absolute level of sales now starts to decline, and customers start moving toward other products and substitutes.

The slow rate of demand growth and overcapacity leads to intense competition for market share. Consumers are more cost conscious and technically knowledgeable. Sophisticated cost analysis is needed to provide data required to identify and prune unprofitable services from the broad service line initiated during the growth stage. Also, correct pricing is essential because cross-subsidization, through average cost pricing, may not be possible. Service delivery innovation is directed toward identifying lower-cost delivery methods.

Defending the remaining market share that an organization possesses is important. Existing consumers are encouraged to increase their use of the scope of services offered by the institution, an approach that is less costly than winning new consumers. Providers become more selective in terms of the groups to whom they will provide services.

The final phase, *decline*, is evidenced by a significant drop in demand. This reduction may occur rapidly or gradually. There will be uncertainty as to whether this downturn is permanent or a short-term condition that will self-correct. If the downturn represents a sharp movement toward market extinction, management must withdraw as soon as possible to prevent significant losses. Gradual decline suggests that management might be able to harvest some profits from the market by controlling service delivery costs and efficiently providing services. Alternatively, pockets of demand may remain that allow highly selective marketing to be initiated toward those niches. Finally, decline may be temporary, and aggressive marketing tactics could renew demand.

Strategy Identification and Selection

The above methods for analyzing portfolios contribute to management understanding of the organization–environment interface. These conceptual tools, combined with important data on market conditions and internal capabilities, are valuable aids in determining future directions for health care organizations. Decision algorithms have been developed to augment the previously described portfolios.

Strategic decisions for business areas of organizations are facilitated by the BCG Business Grid. Because market growth rate is beyond the control of management (Abell & Hammond, 1979), focus shifts to market share and allocation of funds. One successful long-term strategy is financing efforts to increase market share of question marks from cash generated by cash cows. This produces stars that eventually become cash cows. Question marks not in an adequate competitive position to become stars should not receive infusions of cash and should be allowed to descend with the decline in market growth rate to become dogs.

The Product Life-Cycle Matrix provides direction for managers interested in strategy formulation. Hillestad and Berkowitz (2004) suggest a *strategy action match* to match the organization's life cycle with the marketplace life cycle to determine appropriate managerial action. This match is illustrated in Figure 3.6. During the service introduction, an organization should "go for it" and strive for overall market leadership, limit service variations, concentrate on quality, establish high prices, and make related moves.

"Differentiation" is attempted during the growth stage. At maturity, a "necessity" approach is used if the organization must initiate a service for competitive reasons, does not currently provide it, and will not obtain market leadership. "Maintenance" is an attempt to retain market share without undue investment of funds. Finally, the decline stage suggests that an organization either harvest or divest the service. Interestingly, Porter (1980) suggests that a firm may not only harvest or divest during

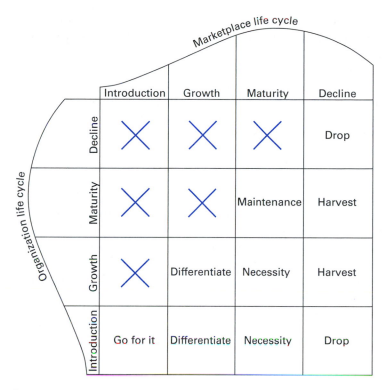

Legend
✗ = Position cannot occur

Figure 3.6. **Strategy Action Match Matrix**

SOURCE: Reprinted from *Health Care Marketing Plans: From Strategy to Action, 2nd Ed.,* by S. Hillestad and E. Berkowitz, p. 123, with permission of Aspen Publishers, Inc., © 1991.

decline but also may attempt to find a defensible niche or maintain a market share leadership position if conditions warrant.

ORGANIZATIONAL STRATEGY AND HUMAN RESOURCES MANAGEMENT

Human resources functions should have a direct supportive relationship to the formulation and implementation of organizational strategy. *The strategic management of human resources is concerned with designing and implementing internally consistent policies and practices to achieve an organization's business goals* (Huselid, Jackson, & Schuler, 1997). Hence, strategic management is different from traditional human resource (HR) management in its focus on financial performance and integration of various HR functions to achieve organizational business objectives (Welbourne & Andrews, 1996). In order to achieve these goals, qualifications for operation of the units must be determined; appropriate personnel must be recruited and selected; development of manpower to meet future needs must occur; and adequate rewards must be provided to attract and retain valuable employees. Recent research indicates that the link between some HR practices and business value is stronger than ever (*Watson Wyatt's Human Capital Index*, 2002). Over 600 companies participated in this 2002 European study. The results demonstrate that aligning HR strategies with business strategies is associated with additional shareholder value in the range of 7.2%. Firms that have effective delivery of HR services see higher shareholder value in the range of 9.6%. Rewarding employees for good work has a dramatic impact on shareholder value (21.5% higher market value). It is also found that having progressive staffing strategies is associated with 6.5% market value. Unfortunately, only a few progressive organizations seek to include human resources management activities in the strategy planning process. Briggs and Keogh (1999) studied strategic HR practices among technology-based small–medium companies and found that the majority of the respondent businesses had no strategic approach to HR. A survey of North Carolina county social service professionals revealed only moderate use of strategic HR concepts (Daley, Vasu, & Weinstein, 2002). The general role that human resources functions should play in the strategy of health care organizations is discussed in the following section. Then, the relationship of these functions to the portfolio of services managed by the organization is described.

Recruitment and Selection

Recruitment and selection are concerned with methods for hiring individuals and the internal movement of personnel to positions. Matching qualified individuals to appropriate jobs is crucial for organizational performance. Health care organizations must design selection systems that support the organization's strategy. For example, if an organization plans to diversify, management must have careful analysis of types of persons needed to staff and manage the new enterprise. Diversification by large health care systems may be hindered if new products or services that are developed are not well-managed. Early development of selection criteria and hiring of individuals for the diversification will ensure that staff is in place when the new venture is initiated. Vast empirical evidence shows that companies that invest in human resource planning and hiring practices are more likely to have higher labor productivity (Koch & McGrath, 1996) and enjoy higher performance (Hatch & Dyer, 2004). As mentioned above, having progressive staffing strategies is associated with 6.5% increased market value (*Watson Wyatt's Human Capital Index*, 2002). The organization also must monitor the internal flow of individuals and identify persons who have attributes that match those required for the emerging business strategies. Skills that mark persons as upwardly mobile may change if shifts occur in the strategic thrust. Inpatient acute care managers need the ability to work well with the medical staff, numerous community groups, and others. Determining who is eligible for career advancement in this situation requires assessment of interpersonal abilities (along with other skills). Thus, the types of data used to identify persons for advancement and the priority weights attached to the measures may change with different market thrusts. Comparably, health care organizations must match their key executives to business units that may be pursuing strategies that require unique skills. The advent of portfolio management in health services means that organizations offer an array of services that are situated at different stages of the life cycle. As discussed later, services at different stages of development require distinct managerial capabilities. Individuals should be placed with services at development stages that match their competence.

Development

Identification of needed skills and active management of employee learning for the future in relation to explicit corporate and business strategies contributes to organizational stability and higher employee productivity (Hatch & Dyer, 2004). The process of enhancing an individual's present and future skills most frequently occurs through training on the job. Health care organizations must develop early career developmental tracks aimed at producing people capable of handling key positions.

One approach for identifying personnel with high managerial potential and for developing these persons is succession planning (Hernandez, et al., 1991). This type of program frequently begins with a review process that evaluates the current management skills of persons in supervisory positions. Organizations involved in succession planning are thus able to evaluate and develop managers and have available "promotability ratings" that allow comparison of candidates for management vacancies. Succession planning should be in accord with corporate and business strategies. However, in many organizations succession planning is still not strongly linked to strategy; this conclusion is based on the responses from executives representing 13 large businesses, including one pharmaceutical company (Karaevli & Hall, 2003). Health care systems that have competed exclusively in one market segment (e.g., inpatient acute care) have specific types of experiences planned for developing executives. With the emergence of alternative service delivery systems and diversification into services only tangentially related to health care, human resources managers must devote considerable attention to planning early career experiences for management personnel who will operate these new ventures.

Appraisal

Appraisal is concerned with systematic examination and evaluation of positions and employees. Obviously, the entire human resources planning system depends on valid, reliable appraisals. Recruitment, selection, and placement require that the skills needed in positions be accurately described. Then, the capabilities of candidates for those positions must be assessed to ascertain that an appropriate match is achieved. Compensation systems require support from valid appraisal methods. The reason for this requirement is that rewards can be allocated on the basis of performance only if performance standards for a job have been established and if the performance of the incumbent can be measured. Finally, management development depends on accurate data from the performance appraisal system. Summary information on the strengths and weaknesses of managerial personnel can be analyzed to surface training and development needs.

Compensation

To be effective in securing behaviors that are desired from managers, compensation must be tied to the performance needed by the organization. Compensation systems appear to influence several factors that subsequently affect organizational outcomes. For instance, Murray and Gerhart (1998) examined different pay systems and their impact on productivity and labour costs and found that merit-based systems were associated with higher productivity, decreased labor costs, and better quality outcomes compared with traditional pay systems. In the health care field, pay satisfaction affected the turnover intentions of pediatric nurses (Lum, et al., 1998).

As mentioned above, current research indicates that rewarding employees for good work has a powerful impact on shareholder value, resulting in a 21.5% higher market value for the organization (*Watson Wyatt's Human Capital Index*, 2002).

A major consideration for individuals responsible for designing compensation systems is that the systems drive managers toward long-term goals. If rewards are tied to short-term results, it will be difficult to get managers to focus on long-term goals for which results may not be known for years. The difficulty of designing compensation systems to accomplish this task is discussed in the next section of this chapter.

PORTFOLIO ANALYSIS AND HUMAN RESOURCES MANAGEMENT

The portfolio analysis methods that were described previously have positive and negative attributes in terms of their ability to guide the human resources management process of health care organizations.

The BCG Business Grid does an excellent job of guiding the suggested flow of funds among business unit choices. However, it does not lend itself to clarification of human resources planning requirements.

The Product Life-Cycle Matrix has more intuitive appeal. The stages of the cycle of development for services suggest market conditions that lead to critical issues that must be faced by senior management. These issues, in turn, require that selected elements of the human resources system be used to address the issues that are raised. In addition, the skills required of managers vary based on the stages of the life cycle of the services being managed. Identification of the competencies needed assists in development of criteria for selection, appraisal, compensation, and development of managerial personnel across the business units of the organization.

Each of the four stages of the life cycle is examined to identify the management issue that must be faced. The human resources function or tactic that is critical during the stage is noted. Finally, the managerial skills most important for handling business units during that stage of the life cycle are listed.

Introduction

As previously noted, during the introductory stage of the life cycle, the service is not widely known and considerable time must be devoted to identification and development of markets. Because the best methods for producing the service are relatively unknown, the scope of services offered must be limited and concentration must be placed on maintaining the quality of services offered. The dominant competitive issue that must be faced by the organization is associated with identifying methods to be employed to *develop the market.*

Because this is a new venture for the institution, the major concerns for the human resources management system are *recruiting and selecting* competent managerial personnel to staff the enterprise. Additionally, other individuals must be recruited to staff all of the positions required for the new unit

to be able to deliver services. Internal or external sources of personnel must be considered. Criteria for selection of appointments must be developed.

Because of the uncertainty associated with the technology required to deliver the service, the managers responsible for these new ventures must be able to handle ambiguity well. Rapid changes in the methods used to provide the service or in the expectations placed on employees means that these managers also must have good interpersonal skills to handle the disturbances that are likely to occur.

Managers and other employees of the health services organization must be entrepreneurial and exploit new markets or variations in service delivery techniques that improve operations. Knowledge of new services marketing tactics is critical. Skills in financing the new services or in budgeting and projecting the economic results of business unit operations are required.

Growth

The growth stage is characterized by increase in consumer knowledge of the service and rise in consumer demand. The largest shifts in relative market share occur during the growth stage. Improvements in quality and in the availability of differentiated services provide a competitive edge for health care organizations that are able to institute these enhancements. Thus, the significant managerial issue that must be handled during the growth stage relates to the ability of the organization to *meet market demand* for the service.

The ability to respond to rapid changes and to maintain or increase market share is improved by the organization having managers and other health professionals within the institution who are exceptionally knowledgeable about opportunities occurring in the market and who have technical knowledge of the production capabilities of their units. The human resources function that takes on increased importance during this stage is concern for *management development* activities.

Improving the current and future effectiveness of managers during the growth stage is critical for several reasons. First, managers who were selected to operate these business units may have general management training but little knowledge of health services, or they may be health professionals without formal training in business and marketing principles. During this stage managers must have both technical product knowledge and marketing/management competence. Marketing skills that are required include methods to increase market share or begin market penetration tactics. Thus, a concern for human resources management is ensuring that either experiential or technical training activities are planned to develop expertise necessary in this type of market.

As demand for the service increases, more organizations will enter the market and current providers will expand operations. Thus, a second reason that management development is critical for this stage is that demand will grow for managers knowledgeable about operation of these units. For example, as managed care and health maintenance organizations (HMOs) increased in importance in the 1990s, new sites to begin future operations were sought. Large HMO systems devoted inadequate attention to identifying and developing individuals to manage the new sites. Thus, a seller's market existed for managers with HMO experience. Corporations interested in expanding their managed care activities need to develop individuals for projected growth or they will be unable to implement their plans successfully.

Maturity

During maturity, the rate of increase in growth of demand drops sharply. Consumers are more cost conscious and knowledgeable about service features. The scope of services that was broadened during the growth stage may be a liability now and pruning of services occurs. *Competition* is the dominant competitive issue facing the organization. Cost analysis and cost-cutting methods are required to keep the services of the organization competitively priced. Defending market share in a mature-to-declining market is essential for continued survival.

Appraisal and *compensation* are crucial functions performed by human resources managers during this stage. The character of compensation systems changes from loose, informal methods appropriate for a rapidly changing environment to a more structured, formal approach as industry maturity takes place. Human resources personnel must spend greater time and effort developing and fine-tuning this formal system to ensure that equity is engineered into the process. Compensation also may take on increased significance to managers of mature service units because less intrinsic satisfaction may be derived from managing these units during periods of increased competition.

Valid appraisal of managerial performance is important because the reduction in demand for an organization's services may result from overall market conditions, or it might arise from judgmental errors by management. Additionally, managers of business units may be eligible for promotion into senior, general management positions. The appraisal system and succession planning system must be able to identify successful managers at the business unit level so that compensation will be equitable and simultaneously identify individuals who have talents needed for higher levels of management or for corporate positions.

Decline

The final stage of market conditions is associated with significant drops in consumer demand. An organization may decide to divest itself of the business, remain in the market for an extended period and harvest profits from the service, identify a suitable market niche for the organization, or attempt to maintain a market share leadership role if it is believed that demand for the service will be relatively enduring. The dominant issue or concern facing management will depend on the strategic decision that is made. Divestment simply means that a suitable buyer for the service is found or that the business unit is terminated. Attempting a harvesting position suggests that *cost control* must occupy managerial attention. Conversely, finding a

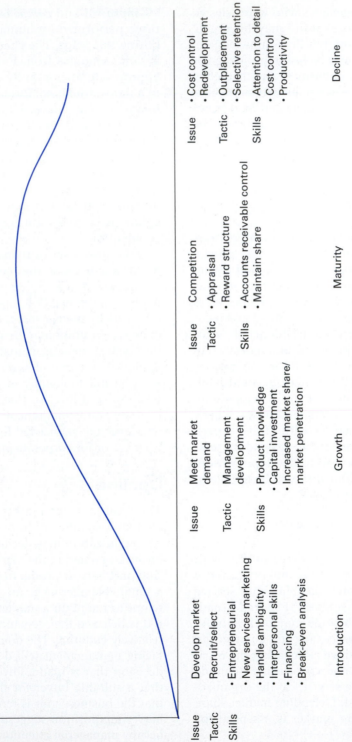

Figure 3.7. Integration of the Human Resources Management Process into a Life-Cycle Model

market niche or attempting to maintain leadership suggests that *redevelopment* is to occur.

Given the decline in demand for services, fewer business units may be operated and cost reduction strategies are in order. Thus, the major activities for the human resources manager concern performing *outplacement* services for individuals who will not be retained or in engineering *selective retention* of personnel and their replacements in other operating units of the organization.

Human Resources Management

The above discussion described the management issues during each stage of the life cycle of a product and the human resources function or tactic critical during the stage and suggested managerial skills required for handling business units at various stages of growth. This information is illustrated in Figure 3.7. The association of a human resources function or tactic with each stage of the life cycle does not mean that other functions are not necessary during that stage. This illustration is used to identify the activity that is *most critical* during the listed stage.

This material serves as a guide to suggested interrelations that should exist between human resources management functions and strategic planning and management activities within health services organizations.

SUMMARY

The major planning approaches used in the health services sector were reviewed in this chapter. Emphasis was placed on the types of strategies available to health care organizations. The detailed processes used for strategy formulation were reviewed and the value of involving health resource executives in the formulation process was provided.

MANAGERIAL GUIDELINES

The following are managerial guidelines to formulating an organizational strategy for health services organizations:

1. *Several planning approaches have been used by health services organizations, but an emphasis must be placed on strategic planning and strategic management in today's competitive marketplace.* Organizational strategies that might be used by health services institutions require determining the "business" of the organization and the methods that will be used to compete in those businesses.

2. *The formulation of the organization's strategy begins with a well-articulated mission statement.* Analysis of external opportunities and threats, as well as internal strengths and weaknesses, provides input in determining the alternative services that a health services organization should include in its portfolio. Portfolio analysis also suggests strategies that should be followed for the services that the organization decides to provide.

3. *Relationships exist among business strategies, stages of product life cycle, and human resources functions.* Life-cycle stages suggest critical issues that must be handled under different market conditions. These issues require that varying elements of the human resources system be used to address the issues and that the skills required of managers vary based on the stages of the life cycle of the service. Identification of the competencies needed assists in development of criteria for selection, appraisal, compensation, and development of managerial personnel across the business units of the organization.

DISCUSSION QUESTIONS

1. Compare and contrast strategic planning and strategic management. Of the two approaches, which one do you think is more difficult for management to realize? Why?
2. Three approaches to achieving competitive advantage for a business are cost leadership, differentiation, and focus. Is it possible for a community general hospital to use both a cost leadership and differentiation method with separate services in the hospital? Explain your response.
3. A variety of tools is available for analyzing a portfolio of strategic business units. Which of these tools would you suggest health services managers use when attempting to gain insight into the aptitudes and skills required for the manager of a soon-to-be-developed business unit? Explain your selection.
4. Describe the approach you would take to determine the stage of Product Life Cycle for the following services: (1) coronary artery bypass graph, (2) in-vitro fertilization, and (3) home health care.

CASE

Lakeview Medical Center was founded in 1895 when civic leaders in a midwestern town united to establish a home for the sick poor. Over time, the scope of services was expanded to include maternity care, sick infants and children, and a full array of health services needed by the community. The Medical Center increased in size to become a 577-bed, acute care hospital with numerous affiliated activities. The foundation that controls the hospital also controls a family practice center, a fitness and sports medicine program, a health promotion center, three urgent care centers, a hospice, two skilled nursing facilities, and a patient transport service with several helicopters and ground ambulance capabilities.

There is a feeling among some of the administrative staff that the organization has become "overstretched" in its attempt to provide the number of services that it does. Additionally, numerous opportunities arise to develop new service ventures at the Medical Center. The management team is in the process of considering methods that can be used to prioritize the services currently provided as well as to help in the process of considering new ventures. The team's concern is that each of the services currently offered makes a somewhat different contribution both to the Medical Center and to the community. Additionally, numerous stakeholders have desired outcomes that are achieved by the operation of some services and not others.

CASE DISCUSSION QUESTIONS

1. Describe the method or methods you would use to determine priorities for both existing and potential services that the Lakeview Medical Center might offer.
2. What criteria would you choose for selecting among the various services and how would you choose the criteria?
3. The business units of the Medical Center provide services at different stages of the product life cycle. What implications does this situation have for the human resources functions of the Medical Center?

REFERENCES

Aaker, D.A. (1984). *Developing Business Strategies.* New York: Wiley.

Abell, D.F., & Hammond, J.S. (1979). *Strategic Market Planning.* Englewood Cliffs, NJ: Prentice-Hall.

Ansoff, H.I. (1977). The state of practice in planning systems. *Sloan Management Review, 18*(2), 1–24.

Ansoff, H.I., & McDonnell, E.J. (1990). *Implanting Strategic Management* (2nd ed). Englewood Cliffs, NJ: Prentice-Hall.

Bonn, I. (2001). Developing strategic thinking as a core competency. *Management Decision, 39*(1): 63–70.

Brigg, S., & Keogh, W. (1999). Integrating human resource strategy and strategic planning to achieve business excellence. *Total Quality Management, 46*(3490): 46–51.

Bryson, J.M. (2004). *Strategic Planning for Public and Nonprofit Organizations: A Guide to Strengthening and Sustaining Organizational Achievement* (3rd ed.). San Francisco, CA: Jossey-Bass Publishers.

Camillus, J. (1997). Shifting the strategic management paradigm. *European Management Journal, 15*(1): 1–7.

Daft, R.L. (2007). *Organization Theory and Design* (9th ed.). Mason, OH: South-Western Press.

Daley, D., Vasu, M., & Weinstein, M. (2002). Strategic human resource management: Perceptions among North Carolina county social service professionals. *Public Personnel Management, 31*(3): 359–375.

Drucker, P.F. (1974). *Management: Tasks, Responsibilities, Practices.* New York: Harper and Row.

Fabrizio, N., & Hertz, K. (2005). Strategic planning and budgeting. *Urologic Clinics of North America, 32*: 291–297.

Gractz, F. (2002) Strategic thinking versus strategic planning: towards understanding the complementarities. *Management Decision, 40*(5): 456–462.

Griffith, J.R., & White, K.R. (2006). *The Well-Managed Healthcare Organization* (6th ed.). Chicago, IL: Health Administration Press.

Hall, W.K. (1980). Survival strategies in a hostile environment. *Harvard Business Review, 58*(5), 75–85.

Hatch, N., & Dyer, J. (2004). Human capital and learning as a source of sustainable competitive advantage, *Strategic Management Journal, 25*: 1155–1178.

Hax, A.C., & Majluf, N.S. (1984). *Strategic Management: An Integrative Perspective.* Englewood Cliffs, NJ: Prentice-Hall.

Heldey, B. (1977). Strategy and the business portfolio. *Long Range Planning, 10*(1) 9–15.

Henderson, H. (2003a). Budgeting: Part one. *Nursing Management, 10*(1): 33–37.

Henderson, H. (2003b). Budgeting: Part two. *Nursing Management, 10*(2): 32–36.

Heracleous, L. (1998). Strategic thinking or strategic planning? *Long Range Planning, 31*(3): 481–486.

Hernandez, S.R., Haddock, C., Behrendt, W.M., & Klein, W.F. (1991). Management development and succession planning: Lessons for health service organizations. *Health Care Management Development, 10*(4), 19–30.

Hillestad, S.G., & Berkowitz, E.N. (2004). *Health Care Marketing Strategy: From Planning to Action.* Subury, MA: Jones and Bartlett.

Hofer, C.W., & Schendel, D. (1978). *Strategy Formulation: Analytical Concepts.* St. Paul: West Publishing.

Hoskisson, R., Hitt, M. Wan, W., & Yiu, D. (1999). Theory and research in strategic management: Swings of a pendulum, *Journal of Management, 25*(3): 417–456.

Huselid, M., Jackson, S., & Schuler, R. (1997). Technical and strategic human resource management effectiveness as determinants of firm performance. *Academy of Management Journal, 40*(1): 171–188.

Karaevli, A., & Hall, D. (2003). Growing leaders for turbulent times: Is succession planning up to the challenge? *Organizational Dynamics, 32*(1): 62–79.

Koch, M., & McGrath, R. (1996). Improving labor productivity: Human resource management policies do matter. *Strategic Management Journal, 17*: 335–354.

Kotler, P., & Keller, K. (2006). *Marketing Management* (12th ed.). Englewood Cliffs, NJ: Prentice-Hall.

Liedtka, J. (1998). Strategic thinking: can it be taught? *Long Range Planning, 31*(1): 120–129.

Lum, L., Clark, J., Reid, F., & Sirola, W. (1998). Explaining nursing turnover intent: Job satisfaction, pay satisfaction, or organizational commitment? *Journal of Organizational Behavior, 19*: 305–320.

McVay, G., & Cooke, D. (2006). Beyond budgeting in an IDS: The Park Nicollet experience. *Healthcare Financial Management,* October: 100–110.

Mintzberg, H. (1994). The Fall and Rise of Strategic Planning. *Harvard Business Review,* January-February, 107–114.

Mobley, W.H. (1982). *Employee Turnover: Causes, Consequences, and Control.* Reading, MA: Addison-Wesley.

Murray, B., & Gerhart, B. (1998). An empirical analysis of a skill-based pay program and plant performance outcomes. *Academy of Management Journal, 41*(1): 68–78.

Nag, J., Hambrick, D., & Chen, M. (2007). What is strategic management, really? Inductive derivation of a consensus definition of the field. *Strategic Management Journal, 28*: 935–955.

Nutt, P.C. (1984). *Planning Methods for Health and Related Organizations.* New York: Wiley.

Pearce, J.A. (1982). The company mission as a strategic tool. *Sloan Management Review, 23*(1), 15–24.

Perlin, M.S. (1976). *Managing Institutional Planning.* Germantown, MD: Aspen Systems.

Pettigrew, A., Thomas, H., & Whittington, R. (eds) (2002). *Handbook of Strategy and Management.* London, UK: Sage Publications Ltd.

Porter, M.E. (1980). *Competitive Strategy.* New York: The Free Press.

Porter, M.E. (1985). *Competitive Advantage.* New York: The Free Press.

Rickards, R. (2006). Beyond budgeting: Boon or boondoggle? *Investment Management and Financial Innovation, 3*(2): 62–66.

Samli, C., & Shaw, E. (2002). Achieving managerial synergism: Balancing strategic business units and profit centers. *Journal of Market-Focused Management, 5*: 59–73.

Steiner, G.A. (1979). *Strategic Planning.* New York: The Free Press.

Swayne, L.E., Duncan, W.J., & Ginter, P.M. (2006). *Strategic Management of Health Care Organizations* (5th ed.). Malden, MA: Blackwell Publishing.

Thompson, A.A., Strickland, A.J., & Gamble, J. (2008). *Crafting and Executing Strategy* (16th ed.). New York, NY: McGraw-Hill.

Watson Wyatt's Human Capital Index. (2002). European Survey Report 2002. Retrieved October 15, 2004, from http://www.watsonwyatt.com.

Webber, J.B., & Peters, J.P. (1983). *Strategic Thinking: New Frontier for Hospital Management.* Chicago: American Hospital Publishing.

Welbourne, T., & Andrews, A. (1996). Predicting the performance of initial public offerings: Should human resource management be in equation? *Academy of Management Journal, 39*(4): 891–919.

Wilson, R., & Gilligan, C. (2005) *Strategic Marketing Management: Planning, Implementation and Control.* Boston: Butterworth-Heinemann.

Wind, Y.J. (1982). *Product Policy: Concepts, Methods, and Strategy.* Reading, MA: Addison-Wesley.

TWO

Organizing for Human Resources

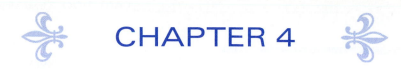

CHAPTER 4

The Health Care Workforce

Stephen N. Collier, PhD

LEARNING OBJECTIVES

Upon completing this chapter, the reader will be able to:

1. Describe, in general, the Bureau of Labor Statistics' projected growth for the health care workforce as compared to the economy as a whole
2. Describe the major factors that have led to a shortage of physicians and nurses
3. Identify the primary purposes of regulation of health personnel
4. Describe the effects of changing gender composition at the upper levels of the health workforce
5. Identify the persistent causes of health workforce shortages at various training levels

KEY TERMS

Accreditation

Balanced Budget Act of 1997

Bureau of Labor Statistics

Certification

Degree Creep

Licensing

Medical Assistants

Workforce Regulation

INTRODUCTION

In recent alternate years, the U.S. **Bureau of Labor Statistics** (BLS) has produced a ten-year projection of employment in many areas of the U.S. economy, including the health professions and occupations. The report for 2006–2016 is the most recent, released in November 2007, and includes the number of individuals employed in 2006 with projected employment to 2016. It is anticipated that by 2016, health care will provide over 20% of new jobs in the economy, and a majority of the 20 fastest-growing occupations in the U.S. economy are in health areas. The growth in all occupations in the U.S. economy between 2006 and 2016 is estimated to be 10.4%, compared to a growth rate of 19.8% for the category of "health care practitioners and technical occupations" and 26.8% for "health care support occupations" (Dohm & Shniper, 2007).

As shown in Table 4.1, there is strong employment growth in many health care professions, with the largest growth being in the number of nursing positions. Nursing for many years has been, and continues to be, the largest health care profession. The occupations with the largest growth on the basis of percentage change are found at the lower end of the training continuum and include home health aides and **medical assistants.** At a higher training level, strong percentage growth, between 20 and 30%, is anticipated for a number of what may be considered the mid-level health professions. This includes a number of disciplines that address rehabilitation care, some of which in recent years have

Table 4.1. Health Workforce Employment 2006–2016

Occupation	Employment Number		Change		Total job openings due to growth and net replacements, 2006–2016
	2006	2016	Number	Percentage	
Registered nurses	2,505	3,092	587	23.4	1,001
Physicians and surgeons	633	723	90	14.2	204
Dentists	161	176	15	9.1	46
Pharmacists	243	296	53	21.7	95
Optometrists	33	36	4	11.3	9
Medical and health services managers	262	305	43	16.4	92
Physician assistants	66	83	18	27.0	27
Dental hygienists	167	217	50	30.1	82
Physical therapists	173	220	47	27.1	68
Occupational therapists	99	122	23	23.1	37
Respiratory therapists	102	126	23	22.6	38
Radiologic technologists and technicians	196	226	30	15.1	56
Clinical laboratory technologists and technicians	319	362	43	13.6	92
Medical assistants	417	565	148	35.4	199
Home health aides	787	1,171	384	48.7	454

Numbers listed are in thousands of jobs.

SOURCE: Table prepared by Stephen N. Collier using data from the Bureau of Labor Statistics: Occupational employment projections to 2016, *Monthly Labor Review*, November 2007.

moved to the clinical doctoral level in their educational preparation.

Employment for physicians and surgeons is expected to increase by a little over 14% during this time period, which represents a large total number—an additional 90,000 individuals. However, if positions due to growth in demand and replacements due to retirements and other factors are included, the number of additional physicians and surgeons needed by 2016 rises to 204,000 individuals.

IMPENDING CHANGES IN THE HEALTH WORKFORCE

As the U.S. population is aging and becoming more diverse, so is the overall workforce, including the health workforce. The retirement of individuals born during the baby boom will have a large impact on the number of jobs in the economy. Growth in the labor force is expected to slow during the 2006–2016 period. In addition, according to the BLS, assuming that current immigration policy and levels of immigration remain the same as at present, the percentage of women in the labor force has already peaked (Dohm & Shniper, 2007). Since women make up the vast majority of workers in health care, reduction in their numbers and the consequences of retiring baby boomers in general could signal the potential for long-term shortages in many areas of the health workforce.

The need for workers in health care is expected to grow faster than most other areas of the economy. According to the BLS, "The 55-years-and-older group consumes significantly more health care and social assistance services than any other age group. As a result, jobs in health care and social assistance are expected to have the fastest rate of growth over the next 10 years, adding a projected 4.0 million new wage and salary jobs, or 27% of all new nonagricultural wage and salary jobs.... To reduce labor costs, some jobs are being sent offshore while others are being replaced by technology or are being filled with lower cost

workers. As a result, information technology-related jobs are expected to be among the fastest and largest growing jobs in the economy, and the category of health care support occupations, for example, will grow faster than health care practitioner and technical occupations" (Dohm & Shniper, 2007, p. 89).

Growth is expected to be strong in most all components of the health care industry. However, due to efforts to contain cost, the fastest growth is projected to be in those health occupations that assist health care practitioners.

While larger-than-average growth is occurring in most fields involved in health care, the disproportionate growth at the lower end of the training continuum is exemplified by the medical assistant occupation. Medical assistants are largely unregulated, but are becoming an increasingly important part of primary care. They are involved in both back office (clinical) functions such as drawing blood, giving shots, and conducting other basic clinical procedures and front office (administrative) tasks such as scheduling patients and billing for insurance payments.

Several factors have precipitated the increased use of medical assistants. Physician office practices have become more complex, there are shortages in the nurse workforce, and personnel costs favor the use of medical assistants as substitutes for other workers when it is appropriate and allowed by law (Tache & Chapman, 2006). According to June 2006 data from the BLS, mean annual earnings for medical assistants were $26,843, well below the salaries for nurses, radiologic technologists, and clinical laboratory technicians. So, if medical assistants can conduct both basic clinical tasks and needed administrative tasks, it is less expensive for a physician or clinic practice to hire them rather than more expensive personnel, particularly if they can perform functions that would require the hiring of multiple individuals from different fields. Unless prescribed by state statute, the responsibilities carried out by medical assistants are permitted under the license of a supervising physician.

The preceding example of the increased utilization of medical assistants also holds true for many other fields. In an effort to contain costs or increase profitability, employers generally strive to use the least-trained or lowest-paid individual to accomplish a task while maintaining an appropriate level of quality, safety, and job stability.

HEALTH CARE AS ECONOMIC DEVELOPMENT

The growth in health care has been pointed out in a number of sources. One dramatic illustration appeared in a 2006 *Business Week* article in which it was shown that between 2001 and 2006, 1.7 million new jobs were added to health care (*Business Week,* September 16, 2006). This figure also includes other health care services, such as health insurance and pharmaceuticals. The article goes on to state that the number of private sector jobs other than those in health care did not grow during that five-year period. Some areas of the workforce grew; but overall, outside of health care, growth was offset by reductions in other areas. Therefore, health care has become the primary job growth area in the U.S. economy.

According to the Bureau of Labor Statistics, of the 30 fastest-growing occupations, 13 are in health care—related to either physical or mental health. They include personal and home care aides, home health aides, medical assistants, substance abuse and behavioral disorder counselors, physical therapists and physical therapy assistants, pharmacy technicians, dental hygienists and assistants, mental health counselors, and physician assistants. The fastest-growing health care jobs are in fields requiring, in general, lesser amounts of postsecondary training. While the preceding are fields with the largest percentage growth, or rate of change, they do not necessarily indicate the fields where the largest number of additional jobs will be added to the economy. The occupations with the largest job growth in the economy also contain several of the fastest-growing health fields, namely personal and home care aides and home health aides. However,

the occupation that trumps all others, not only in health care but in the economy as a whole, is nursing, with an estimated 587,000 growth in jobs (Bureau of Labor Statistics, "fastest growing occupations," Table 2 and "occupations with the largest job growth," Table 3, 2007).

A number of states have experienced a transition in their economies, with a shift from manufacturing to the service sector. For example, in North Carolina in 1990, the manufacturing sector accounted for 27% of the state's jobs. By 2004, the manufacturing workforce had dropped to 15%. However, the loss in manufacturing jobs was offset to a large degree by a corresponding increase in health and human service jobs (University of North Carolina at Chapel Hill, 2006). Research and analysis done in the state has shown that between 1990 and 2005, North Carolina lost 255,971 manufacturing jobs but gained 230,476 jobs in health care services and social assistance. The loss in manufacturing jobs was more pronounced in rural areas of the state (The Council for Allied Health in North Carolina, 2005).

In the auto manufacturing state of Michigan, many auto workers have taken buyouts to move into various health care training programs, including nursing, radiologic technology, dental hygiene, and other fields. With a projected shortage of 18,000 nurses by 2015, the employment demand for nurses is widespread and every school has a waiting list. Health care is a growth sector in Michigan and is the industry-in-demand in that state (*The Wall Street Journal Online,* September 11, 2007).

States are becomingly increasingly aware of the importance of the health workforce to the economic viability of their state. As a result, many states have on occasion conducted studies to determine the ability of their educational system to produce the numbers of health professions graduates necessary to meet the needs of their citizens (State of Georgia Department of Community Health, 2002). The federal government, in conjunction with the states, monitors and analyzes various components of the labor force, including the health workforce.

An example of the attention that the health workforce is receiving regarding its relation to a state's economy can be found in a report from

Oklahoma's Governor's Council for Workforce and Economic Development: "As one of Oklahoma's most important industries, health care continues to be a key element in the state's ability to recruit and retain new and expanding businesses.... In 2004, health care was the second largest employing industry in Oklahoma, comprising 14% of the state's total employment" (2006). The importance of the health workforce to the economic clout of any state is becoming clearer in the minds of state governmental officials and policymakers.

Local communities and states are beginning to see health care as part of the economic development for their areas. For each dollar spent on health care, there is a large multiplier effect on the local economy. Since health care is in large part a local market, not many of the jobs can be moved offshore. That is particularly true for most of the clinical tasks, although some nonclinical functions can be accomplished in locations other than the local geographic area.

RIGHTSIZING THE WORKFORCE

The supply and demand for personnel in the health professions has traditionally been cyclical. An actual or anticipated shortage of workers leads to expansion of educational programs and graduates, which then may create an oversupply. If economic conditions change, or employment opportunities become more attractive in other fields, individuals may leave the profession and a shortage of workers may be created. The waxing and waning of the workforce may occur over a period of years, or circumstances may cause a more rapid shift in supply and demand. Regardless of the speed of the shift, an imbalance may cause problems for employers, for educational programs, and for potential students, as well as the health care consumer.

The difference between the current shortage of health care personnel and those in the past is that the current situation is not being viewed as just a cyclical event as in previous periods—a much

longer period of shortage is currently anticipated by most observers, although not all agree with such an assessment (Benton, 2007). Generally, employers would like there to be an oversupply of potential workers so that they can pick and choose the best qualified among those seeking jobs. The competition for a limited number of positions also aids employers in keeping salary levels within acceptable ranges based on education and experience.

In a similar fashion, educators like to have more applicants to programs than spaces available so that they can choose the most academically qualified and reduce attrition from the programs. Because of the lockstep nature of most health professions programs, it is not possible to replace a student in a cohort once someone drops out of a program. Therefore, from an economic perspective, particularly since health professions programs are more expensive to conduct than many other forms of higher education programs, it is desirable to have a good match between supply and demand.

HOW THE PHYSICIAN AND NURSING WORKFORCE HAS CHANGED OVER TIME

Medicine

The Association of American Medical Colleges (AAMC) has called for a 30% increase in enrollment in medical schools by 2015 as compared to the 2002 enrollment levels. This is to meet a projected shortage of physicians. A survey during the fall of 2006 indicated significant growth in enrollment numbers already underway (Association of American Medical Colleges, 2007).

In 1970, there were an estimated 149 active physicians per 100,000 population in the United States. Thirty years later that ratio had increased to 264 active physicians per 100,000 population (U.S. Department of Health and Human Services, 2002). The demand for physician and other health personnel services will grow as the population ages, and it is an open question as to what a desired ratio should be. About one in four physicians in residency programs graduated from a foreign medical school, a figure that has remained fairly constant in recent years. Much of the need for foreign trained physicians comes from a demand for physicians in primary care in rural areas and in specialities such as psychiatry. U.S. medical graduates tend to not enter those specialities to the extent necessary, thus creating a need that is being met by medical graduates from other countries. Some of those foreign trained physicians are U.S. citizens who go to school in other countries because of space limitations in U.S. schools.

In addition to allopathic medical schools increasing their numbers of graduates, the field of osteopathy has increased its graduates by expanding the number of osteopathic medical schools. In 1968, there were 5 osteopathic medical schools in the United States, but by 2007 there were 23, with 3 new provisionally accredited schools enrolling students in 2007 (Association of Academic Health Centers, 2008).

Because of the length of time required to train new physicians and modify the educational infrastructure, accurate projections of physician supply and concomitant requirements must be made as much as a decade in advance of their need in the workforce. Although other health professions have a shorter training period than physicians, effective workforce planning still needs to be made well in advance of the individuals actually entering the workforce. While there is debate about whether a physician shortage already exists or will be present within a few years, "a growing consensus is that over the next 15 years, requirements for physician services will grow faster than supply—especially for specialist services and specialties that predominantly serve the elderly" (U.S. Department of Health and Human Services, 2006, p. 3).

Nursing

A nursing shortage has been widely reported, and it is projected to be long-term. The economic viability of hospitals and many other health care institutions depends on an adequate supply of nurses.

The federal government over the last 30 years has conducted a sample survey of the nation's registered nurses (RNs). According to the most recent survey of March, 2004, there is a total estimated number of RNs in the United States of almost 3 million. Of that number, 83.2% were employed in nursing in 2004. Of those employed, approximately 58%, or 1,696,916, were working full time, almost 25% were working part time, and 17% were not employed in nursing (U.S. Department of Health and Human Services, 2004).

There are several characteristics of the registered nurse population that give concern to those who monitor the nursing workforce. The average age of RNs has increased markedly over the last 20 or so years. It is estimated that at the time of the March 2004 survey, the average age of the RN population was 46.8 years. Less than ten years prior to that, in 1996, the average age was 42.3 years. In 1980, 40.5% of RNs were under 35 years of age, compared with 16.6% in 2004 (U.S. Department of Health and Human Services, 2004). The increase in the average age of nurses means that many will be retiring within the coming decade, suggesting that the shortage may increase dramatically after about 2010.

International nursing graduates have helped to alleviate the shortage in some settings in recent years, but most observers believe that international graduates are not a sustainable solution to the shortages. In 2005, international nursing graduates constituted 13% of all newly licensed nurses in the United States (PriceWaterhouseCoopers, 2007). A limiting factor on the ability of the U.S. educational system to greatly increase enrollment in programs, or develop new programs, is a shortage of qualified faculty.

EDUCATIONAL RESPONSE TO WORKFORCE CHANGES

Of great concern to policymakers at both state and federal levels is whether the educational system is adequate to meet the demand for growth in health care professions that is currently evident, as well as that projected for the future. Workforce changes generally occur more quickly than the educational system and its institutions can respond to in terms of modifying the number and size of programs or modifying the curriculum.

The health workforce is susceptible to changes in federal or state governmental policy, especially changes in reimbursement policy. Changes in reimbursement policy can create extraordinary changes both in employment and demand within a short period of time. As an example, the federal **Balanced Budget Act of 1997** placed a cap on reimbursement for the rehabilitation professions. Though passed several years earlier, the reimbursement change became effective in January 1999 and resulted in depressing the employment market for physical therapists, occupational therapists, and speech-language pathologists. When prospective students learned of the change in the employment market, applications to educational programs in the rehabilitation disciplines declined significantly.

If the employment demand projections by the Bureau of Labor Statistics are accurate, the capacity of programs in the health professions to graduate sufficient numbers to meet the future requirements is lacking. While the high job vacancy rates in some health care fields in the 2000–2005 period have eased somewhat, perhaps leading to diminished concern on the part of some employers and educators, the vacancy rates are still high in many disciplines. What is particularly troubling is the anticipated high rate of retirements from the workforce expected to begin around 2010. Like the overall society in which it is found, the health workforce is aging. In addition, many individuals employed in clinical roles retire from health care employment at an earlier age than their counterparts in other industries.

If one compares the Bureau of Labor Statistics projected employment demand for future years with existing program capacity and level of graduates, a large gap is found in most of the health professions. Even though educational institutions try to be responsive to workforce needs, there is a delay between when a shortage is apparent and the creation or expansion of programs to meet the need.

Regardless of the degree level, a professional program of two years or longer may take four or more years to identify the required financial resources, proceed through the approval processes of the educational institution and/or the state higher education agency, recruit and hire faculty, obtain preliminary **accreditation** approval for the program, plan the curriculum and enroll students, and graduate the first students from the program. The existing program capacity nationally in most health professions, especially in nursing and many allied health professions, appears to be seriously lacking when comparing current graduates with the BLS projections (Collier, 2006).

The adequacy of the supply of the health workforce is not a new issue. With swings between periodic undersupply and oversupply over the years, it has been an issue of continuing debate and concern on the part of governmental and educational policymakers. Just as observed some 25 years ago, the cyclical and troubling nature of the issue requires a broad response if a solution is to be found. "It seems clear that simply increasing further the number of professionals will do only a little to solve these problems, and may aggravate them, unless other more definite actions are taken. Solutions require sophisticated combinations of action by the health professions schools, higher education agencies, elected officials, third-party payers, **licensing** boards, and the professional societies. Single strategies have a poor record of success" (Southern Regional Education Board, 1983, p. 2).

HEALTH WORKFORCE TRENDS AND ISSUES

Workforce regulation

There is always a tension between attempting to assure quality that will provide a means of protection for the public and rigidifying the workforce. **Workforce regulation** may be voluntary or self-imposed by the profession, or it may be governmental at either the federal or state level. Much of the regulation, such as licensure, occurs at the state level.

The specific intent of health workforce regulation is to provide protection for the public against unscrupulous or unqualified individuals. If the controls placed on individuals are too strict, then a monopoly may be created, which can restrict the delivery of services and inflate costs. If the controls are too lax, then unqualified individuals can provide services that place the public at serious health risk or take advantage of them economically without providing the desired health benefits.

Across the continuum of levels and kinds of training, what is the appropriate mix of health professionals and workers needed in the U.S. health care system? Answering the question will ultimately address the effects of the various forms of regulation and credentialing on the health workforce. Related to this fundamental question is a host of others concerning the effects of credentialing on quality of care, salaries and wages of health personnel, educational preparation, and rigidity or flexibility within the health care system.

The various forms of credentialing, here meaning primarily licensure, **certification,** and accreditation, comprise both governmental mandates and voluntary processes. Even within the governmental parameters, the licensure boards are controlled principally by individuals within the profession who are acting in a voluntary capacity. Since the governmental authority is designed to serve the public interest, it raises a public policy question of whether the professions have the ability to govern themselves and also represent the public interest, or whether other mechanisms might be more effective in protecting the public interest. It also raises the question of the effectiveness of a largely voluntary system in many respects.

Since licensure has the power of law, it may be considered one of the more powerful forms of credentialing. It is also a state-level function, raising the likelihood of variance from one state to another. Coordination and communication across the states can pose problems, especially when a uniform standard of care is desired.

Gender

Women comprise the majority of the health workforce. Nursing, the largest health profession; most

of the allied health professions; and the frontline health occupations employ many more women than men. The traditional doctoral health professions of medicine, dentistry, and others have historically attracted more males, but that is changing. The shift in gender representation is true not only for the health professions, but also for higher education overall at undergraduate, graduate, and professional levels. Women made up 57% of the total of over 17 million students enrolled in colleges and universities in 2004, including graduate and professional fields (Chronicle of Higher Education, 2007).

When viewed over the last three decades, the shift is striking. Table 4.2 shows the changes in enrollments for both graduate and first-professional students.

In the first half of this decade, first-professional students increased 17% for females and only 4% for males. There is a lag of several years between the year of graduation and its compilation and report by the National Center for Educational Statistics. The most recent results of the NCES graduation data are shown in Table 4.3.

A frequently mentioned characteristic of women health professionals is that due to child responsibilities during the child bearing and rearing years, they tend to work fewer hours per week collectively on average than males. If so, then greater numbers of health professionals are needed to achieve the same units of output than previously. Another factor being observed, though, is what appears to be a generational shift in the values and attitudes of men in the health professions. Men in professional roles appear to increasingly be willing to do without higher income for more discretionary time. An ongoing gender shift in the composition of the health professionals at the highest level, along with a possible shift in career expectations and values for both men and women, appears to be occurring. The long-term implications of these changes deserve further examination.

Divergence in Training Levels

The U.S. health care workforce is becoming increasingly bimodal in regard to training levels. This is seen both in greater numbers of individuals

Table 4.2. Graduate/First Professional Enrollment: Graduate and first professional enrollment in degree granting institutions in 1976 and 2005 and percentage increase between the two years, by sex.

Characteristic	Graduate Enrollment			First Professional Enrollment		
	1976	2005	Percent Change	1976	2005	Percent Change
Total	1333	2186	64	244	337	38
Sex						
Male	714	877	23	190	170	−11
Female	619	1309	112	54	167	207

(Enrollment in thousands)

SOURCE: Trends in Graduate/First Professional Enrollments. The condition of Education 2007. U.S. Department of Education.

Table 4.3. Earned degrees, first-professional programs 2003–2004.

Professional degrees	Men	Women	Total
Dentistry	2532	1803	4335
Medicine	8273	7169	15442
Optometry	543	732	1275
Osteopathic Medicine	1567	1155	2722
Pharmacy	2711	5510	8221
Podiatry, Podiatric Medicine	221	161	382
Veterinary Medicine	569	1659	2228
Chiropractic	1868	862	2730
Law	20332	19877	40209
Theology	3511	1821	5332
Other	42	123	165
All Fields	42169	40872	83041

SOURCE: U.S. Department of Education.

trained at lower levels along with increases in those prepared at higher levels. At the same time, there is a decline, in a relative sense, of individuals prepared for health careers at the baccalaureate degree level.

While the public may believe that health care jobs consist mainly of physicians and nurses, the majority of jobs are located at the lower end of the training continuum and require an associate degree or less. Economic realities are pushing the training continuum in both directions—creating both the demand for higher levels of training at the graduate and professional levels, and lower levels at the associate degree and below, shrinking the proportion of individuals who previously were educated at the baccalaureate and post-baccalaureate certificate level.

A number of fields that previously had their entry level to practice at the bachelor's degree level, such as physical therapy and occupational therapy, have moved to the master's or clinical doctoral level. Other areas representing large numbers of workers, such as radiologic technologists, (182,000 employed in 2004) and respiratory therapy (94,000 employed in 2004), have not yet increased their entry level to practice (Berman, 2005). While in recent years there have been discussions within the professional organizations representing these fields attempting to raise the level of education, there have not been significant changes in the proportion of programs that prepare individuals at the associate degree level rather than the baccalaureate level.

The push for higher and lower degree levels is driven by both the desire of professional organizations to advance their professions and the desire by employers to control personnel costs.

These opposing forces are creating a movement in both higher and lower levels of training.

Other factors also contribute to a bifurcating educational level of the health workforce. *FutureScan*, a study by the American Society of Radiologic Technologists (2006), found that technological advances are creating a situation in which some imaging procedures can be done faster, using smaller equipment, and at a cheaper price than in the past. There is also a need by physician radiologists to have some assistance at a more complex and higher level than provided by associate degree-trained radiographers. These two kinds of needs within the same overall field are causing the educational preparation in medical imaging to expand in opposing directions.

Increasing centralization of some components of the health services industry is also contributing to a more divergent workforce. The movement toward larger and more centralized clinical laboratories outside of the hospital setting has created a new economy of scale for conducting many lab tests. In combination with advances in technological equipment, many lab tests that previously had to be conducted by higher-trained individuals now are more automated and can be conducted by lower-trained individuals. Centralization and new economies of scale due to technological and other improvements are also occurring in other areas of the health care system, such as in the pharmacy. There is increasing use of automated equipment to assist in filling prescriptions. A movement to mail-order pharmacies also helps to increase production and limit costs.

Increased Degree Levels

In recent years, employers and higher education leaders have expressed concerns about increasing degree levels in a number of health professions. This trend is sometimes referred to as **"degree creep."** There is uneasiness about the effects that increases in requirements for a higher degree level of training will have on health care costs and other health system dynamics. The concern is particularly acute in those professions that have moved to the clinical doctoral level. Depending on the profession involved, the clinical doctorate is sometimes also referred to as the professional doctorate or practice doctorate. Even in the absence of a mandate from professional accreditation entities, there has been swift movement to the clinical doctorate in several disciplines, such as physical therapy, due to the market forces of educational programs competing with each other for potential students.

There are pros and cons regarding increasing the level of the educational degree. A variety of parties weigh in on the issue: professional organizations, educators from the affected professions, higher education officials at institutional and state levels, regional accreditation agencies, and, of course, employers. Those in favor of increased degree levels cite an expanding knowledge base and technological progress. They also point out that frequently the programs within the profession have already expanded the number of months of training and the credit hours required for the degree beyond that required for comparable degrees in other fields. Those who oppose the clinical doctorates state that the move to the doctoral level is professional aggrandizement rather than a response to market demand. They also assert that the educational programs train their students beyond the scope of practice authority permitted in many states and settings. Moreover, the lengthened educational process creates additional expense for both the student and society.

Employers are apprehensive that increased degree levels in a discipline may make staffing more expensive and difficult to obtain. Third-party payers reimburse for the services provided and not the degree level of the provider. As a result, it is not possible to differentiate between the services provided by professionals holding different levels of degrees.

The Frontline Workforce

At the other end of the continuum from the doctorally prepared health workforce is the "frontline" workforce, which consists of over 4.5 million out of a total of more than 12 million people employed in health care (Berman, 2005). The frontline category is a relatively new term, and is used to group together heath care workers who have substantial patient contact, are educated at the baccalaureate degree or below, and earn less than $40,000 annually.

While the category includes those health care workers with associate and bachelor's degrees in fields with rigorous credentialing criteria, the majority of individuals in the frontline group have minimal levels of health-specific training, and most of that is either short-term or received on the job. Many in the frontline workforce are home health aides, nursing aides, and related occupations. Approximately 80% of frontline workers are women and over 30% are African American or Hispanic (Robert Wood Johnson Foundation, 2006). Their jobs are found in hospitals, long-term care institutions, and in organizations that provide health care in a home setting. In the past, the grouping has been referred to as the health care auxiliary workforce, and it has been a frequently overlooked, but very large, component of the total health care system (Ruzek, et al., 1999).

Especially at the lower training levels, this set of occupations has some frequent characteristics that are troublesome for the provision of quality health care and an environment in which the various components of the health system are well integrated. The occupations have relatively low wages and benefits and a high stress-level environment for the workers. As a result, there is high job turnover, with individuals leaving the field to work in other occupations or moving within the field to make a small additional increment in salary. With the shortages in this component of the workforce, high turnover, and projected high growth needs, these circumstances present considerable challenges for health care human resource managers.

PERSISTENT CAUSES OF WORKFORCE SHORTAGES

Many factors contribute to personnel shortages. Some exist in the education sector; some are the result of employment characteristics and the work

setting; some are created by professional organizations, principally as they influence educational program accreditation (and therefore the supply of graduates) or personnel credentialing mechanisms; and some are the result of governmental and third-party payer policies.

Factors influencing the frontline workforce are often poor pay relative to other occupations requiring the same level of training and physically and emotionally stressful jobs with little assistance in dealing with the stress. In many cases there is poor to no career advancement, thus creating high job turnover and workforce attrition. This, in turn, creates a demand for many additional people in this part of the workforce to address not only job growth but also the considerable need for job replacements.

Within one-year technical training programs and two-year associate degrees in many health care programs there are too few applicants who are adequately prepared to take on the academic difficulty of the curriculum, resulting in high attrition in many programs. Weak high school preparation or poor aptitude, particularly in science and math, are often seen as the main reasons for attrition from health occupational programs.

At higher levels of education, particularly at the graduate and professional levels, the time required to complete the educational program and be eligible for practice may be an obstacle to many. Also, the cost of a health professions educational program frequently results in high levels of debt upon graduation. This is especially common in medicine, which has a very long educational process, but it is also true, even if to a lesser extent, in many other health professions areas.

Professional organizations may also contribute to the shortage of workers. Because of their association with establishing or enforcing credentialing standards, particularly with regard to personnel certification or licensure and program accreditation, they exert a strong influence on workforce supply and the work environment. The capability of health professional organizations to mandate workforce dynamics without effective counterbalances gives them the ability to be overly influential, to the potential disadvantage of health system effectiveness and the optimal benefit to the public. The root causes of health workforce shortages are complex, varied, and intertwined.

SUMMARY

The trends that are occurring in the U.S. health care system are frequently dichotomous and are characterized by a multiplicity of causes with no single point of control or influence. An increasing concern for quality would imply stricter measures and credentials for those engaged in health care. The occupations with the greatest growth, however, are found at lower levels of training and have either weak or no credentialing. The increase in the numbers of workers at the lower levels is an attempt to contain cost and create greater efficiency among the higher-trained individuals. However, without more effective management and coordination among all who work in inpatient and outpatient settings, both quality and efficiency of health services may be compromised.

Some health professions have moved to a higher degree level for entry into practice. With others considering such a move, an extended educational process may increase overlap in scope of practice among the health disciplines. Moving to a higher degree level may also create more encouragement for greater independence. Whether this results in greater service to the public, or just greater competition and conflict within the health system, is an issue of debate and possible regulation through governmental and other public policy processes.

Health professional organizations perform the twofold role of serving the members of their profession and also of benefiting the public. As a normal result of organizational advocacy and professional aspiration, each profession tries to enlarge its market share relative to the other health professions and expand its scope of practice. The most frequent way of justifying an expanded scope of practice is to increase the amount of training in the profession.

In another consistent trend, there has been a steady increase in the percentage of women receiving degrees in higher education, particularly at the graduate and professional level. Some health professions that previously had a preponderance of men entering the workforce now have a majority of women graduates. Previous measures of productivity are changing for both men and women health professionals who want to limit their work hours and achieve a greater balance in life. As a result, there will be greater numbers of health professionals needed to conduct the same amount of work

States are realizing the importance of the health workforce to their state's economy. This is true in terms of having an adequate health workforce to serve the state's residents as well as the related impact on economic strength and tax revenues. However, health professions programs have higher-than-average costs to educate individuals when compared to many other types of education. Competing demands for state dollars and increases in nondiscretionary areas of state spending may result in fewer dollars being available for education in the higher-cost health professions.

At the lower end of the employment range, the frontline workforce is likely to continue to experience significant personnel turnover, characteristic of some other lower-paying jobs. If other areas of the U.S. economy are strong, the worker turnover may increase as workers move from one setting to another, seeking higher pay and a less demanding work environment. Increased personnel turnover results in higher costs of training and retraining and disruptions in the workplace. With a push to contain health care costs, particularly personnel costs, hiring of noncredentialed or minimally credentialed personnel is likely to occur. This may include greater numbers of foreign-born individuals who are willing to emigrate to take the lower-paying jobs.

Health system regulation involves both voluntary and governmental processes. Health care reimbursement is profoundly influenced by governmental policy. The regulation of health care personnel is in essence a quasi-voluntary process controlled by the professions being regulated. The capability of the professions to govern themselves and balance their self-interest with the public interest is an issue of continuing debate. Thus far, because of the pluralistic nature of American governance, there is a dependence on many voluntary and self-regulating mechanisms.

Recent years have seen a shortage of health care personnel in the U.S. While enrollments have expanded in nursing and a number of other programs, shortages have persisted and are expected to continue in the coming years. The ability of the health care system to deliver needed services at the level of quality desired and expected will be a challenge for all concerned.

MANAGERIAL GUIDELINES

1. In response to a shortage in the health care workforce, numerous health care organizations employ foreign health care professionals. While this may answer the supply side of the equation, U.S. health care managers must consider a number of issues associated with this strategy, such as current immigrant policy, the growing concern about outsourcing, and the effects of English language deficiency on patient satisfaction and quality of care.

2. Another cost-containment strategy used by health care organizations is the employment of medical assistants. This trend is occurring not only in the field of medicine but also in other health care fields such as dentistry, pharmacy, and physical therapy. While health care organizations may benefit from controlling costs and therefore an increase in profitability, managers must ensure that this strategy does not undermine the quality of patient care or the relationship between other health care professionals and the organization.

3. Trends indicate that the health care sector has created great employment opportunities and significant contributions to economic development. However, this also reflects higher competition among health care organizations within this sector. Therefore, the ability to secure and leverage an effective health care workforce is one of the critical tasks of health care managers.

4. Health care delivery organizations can play a major role in keeping a balance between the supply and demand of health care professionals. Their involvement in the educational processes can provide opportunities for the development of a proficient health care workforce.

5. When conducting strategic planning, health care managers must analyze government legislation and regulations that may have an impact on different parts of the health care workforce, such as reimbursement, an expansion of educational programs, and requirements in competencies.

DISCUSSION QUESTIONS

1. The health care workforce appears to be evolving in a bifurcated manner. What are the forces that are influencing this development?
2. What are some of the major factors that may cause the health workforce supply/demand balance to wax and wane over a period of years?
3. As the economy shifts away from manufacturing to service jobs, why is health care seen as increasingly important to a state's economy?

REFERENCES

American Society of Radiologic Technologists. (2006). *FutureScan.* Albuquerque, NM.

Association of Academic Health Centers (2007). *Issues and Priorities.* Retrieved January 24, 2008, from http://www.aahcdc.org.

Association of American Medical Colleges. (2007). *Medical School Expansion Plans: Results of the 2006 AAMC Survey.* Center for Workforce Studies, February 2007. Washington, DC.

Benton, T. (2007). The Annual Labor Shortage Hoax. *The Chronicle of Higher Education, 54,* Issue 2, September 4, 2007, C2.

Berman, J. (2005). *Industry Output and Employment Projections to 2014, Monthly Labor Review.* November, 2005. Washington, DC: U.S. Bureau of Labor Statistics.

Business Week Online. (2006). What's Really Propping Up the Economy. September 16, 2006 from http://www.businessweek.com.

Chronicle of Higher Education. Almanac of Higher Education 2006–2007, Volume 53, Issue I, 15. *College Enrollment by Racial and Ethnic Group, Selected Years.* Washington, DC. Retrieved June 14, 2007, from http://chronicle.com.

Collier, S. (2006). How Well Prepared Are Allied Health Schools to Meet Future Workforce Demand? *Trends*, May 2006, Washington, DC: Association of Schools of Allied Health Professions. 5–6.

The Council for Allied Health in North Carolina. (2005). The State of Allied Health in North Carolina. May 2005.

Dohm, A., & Shniper, L. (2007). Occupational employment projections to 2016. *Monthly Labor Review,* November, 86–105.

Health Workforce Solutions LLC. (2006). *Workers Who Care: A Graphical Profile of the Frontline Health and Health Care Workforce.* November 2006. Princeton, NJ: Robert Wood Johnson Foundation.

Oklahoma Department of Commerce. (2006). *Industry Report on Health Care 2006.* April 10, 2006. Governor's Council for Workforce and Economic Development. Retrieved May 23, 2007, from http://www.okoha.com.

PriceWaterhouseCoopers. (2007). *What Works: Healing the Healthcare Staffing Shortage.* PriceWaterhouseCoopers Health Research Institute. Retrieved November 15, 2007, from http://www.pwc.com.

Ruzek, J., Bloor, L., Anderson, J., Ngo, M., & UCSF Center for the Health Professions. (1999). *The Hidden Health Care Workforce: Recognizing, Understanding and Improving the Allied and Auxiliary Workforce.* San Francisco, CA: UCSF Center for the Health Professions.

Southern Regional Education Board. (1983). *Health Professionals for the South: Supply and Cost Issues Needing State Attention.* Atlanta GA.

State of Georgia Department of Community Health. (2002). *What's Ailing Georgia's Healthcare Workforce? Serious Symptoms, Complex Cures.* Healthcare Policy Advisory Committee. Atlanta, GA: August 2002.

Tache, S., & Chapman, S. (2006). The Expanding Roles and Occupational Characteristics of Medical Assistants: Overview of an Emerging Field in Allied Health. *Journal of Allied Health*, Winter 2006, 35, Number 4, 233–237.

University of North Carolina at Chapel Hill. (2006). Carolina Context. *The Program on Public Life, Center for the Study of the American South*, 2, October 2006, Chapel Hill: University of North Carolina.

U.S. Bureau of Labor Statistics. (2007). "Fastest growing occupations," table 2 and "Occupations with the largest job growth," table 3. Retrieved December 15, 2007, from www.bls.gov/emp.

U.S. Department of Health and Human Services. (2002). *U.S. Health Workforce Personnel Factbook, table 202.* National Center for Health Workforce Analysis. Rockville, MD. Retrieved January 24, 2008, from http://bhpr.hrsa.gov.

U.S. Department of Health and Human Services (2004). *The Registered Nurse Population: National Sample Survey of Registered Nurses, March 2004, Preliminary Findings.* Health Resources and Services Administration. Rockville, MD.

U.S. Department of Health and Human Services (2006). *Physician Supply and Demand: Projections to 2020.* Bureau of Health Professions, October, 2006. Rockville, MD.

The Wall Street Journal Online. (2007). In Shift, Auto Workers Flee to Health-Care Jobs. September 11, 2007. Retrieved September 11, 2007, from http://online.wsj.com.

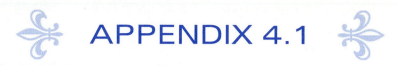

APPENDIX 4.1

Health Care Workforce Data Resources

While any report providing health workforce data is a snapshot in time, there are sources that provide periodic or continuous monitoring of various aspects of the workforce. Included are the health professional associations and various governmental agencies. Foremost among these are the U.S. Bureau of Labor Statistics and its counterpart agencies in each of the states. Following is a listing of sources of health care workforce data that may be accessed and used for various types of planning purposes. As pointed out earlier, due to substantial variance, data at the national level may be of limited use for local or regional planning. Other sources, such as those provided by state agencies, hospital associations, and the U.S. Census Bureau for local data, may be more relevant for local planning purposes.

State Hospital Associations

http://www.americanhospitals.com
http://www.pohly.com

State Boards of Nursing

https://www.ncsbn.org

Bureau of Labor Statistics

http://www.bls.gov

National Center for Health Workforce Analysis (HRSA)

http://bhpr.hrsa.gov/healthworkforce

Census Bureau (American FactFinder)

http://factfinder.census.gov

HRSA Geospatial data warehouse

http://datawarehouse.hrsa.gov

National Center for Health Statistics (CDC)

http://www.cdc.gov

National Center for Education Statistics

http://nces.ed.gov

IPEDS

http://nces.ed.gov

AHA

http://www.hospitalconnect.com

Regional Centers for Health Workforce Studies

http://chws.albany.edu
http://futurehealth.ucsf.edu
http://depts.washington.edu

http://www.uic.edu
http://www.healthworkforce.unc.edu
http://www.uthscsa.edu

CHAPTER 5

Using Health Care Competencies in Strategic Human Resource Management

G. Ross Baker, PhD and Louise Lemieux-Charles, PhD

LEARNING OBJECTIVES

Upon completing this chapter, the reader will be able to:

1. Describe the nature of competencies and their relationships to individual skills, knowledge, and attitudes as well as the broader organizational context.
2. Describe and discuss how competencies inform and align the Strategic Human Resource Management System.
3. Discuss the tension between competencies defined by professional groups and those used in health care organizations.
4. Identify how competencies contribute to overall health care organization performance.

KEY TERMS

Competence
Competency
Competency Clusters
Competency Code Book
Competency Models
Core Competencies
Job Family Competencies
Level Competencies
Organizational Core Competencies
Organizational Learning Perspective
Single-Job Competency Model Approach
Technical Competencies

INTRODUCTION

Effective health care organizations face growing challenges in recruiting and developing human resources. The growing complexity of health care services requires a broad range of knowledge and skills, both the technical skills needed to deliver safe, effective, and patient-centered care and the aptitudes needed by all staff to learn quickly, communicate effectively, collaborate with others, and implement improvements in care. Health care organizations need to identify the job-related skills necessary for effective work. But selecting staff based on current job characteristics may be insufficient when changes in health care practice and rapidly changing organizational environments require staff to master new skills and work in different ways. The full range of competencies needed to perform work in a unit or organization includes attitudes and values that will provide the capability to meet the needs of a changing environment and emerging strategic directions. Defining the competencies needed at an individual, team, and organizational level is a critical component of strategic human resource management. Knowledge of the **core competencies** guides assessment and selection, training and development, performance management, and succession planning. In this chapter we explore how developing and using the full range of competencies provides a useful approach to strategic human resource planning and management.

HISTORICAL BACKGROUND

The development of a competency-based methodology to human resources management was pioneered by Harvard psychologist David McClelland. In the early 1970s, McClelland questioned whether intelligence tests measured the abilities responsible for job success. He argued instead that success was determined by specific competencies, and he began to test for **competence** rather than intelligence. He defined competence as "an underlying characteristic of a person which enables them to deliver superior performance in a given job, role or situation" and which can be learned over time (McClelland, 1973). This definition suggests that if competencies are made visible and training is accessible, individuals can understand and develop the required level of performance. In this approach, **competency** is not about detailed job characteristics but rather the more generic underlying personal characteristics that contribute to successful performance (Elkin, 1990). These macro or generic characteristics include the essential skills, knowledge, and personal traits needed by an employee that determine effective performance.

In 1982, Boyatzis outlined competence as applied to managerial work and popularized the term "competency," while John Raven (1984) published *Competence in Modern Society* in the United Kingdom. These two publications popularized the concept of competency and helped to spread the use of competencies in the work of managers, consultants, and human resource managers.

WHAT ARE COMPETENCIES?

The term competency has been used in many different ways, which can create confusion. Zemke (1982) noted that the terms competency, competencies, **competency models,** and competency-based training are often used interchangeably without much agreement on their meaning. In this chapter, we refer to competencies as "a set of observable performance dimensions, including individual knowledge, skills, attitudes and behaviors as well as collective team, process and organizational capabilities that are linked to high performance, and provide the organization with sustainable competitive advantage" (Athey & Orth, 1999). Several aspects of this definition are critical for understanding the nature and use of competencies. Competencies are *observable* performance dimensions, meaning they are measurable. The capabilities of staff can be assessed in these dimensions, allowing their use in hiring, training, and performance management. While many competencies are related to specific jobs, some are common across job families (groups of related jobs) or the organization as a whole. Competencies are linked to high performance, both at an individual and organizational level. Thus success in developing competencies is a critical component of organizational capability. Identifying critical competencies and building this knowledge, skill, and other attributes is key to achieving organizational goals.

Competency experts frequently refer to the varying components of competency as including knowledge, skills, abilities, and other personal characteristics (KSAOs) (Harvey, 1991). Knowledge includes the information and understanding of critical rules, concepts, and work processes necessary to perform tasks (Marrelli, 2001). Skills are the capacities to perform mental or physical tasks to achieve desired outcomes. Abilities include the underlying cognitive or physical capabilities required in order to fully perform a task (e.g., physical strength, analytical reasoning abilities, etc.). Other personal characteristics related to competencies might include attitudes, values, and behaviors necessary to perform effectively. For example, having a positive attitude to collaborating on care plans with other staff.

Therefore, competencies consist of clusters of knowledge, attitudes, and skills that affect an individual's ability to perform. Behavioral indicators enable recognition of that competency in the workplace. Those behaviors are demonstrated by excellent performers on the job much more consistently than average or poor performers. Competencies are determined by identifying the behaviors that are exhibited by high-performing individuals and then identifying the knowledge, skills, attitudes,

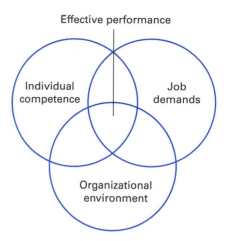

Figure 5.1. **Boyatzis's Model for Competencies and Effective Performance**

and other personal characteristics that underlie those behaviors.

Competencies are not determined by individual characteristics alone. Rather, as Richard Boyatzis has noted, competencies are determined by those characteristics in relation to job demands and the organizational environment (see Figure 5.1). Thus, competencies are more than individual knowledge, skills, and abilities; they must be demonstrated in the work environment. This model suggests that individuals with skills, knowledge, and abilities are able to perform effectively in some jobs or in some organizations, but may struggle when they assume different roles, or even the same role in another organization.

To understand what competencies look like, examine the following two examples of competencies, which were defined for a government service-level position (Table 5.1). Each example includes a general definition and some samples of behaviorally specific performance statements that reflect how the competency is demonstrated in this workplace. In developing competencies it is important to reflect *both* the specific job requirements *and* the organizational factors such as strategy and culture that determine what skills, attitudes, and values are critical for success.

Table 5.1. Examples of Competency Definitions and Behaviors

Competency Label—Customer Focus

Description
Build and maintain internal and external customer satisfaction with the products and services offered by the organization.

Performance Statement Examples
- Customer priority: Put the customer first, making excellent customer service a high priority.
- Customer knowledge: Know customers and their expectations; anticipate, assess, and respond promptly to changing customer needs.
- Exceed expectations: Consistently go beyond basic service expectations to help customers implement complete solutions.
- Solicit feedback: Regularly take action to solicit feedback and ensure that needs have been fully met.
- Customer communication: Provide status reports and update on progress to customers.
- Achieve outcomes: Consistently help both internal and external customers achieve desired outcomes.
- Improve efficiency/effectiveness: Search out ways to enhance customer satisfaction by improving efficiency and effectiveness of service delivery.
- Gain customer confidence: Gain customer confidence and trust by making sure that long-term needs are met.
- Develop alternatives: Recognize adverse customer reactions and develop better service alternatives.
- Customer service experience: Share customer service lessons with others within organization.
- Team player: Emphasize the team approach to providing excellent customer service.

Competency Label—Accountability

Description
Accept personal responsibility for the quality and timeliness of work. Possess the ability to be relied upon to achieve results with little need for oversight.

Performance Statement Examples
- Productivity: Meet productivity standards, deadlines, and work schedules.
- Goal measurement: Understand, communicate, and measure goals accurately.
- Focus: Stay focused on tasks despite distractions and interruptions.
- Time efficiency: Make the best use of available time and resources.
- Balance quality & deadlines: Appropriately balance quality of work with ability to meet deadlines.
- Bottom line: Clearly see the "bottom line" of customer expectations and ensure that work products meet that bottom line.
- Acknowledge & correct mistakes: Do not make excuses for errors or problems; acknowledge and correct mistakes.
- Assume responsibility: Do not attempt to diffuse blame for not meeting expectations; face up to problems with people quickly and directly.

TYPES OF COMPETENCIES

Competencies are frequently defined at an individual level in terms of specific jobs or job families (e.g., the competency of diagnosing congestive heart failure in patients or operating a blood analyzer in a lab). **Technical competencies** are those that are specific to a particular job family. Examples include financial analysis skills or information technology skills. Some technical competencies are broadly shared across many different roles. One example in health care is the management of pain. All health care professionals would be expected to know how to keep a patient comfortable and free of pain.

Competencies can also be determined more generally, beyond the specific job requirements associated with the traditional job descriptions, and can be applicable to all staff in certain work units or throughout the organization. These **core competencies** are broader organizational requirements that reflect organizational goals and the strategies developed to respond to changing environments. Examples include effective communication skills, teamwork skills, and a willingness to demonstrate concern and compassion for patients. These competencies are defined at a unit or organizational level and specify the individual or team behaviors necessary for achieving strategic goals and desired organizational outcomes.

The grouping of competencies into **competency clusters** of knowledge, skills, abilities, and other personal characteristics facilitates their use. This approach contrasts with traditional job analysis, which details the many specific elements required for a particular job. A competency cluster such as "analytical thinking," for example, would include distinct skills, knowledge, and abilities such as deductive reasoning, identifying and accessing critical information, classifying and analyzing data, and pattern recognition (Hoge, 2005).

Individual competencies or competency clusters can be combined and organized into competency models. These models specify the competencies needed for effective practice by particular types of staff or jobs. Reflecting the distinction between technical and core competencies made above, competency models sometimes organize competencies into three levels: core competencies that apply to everyone in the organization; **job family competencies** that apply to broad groups of jobs; and **level competencies** that are specific to particular jobs in a job family (Hoge, 2005).

The idea of core competencies can also be applied at the organizational level. In an influential article published in 1990, Prahalad and Hamel argued that successful organizations develop core competencies that address the key technologies and work skills necessary for success in a changing environment. Their article focused on technology and manufacturing firms such as Canon and Honda that have developed core competencies in developing a range of products with features beyond those of their competitors. Core competencies in health care organizations might include the capabilities to transfer in-patient procedures to more convenient outpatient settings while retaining the safety and effectiveness of inpatient care. Another **organizational core competence** is the capability to use staff in more flexible ways across different units. These organizational core competencies are based on the skills, knowledge, and attitudes and other personal characteristics of many different staff. They represent the collective learning skills within the organization and the ability to bring together different technical competencies, including redesigning work based on emerging technologies and customer-focused work processes.

Organizations can use a competency framework as they assess the knowledge, skills, attitudes, and behaviors needed to achieve their strategic goals. Thus competencies become a critical linchpin between organizational level outcomes and the attributes of staff.

DEVELOPING COMPETENCY MODELS

In our discussion above, we noted that competencies are individual, team, and organizational capabilities that distinguish high performance. However, before a person can be judged as competent, there needs to be agreement on what constitutes competence. What will be the scope of any statement of competence, which criteria will be used, and what will be regarded as sufficient evidence of competence?

Answering these questions requires an understanding of the technical requirements of jobs that need to be filled, but this alone is insufficient. These

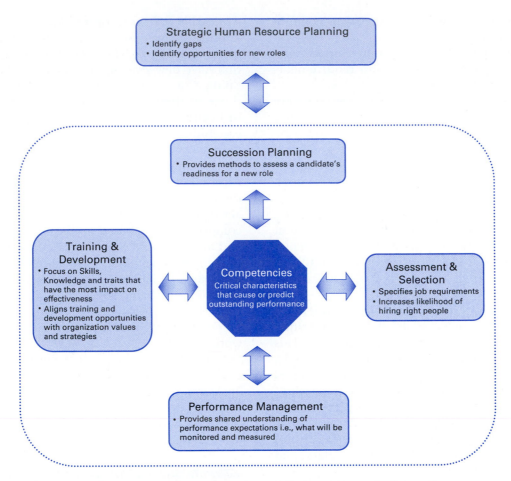

Figure 5.2. The Role of Competencies in Relation to Strategic Human Resource Planning. Adapted from: www.workitect.com, Integrating HR and Talent Management.

questions need to be addressed within an organizational context, including its vision, mission, and value statements; job descriptions; performance expectations; and comparison with similar positions in other successful organizations. Figure 5.2 illustrates how competencies are integrated within the human resource functions.

As Figure 5.2 indicates, the identification of job family and core competencies in an organization informs Assessment and Selection, Performance Management, Training and Development, and Succession Planning activities. Some of the key functions of competencies in each of these activities

are noted in Figure 5.2. A longer list is provided in Table 5.2. Competency development is dynamic. Information derived from developing and implementing training programs appraising performance of current staff and planning for succession helps to identify gaps and new competencies.

The two most common ways of developing competency models are the **single-job competency** and the "one-size fits all" and/or generic model (Mansfield, 1996). As illustrated earlier, a competency model is a detailed, behaviorally specific description of the skills and traits that employees need in order to be effective in a job. The

Table 5.2. **How Competency Models Can Enhance Human Resource Management Systems**

HRM System	Benefits
Selection	Provides a complete picture of the job requirements
	Increases the likelihood of hiring people who will succeed in the job
	Minimizes the investment (both time and money) in people who may not meet the organization's expectations
	Ensures a more systematic interview process
	Helps to distinguish between competencies that are trainable and those that are more difficult to develop
Training and development	Enables people to focus on the skills, knowledge, and characteristics that have the most impact on effectiveness
	Ensures that training and development opportunities are aligned with organizational values and strategies
	Makes the most effective use of training development time and dollars
	Provides a framework for ongoing coaching and feedback
Appraisal	Provides a shared understanding of what will be monitored and measured
	Focuses and facilitates the performance appraisal discussion
	Provides focus for gaining information about a person's behavior on the job
Succession planning	Clarifies the skills, knowledge, and characteristics required for the job or role in question
	Provides a method to assess a candidate's readiness for the role
	Focuses training and development plans to address missing competencies
	Allows an organization to measure its "bench strength" (number of high-potential performers)

SOURCE: Adapted from A.D. Lucia and R. Lepsinger (1999).

development of a *single-job competency model* begins with the identification of a single critical job. Data collection proceeds with the assembling of a resource panel of job holders and direct observation of job holders at work. Further data may be collected through interviews with customers and direct reports. The data is then analyzed and aggregated into a competency model that includes, on average, 8–15 competencies with traits, knowledge, or skills, each with a definition and a list of specific behaviors. Table 5.1 describes two competencies—customer orientation and accountability, including their definition and behaviors.

The *"one-size fits all"* or *generic* approach defines competencies for a broad set of jobs (e.g., managerial jobs). In this approach, the various

models available in the field are reviewed, as is the literature in the area. Consulting firms that specialize in competency development and application are also often used to create the competency model for an organization. This approach tends to de-emphasize the technical skills and required knowledge for pecific jobs and provides a more generic set of competencies. The generic approach assumes that specific skills and knowledge will be identified at the work unit level. However, this approach may pose problems when matching individuals to jobs that have important technical requirements beyond these generic competencies.

The development of these competency models can be resource intensive and time consuming.

Mansfield (1996) observes that "the time is ripe for a *multiple-job approach* to building competency models." This approach entails the development of a "job competency menu" (McLagan, 1988) that includes a series of building blocks. This approach facilitates training and development because individual modules can be developed for particular competencies. However, certain technical competencies are still required for particular jobs. For example, an organization might develop a training program in customer focus for all staff, but social workers will also have to have skills in client interviewing and assessment in addition to customer-focus training.

Any competency approach must define a consistent set of levels to distinguish the extent to which a competency is required in different jobs. In addition, the behaviors associated with that level should be described. The competency of "accountability" is one generic competency common across different types of organizations that may be defined differently depending on the type of job. In Table 5.1, the competency of

accountability for a nonmanagerial position is described in detail. The levels and behaviors for this competency can be illustrated using the example of a large university that has defined accountability as one of 14 competencies for its middle-management staff. *Accountability* is defined as the specific behavior of a "manager [who] approaches work in a judicious manner that promotes the University's norms, values, beliefs, policies and procedures. Does not misrepresent self or unit, admits mistakes, displays judgment in the release of information while encouraging openness and promotes the idea of transparency in business engagements." One of the expected behaviors within that competency is the exercise of discretion. Table 5.3 illustrates the levels for that particular competency and the demonstrated behavior of discretion for each level.

For professionals, competency levels may also be defined based on the *scope* and *quality of work*. *Scope* refers to the range of roles, tasks, and situations related to the job, and *quality of work* refers

Table 5.3. Demonstration of Competency Levels for Behavior—Discretion

Unsatisfactory Performance—Lacks Discretion
Did not meet the majority of goals and objectives established. Improvement is needed in most aspects of the job. It is unclear if the employee can develop to the point where all job expectations are met. This needs to be addressed immediately.

Partially Achieving Performance—May not always exercise discretion; occasionally lacks judgment
Partially achieved some quantitative and qualitative goals and objectives; improvement is needed. It is expected that the employee will work to fulfill job expectations in a reasonable period of time—not to exceed one year.

High-Quality Performance—Well-intentioned and committed to the success of the unit
Consistently achieved performance expectations, including protection of confidential information. Work is of high quality in all significant areas of responsibility. Met job expectations, goals, and objectives—both qualitative and quantitative.

Excellent Performance—Goes out of his/her way to protect confidential information
Consistently achieved and frequently exceeded job expectations, goals, and objectives through concerted effort, according to plan. Demonstrated performance of a very high level of quality in all areas of responsibility.

Exceptional Performance—Consistently demonstrates the highest standards of integrity and inspires others.
Consistently and substantially exceeded goals, objectives, and expectations through outstanding achievements in all aspects of the position. This category is reserved for employees who demonstrate exceptional performance of a consistently and distinctly superior level of quality in all areas of responsibility and make significant contributions to the Division/Department and/or University. Those who receive this rating must consistently and substantially exceed all goals as a direct result of concerted effort.

to performance on a continuum ranging from "novices" who are not yet competent in a task to "experts" whose performance is acknowledged by colleagues to be beyond basic competence. Dreyfus and Dreyfus (1982) identified a five-stage continuum of expertise that includes novice, advanced beginner, competent, proficient, and expert. The *novice* is one who rigidly adheres to rules or plans and exercises little discretionary judgment, whereas the *expert* no longer relies on rules or guidelines but has an intuitive grasp of situations based on a deep understanding, uses analytic approaches only in novel situations, and has a vision of what is possible.

Another approach to graduated levels of expertise and expected behaviors that also includes the complexity of work activities and levels of responsibilities is provided by Eraut. (Eraut, 1994, p. 184.) In this approach, Level 5 describes behavioral expectations that are required of an expert.

Level 1   Competence in a range of work activities, most of which may be routine and predictable

Level 2   Competence in a significant range of varied work activities performed in varied work contexts. *Some* activities are complex or nonroutine. *Some* require individual autonomy. Collaboration with others may be required.

Level 3   Similar to Level 2 but *most* activities are complex and nonroutine. Considerable personal responsibility and/or guidance of others is required.

Level 4   Similar to Level 3 but includes a substantial degree of personal responsibility, and responsibility for the work of others and allocation of resources is often present.

Level 5   Involves applications of a significant range of fundamental principles and complex techniques across a wide and often unpredictable variety of contexts, substantial personal autonomy, and often significant responsibility for the work of others and allocation of substantial resources.

COMPETENCIES AND HEALTH CARE PROFESSIONALS

The role of professionals in health care adds an additional dimension to the development of competencies since professional groups typically determine the competencies necessary for practice. Eraut (1994) notes that the public expects that a qualified professional will be competent in normal professional tasks and duties. The professional competence of physicians was recently defined as "the habitual and judicious use of communication, knowledge, technical skills, clinical reasoning, emotions, values and reflection in daily practice for the benefit of the individual and community being served" (Epstein & Hundert, 2002).

The degree of responsibility and autonomy given to health care professionals is usually high because they deal with complex cases where expert knowledge is needed to make decisions. But, as previously discussed, the nature of technical competencies relates not only to job demands and individual competence but also to the goals and needs of the organization. What then is the role of workplace standards in defining competencies for professionals? This is frequently a difficult issue. Debling (1982) noted that responsibility for determining competence is shared between professional bodies and employers:

As far as professional bodies are concerned, nobody has questioned the right of such bodies to define standards of competence for their members, i.e., for the professionals that constitute their membership. Where such bodies by law or practice provide a license to practice, there is no question as to their continued responsibility. Where the membership is self-employed, the professional body is the lead. For some professional bodies members are employed in diverse situations perhaps in different sectors. Under such conditions, it would seem that the prime responsibility would be the employer-recognized organizations. (p. 82)

The challenge faced by employers of health care organizations is the balancing of organizational expectations of professional competencies with those of individual professionals and their professional associations. There are very limited opportunities for human resources departments in health care organizations to influence the definitions of competencies undertaken by professional groups. But collaboration is needed in defining overall organizational expectations of professional staff. This issue is heightened for physicians who are frequently not employees, but instead are granted privileges to practice with an organization. Moreover, beyond the technical competencies required in the practice of medicine, physicians must meet the organization's expectations in terms of such core competencies as teamwork, patient-centered care, and evidence-based practice.

In recent years professional associations have recognized the broader roles that practitioners play in institutional and community-based practice. The Accreditation Council on Graduate Medical Education (ACGME) developed a set of six core competencies that serve as an organizing framework defining the expectations of physicians seeking credentials as specialists. The six core competencies are patient care, medical knowledge, practice-based learning and improvement, interpersonal and communication skills, professionalism, and systems-based practice. While the first two of these general competencies are rooted in the traditional knowledge and skills of physicians, the other four general competencies reflect the broader responsibilities of physicians to participate as team members in the delivery of care, to assess and improve their skills, and to consider their roles in the organizations and practice settings in which they work (Batalden, et al., 2002).

The changing nature of competencies in professional groups may reduce the tension between professional and organizational values and goals. However, senior management must collaborate with the physician (and other clinical) leadership in health care organizations in defining the organization's core competencies and the

relationship of these competencies to professional practice. One approach for doing this suggested by Silversin is to make explicit the expectations that physicians and the administration have for each other and then to work to create a new "compact" that addresses the needs of the organization and the needs of physicians within the organization (Silversin, 2000).

Another issue raised by the nature of professional work is the high degree of specialization within and between professions. What are the core competencies for health care professionals? If each profession specifies different core competencies there may be a lack of consistency in the skills, knowledge, and attitudes demanded by different staff. The calls for action from the Institute of Medicine and other bodies to improve the performance of health care organizations raise issues about who is responsible for the current outcomes. The Institute of Medicine in its report on patient safety, *To Err is Human* (1999), and its later report, *Crossing the Quality Chasm* (2001), suggests that health care delivery organizations have not created systems that ensure efficient and high quality care. Moreover, the Institute has also outlined important needs in the education of health professionals, calling for five general competencies to be developed for all such professionals: providing patient-centered care, working in interdisciplinary teams, employing evidence-based practice, applying quality improvement, and utilizing informatics (Institute of Medicine, 2003).

LEADERSHIP COMPETENCIES

Competencies need to be defined not only for professionals and other staff but also for leaders in health care. The challenges facing health care organizations in the current environment and the difficulties in recruiting effective leadership have stimulated an interest in specifying health care leadership competencies. In *Crossing the Quality Chasm* (Institute of Medicine, 2001), The Institute of Medicine noted

The NCHL model provides breakthrough research and a comprehensive database for defining the competencies required for outstanding health care leadership for the future.

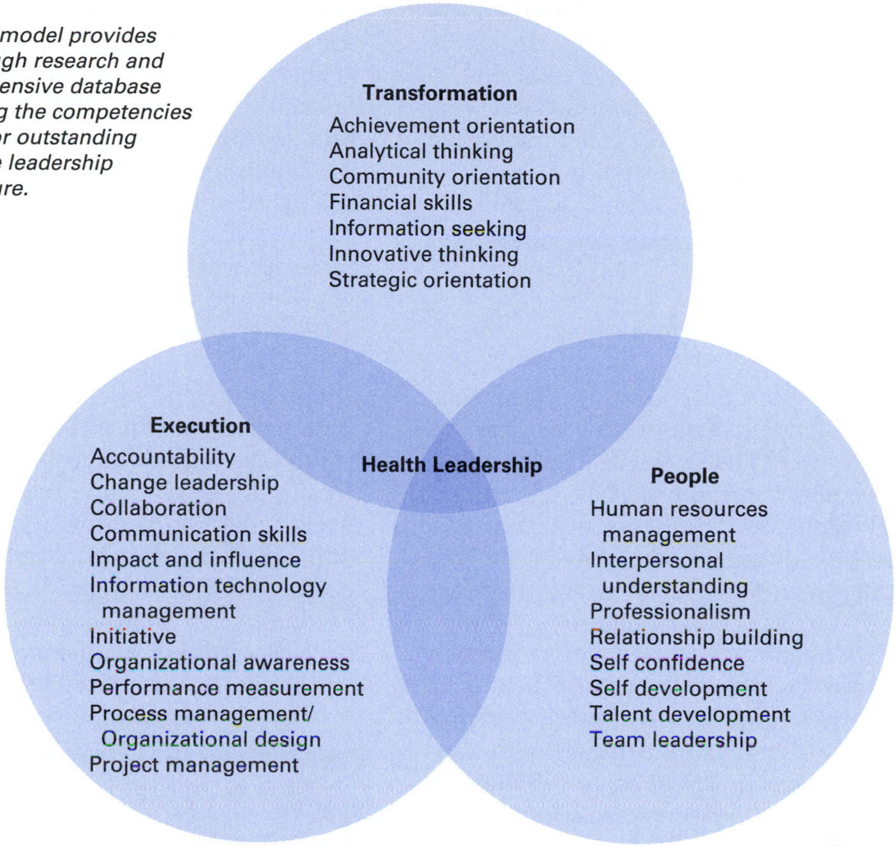

Transformation

Achievement orientation
Analytical thinking
Community orientation
Financial skills
Information seeking
Innovative thinking
Strategic orientation

Execution

Accountability
Change leadership
Collaboration
Communication skills
Impact and influence
Information technology
 management
Initiative
Organizational awareness
Performance measurement
Process management/
 Organizational design
Project management

Health Leadership

People

Human resources
 management
Interpersonal
 understanding
Professionalism
Relationship building
Self confidence
Self development
Talent development
Team leadership

Figure 5.3. **The NCHL Health Leadership Competency Model**
SOURCE: http://www.nchl.org.

the need to provide care that was safe, effective, patient-centered, timely, efficient, and equitable, and they assessed the current health care system as falling short of those goals. This is not simply the responsibility of front line clinicians but also that of leaders who set goals, allocate resources, and have accountability for organizational performance. In addition to the challenge of improving quality and patient safety, leaders are faced with other demands, including maintaining access to services in the light of limited resources; integrating new technologies, including electronic health records; and broadening the diversity of staff groups that are not currently representative of local communities.

Several health care organizations have developed leadership competency frameworks that identify the knowledge, skills, and attitudes needed by individuals in leadership positions. The National Center for Healthcare Leadership (NCHL) has developed a competency framework after reviewing existing competency models and interviewing a cross-section of health care leaders, educators, and others. Consistent with other competency models, the NCHL model identifies those competencies that differentiate outstanding performance from average performance (Calhoun, 2004).

The NCHL Healthcare Leadership Competency Model identifies 26 competencies in three domains: Transformation, Execution, and People. Of the 26 competencies, 8 are technical (knowledge or skill-based). The model is represented in Figure 5.3.

The NCHL Health Leadership Competency Model is now being used in several leadership development initiatives, including an executive team leadership program for current health care executives and the development of curricula for graduate programs in health care administration.

COMPETENCY TRENDS

Athey and Orth (1999) have identified five emerging trends in the development of competencies and competency methods. First is the demand for more participative competency approaches. The competency modeling methods grew out of a statistical assessment of the differences in behavior between a group of high performers and a group of average performers. To collect the data and minimize bias, individuals are often not told to which group they belong. This secrecy can erode trust. As an alternative, some organizations are using more participative approaches to analyzing competencies. One way to achieve this is to assign responsibilities for determining relevant competencies to self-managing teams (Mohrman, Cohen, & Mohrman, 1995).

A second trend in developing competencies is aimed at ensuring that competency models are relevant in rapidly changing organizations. To meet this need, some organizations are using computer-based competency management systems that are more adaptable to changing business requirements and corresponding skill needs (Mirable, 1998).

A third trend is the increasing emphasis on emerging competencies. Since competency analysis is largely based on comparing behaviors of staff who are currently classified as high or average performers, the methods reflect past achievements and behaviors in past critical incidents, not future ones. In order to ensure that assessment, selection, and performance management are oriented toward future needs, organizations are trying to include competency requirements that reflect emerging issues and the skills, knowledge, and personal attributes necessary to address these issues. These core competencies need to be identified as part of the organization's goal-setting or strategic-planning process.

The fourth trend is a shifting focus away from individual competencies and a growing emphasis on team and process competencies. This trend reflects the flattening of organizational hierarchies and emergence of teamwork as a critical component of effective work. Teamwork and the ability to manage processes with many handoffs are critical to safe, effective, and efficient health care. Thus, it makes sense to emphasize competencies that reflect these needs.

The fifth trend reflects the growing transition to an **organizational learning perspective.** As health care organizations become concerned with developing their capabilities to spread improvements across units, or organizations, they become aware of the capabilities necessary to facilitate such learning. As Garvin notes, "a learning organization is skilled at *creating, acquiring, and transferring knowledge*, and at *modifying its behavior*, to reflect new knowledge and insights" (1993, p. 80).

ISSUES

A number of issues have been identified in the development and use of competencies. The first issue addresses the resources needed to develop, use, and maintain a competency framework within an organization. Identifying the technical competencies needed in each job and the core competencies required for all positions demands a considerable investment in time and resources. Some experts have estimated that U.S. businesses spend as much as $100 million per year in developing competency models for specific positions (Athey & Orth, 1999; Spencer & Spencer, 1993).

Some competency frameworks include traits that are so general that they are difficult to assess and thus hard to recruit or train for. Concepts like leadership and professionalism are critical, but these are complex sets of behaviors and skills that need to be specified in a particular context or they have limited value in relationship to human resource performance (see Wrightsman, 1973).

Health care organizations are knowledge-based organizations in which many staff are professionals who resist "being managed" and whose practice is largely governed by licensing bodies. Identifying and creating competencies for this group of workers remains challenging. Some experts argue that health care organizations should be focused on creating favorable conditions for professionals to work, innovate, and excel (Hayton & McEvoy, 2006). Others suggest that health care professionals need to adopt professional roles that include commitment to creating effective interprofessional teams, emphasizing patients' contributions to decisions about their care, and acting as wise stewards of organizational resources. While these goals seem worthwhile, it may be difficult to achieve them all.

In recent years consultants have developed **competency code books** that offer organizations a menu of competencies from which they can select those that are most appropriate. The extent to which these competencies should be adapted to specific organizational requirements is unclear. Adapting these competencies to the organization's unique circumstances provides workers with the opportunity to discuss the relationship of the competency to their goals. These discussions can reduce ambiguity and provide a way of defining and describing agreed-upon behavioral expectations. This shared meaning then gets translated through the competencies (Capaldo, Iandoli, & Zollo, 2006, p. 445).

Competency development requires the collaboration among many groups with different functional expertise. These individuals may have little experience in working together and may have little knowledge about how others' work contributes to the overall organizational goals. In addition, where competencies are future-oriented, long-term employees may fear losing their jobs. Employees must develop trust in the organization to successfully engage in competency development. To do so, the organization will need to be transparent regarding its motivation in using a competency framework.

SUMMARY

Competencies provide a language for identifying the specific work skills and core competencies of the health care workforce. The process of identifying these competencies helps to clarify the goals of an organization. Developing a competency framework provides a mechanism to align assessment and selection, training and development, performance management, and succession processes with those goals. Thus competencies are useful both at an individual level in making human resource management practices transparent and consistent and at an organizational level in translating strategic human resource plans into action. Using competencies in health care organizations is particularly challenging, since health care professionals develop their competencies in educational settings and professionals believe that their first commitment is to their patients. Still, health care leaders must engage in a discussion of specific competencies necessary for high-performing organizations. New tools such as computer-based competency models and menus of competencies provide new approaches for integrating health care competencies into human resource management.

MANAGERIAL GUIDELINES

1. When formulating strategies, planning human resource development, and identifying needs in the recruitment process, health care managers should use a competency-based methodology. Managers must also ensure that there is alignment among competencies, job demands, organizational culture, and structure.

2. Despite the costs and effort to create them, competencies offer considerable value to the

organization and can be a source of competitive advantage for the organization.

3. Different approaches are available for developing competency models. These approaches may be used for different levels of jobs (e.g., laboratory technicians, frontline clinical staff, middle managers, and upper management teams) and job demands. Needs assessment can help health care managers to select the most appropriate approach.

4. Since a competency-based method is an emerging area of human resource management, health care managers must keep competencies updated over time so that the competency method can be properly applied and used, maintaining its effectiveness.

DISCUSSION QUESTIONS

1. In completing your health management education, you will acquire a number of competencies enabling you to work in the health care sector. Identify two competencies you will have mastered, the level at which you expect to have mastered these competencies, and the behaviors associated with each competency.

2. How would freestanding organizations with limited resources select the core competencies that they wanted to use in the hiring of new staff?

3. Customer orientation (or focus) is generally defined as a generic competency that is commonly used in health care institutions. Patient satisfaction surveys are used extensively to assess the extent to which employees are oriented to customer needs. Select one nondirect patient care-delivery employee (e.g., an information management system director) and a direct patient care-delivery employee (e.g., nurse, physical therapist) and discuss how the behaviors associated with the customer-orientation competency would be similar and/or different for both roles.

REFERENCES

Athey, T.R., & Orth, M.S. (1999). Emerging competency methods for the future. *Human Resource Management, 38*(3): 215–226.

Batalden, P., Leach, D., et al. (2002). General competencies and accreditation in graduate medical education. *Health Affairs, 21*(5): 103–111.

Boyatzis, R.E. (1982). *The Competent Manager: A Model for Effective Performance*. New York: John Wiley and Sons.

Calhourn, J.G., Vincent, E.T., et al. (2004). Competency Identification and Modeling in Healthcare Leadership. *Journal of Health Administration Education, 21*(4): 419–440.

Capaldo, G., Iandoli, L., & Zollo, G. (2006). A situationalist perspective to competency management. *Human Resource Management, 45*(3): 429–448.

Debling, G. (1992). Competence and assessment: Five years on and what next? *Competence and Assessment*, Employment Department, London, No.19 quoted in Fuller, A. (1994). New approaches to management training and qualifications. *Journal Management Development, 13*(1): 23–34.

Dreyfus, H.L., & Dreyfus, S.E. (1986). *Mind Over Machine: The Power of Human Intuitive Expertise in the Era of the Computer*. New York: Free Press.

Elkin, G. (1990). Competency-based human resource management: Making sense of the ideas. Working Papers Series. Cranfield School of Management UK: Cranfield University.

Epstein, R.M., & Hundert, E.M. (2002). Defining and assessing professional competence. *Journal of the American Medical Association, 287*(2): 226–235.

Eraut, M. (1994). *Developing Professional Knowledge and Competence*. London: Falmer Press.

Garvin, D. (1993). Building a learning organization. *Harvard Business Review, 71*(4): 78–91.

Harvey, R.O. (1991). Job Analysis. In M.D. Dunnette and L.M. Haugh (eds.) *The Handbook of Industrial and Organizational Psychology vol. 2*, (2nd ed.). Palo Alto, CA: Consulting Psychologists Press.

Hayton, J.C., & McEvoy, G.M. (2006). Competencies in practice: An interview with Hanneke C. Frese. *Human Resource Management, 45*(3): 495–500.

Hoge, M.A., Tondora, J., et al. (2005). The fundamentals of workforce competency: Implications for behavioral health. *Administration and Policy in Mental Health, 32*(5/6): 509–531.

Institute of Medicine. (2000). *To Err is Human.* Washington, DC: National Academy Press.

Institute of Medicine. (2001). *Crossing the Quality Chasm: A New Health System for the 21st Century.* Washington, DC: National Academy of Sciences.

Institute of Medicine. (2003). *Health Professions Education: A Bridge to Quality.* Washington, DC: National Academy of Sciences: 175.

Kierstead, J. (1998). Canada: Public Service Commission of Canada. Accessed December 2007, from www.psagency-agencefp.gc.ca/research/personnel.

Lucia, A.D., & Lepsinger, R. (1999). *The Art and Science of Competency Models: Pinpointing Critical Success Factors in Organizations.* San Francisco: Jossey-Bass/Pfeiffer.

McClelland, D.C. (1973) Testing for competence rather than for "Intelligence." *American Psychologist*, January: 1–14.

McLagan, P.A. (1988). Flexible Job Models: A Productivity Strategy for the Information Age. In J.P. Campbell and R.J. Campbell & Associates (eds.) *Productivity in Organizations: New Perspectives from Industrial Organizational Psychology.* San Francisco, CA: Jossey-Bass.

Mansfield, R.S. (1996). Building Competency Models: Approaches for HR Professionals. *Human Resource Management, 35*(1): 7–18.

Marrelli, A.F. (2001). *Introduction to Competency Modeling.* New York: American Express.

Mirable, R. (1997). Everything you wanted to know about competency modeling. *Training and Development*, August: 73–77.

Mohrman, S., Cohen S., & Mohrman, A. (1995). *Designing a Team Based Organization: New Forms of Knowledge Work.* San Francisco: Jossey-Bass.

National Center for Healthcare Leadership. (2005). *Health Leadership Competency Model Summary.* Accessed January 21, 2008, from http://www.nchl.org

Prahalad, C.K., & Hamel, G. (1990). The Core Competence of the Corporation. *Harvard Business Review, 68*(3): 79–91.

Raven, J. (1984). *Competence in Modern Society.* London: H.K. Lewis.

Silversin, J., & Kornacki, M.J. (2000). Creating a physician compact that drives group success. *MGM Journal, 47*(3), May/June: 54–62.

Spencer, L., & Spencer, S. (1993). *Competence at Work: Models for Superior Performance.* New York: John Wiley and Sons.

Zemke, R., & Kramlinger, T. (1982). *Figuring Things Out: A Trainers' Guide to Task, Needs and Organizational Analysis.* Reading, MA: Addison-Wesley.

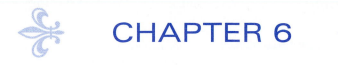

CHAPTER 6

Management of Corporate Culture

Stephen J. O'Connor, PhD, FACHE and E. José Proenca, PhD

LEARNING OBJECTIVES

Upon completing this chapter, the reader will be able to:

1. Define and discuss the role of organizational culture in both the strategic management of human resources and the attainment of organizational goals/objectives.

2. Give examples of health care and nonhealth care organizations where culture and cultural values have played a major role in facilitating or impeding organizational success.

3. Understand how health care executives might develop strong cultures that support organizational goals, match the organizational strategy to the culture, and relate cultural values to such human resource functions as selection, orientation, onboarding, training, performance appraisal, and compensation.

KEY TERMS

Artifacts
Basic Underlying Assumptions
Counterculture
Enhancing Subculture
Hierarchy-Based Rewards System
Motivation Theory
Organizational Culture
Organizational Socialization
Orthogonal Subculture
Performance-Based Rewards System
Strong Culture
Rituals
Values and Beliefs
Weak Culture

INTRODUCTION

Although a great deal of managerial attention is typically given to such activities as planning and marketing, strategy formulation, budgeting, design issues, information systems, operations, and finance, the fact remains that the attainment of organizational objectives can be accomplished only through the activities of its members. Thus, the quality of an organization's employees plays an instrumental role in the proper execution of strategy and in the achievement of stated organizational objectives. How a health care organization goes about recruiting, selecting, socializing, rewarding, promoting, training, and in general, treating these employees through its human resources practices can be traced, in large part, to its corporate or **organizational culture** (Sathe, 1985a). Creating a culture for quality and leadership presented as follows describes how leaders of health care organizations can develop and propagate a consistent culture of quality. The illustration provides an excellent example of how organizational culture can affect health care human resources management practices and vice versa.

Since Pettigrew introduced it to the field of organizational science in 1979, numerous articles and books on organizational culture have appeared in the literature. The 1980s saw interest in the management of organizational culture grow. Books such as *In Search of Excellence* (Peters & Waterman, 1982), *The Art of Japanese Management* (Pascale & Athos, 1981), and *Corporate Cultures* (Deal & Kennedy, 1982) popularized the concept of culture among management practitioners. More recent books such as *Hardwiring Excellence: Purpose, Worthwhile Work, Making a Difference* (Studer, 2003) and *The Baptist Health Care Journey to Excellence: Creating a Culture that WOWs!* (Stubblefield, 2005) detail the practical transformative power of cultural change in health care organizations.

The concept of organizational culture is an important one for health care managers to consider

because of its ability to influence organizational and individual performance. As with all other organizational phenomena, the principal goal of managing culture is to improve performance. The first to assert a connection between culture and performance were Silverzweig and Allen (1976). However, Peter's and Waterman's (1982) *In Search of Excellence* made popular the culture performance relationship. The literature suggests that the incorporation of cultural insights into decision making is helpful in planning mergers and acquisitions (Mirvis & Sales, 1990; Sherer, 1994); in strategic management (Wilkins, 1983); in recruitment and selection (Deal & Kennedy, 1982); in socialization and career planning (Sathe, 1985a); in improving leadership, creativity, and innovativeness (McLean, 2005; Ott, 1989); in fulfilling consumer expectations and sustaining quality management (Rakich, Longest, & Darr, 1992) and patient safety efforts (Runy, 2007; Weinstock, 2007); in improving profitability and market share (Atchison, 1990); in improving productivity (Kopelman, Brief, & Guzzo, 1990); and in improving employee retention and physician relations (Solovy, 2005). In addition, it can influence individual-level performance by its impact on employee satisfaction, morale, pride (Atchison, 1990), commitment (Nystrom, 1993), and turnover (O'Reilly, Chatman, & Caldwell, 1991).

This chapter discusses health care organizational culture. It discusses what it is, what it is capable of achieving strategically, how it can be shaped and controlled through human resources management practices, and how it can be harnessed to realize desired organizational goals.

DEFINING ORGANIZATIONAL CULTURE

The Algonquinian-speaking Indians of North America believed in a concept called *manitou* (Salisbury, 1982). *Manitou* refers to a manifestation of spiritual power (Baraga, 1850), a supernatural strength or metaphysical energy that gave rise to spirits and

⚜ Creating a culture for quality and leadership[1]

Today's fast-changing health care environment requires adept and knowledgeable leadership. Leaders must develop consistent standards across the organization to ensure quality and operational excellence. This will require the adoption of new skill sets and behaviors by clinicians and other employees. Leaders, too, will need to develop new skills and behaviors to effectively implement positive change.

Health Forum convened a group of health care executives and industry experts … to examine how hospital leaders can build and disseminate a consistent quality culture throughout the organization:

Moderator (Richard Wade, AHA): I am sure all of you read the latest management literature—the word "culture" is everywhere. As leaders of organizations you are supposed to create a culture of safety, a culture of transparency, a culture of customer service, and culture of learning. You have to wonder whether it is possible to make all of these cultures fit together.

What struck me about this topic, "Creating a Learning Culture for Quality and Leadership," is that culture can mean different things. How do you define culture? How do you identify what the culture is within your organization? What are the indicators? Once you have identified the culture of the organization, how do you begin to think about how to change it? What kind of process do you use to determine whether a change in culture is needed and how do you go about doing that?

I know I've given you a lot to think about. What are your experiences with the culture within your organization?

David Callender, MD (UCLA Hospital System): Culture is a set of behavioral norms. The norms become a part of the organization and are established over the course of time. In my opinion, culture is played out differently among the different constituency groups that constitute the overall workforce in the organization.

I've been with UCLA for two years. Upon arriving at a new organization, obviously you want to assess the culture of the place. I did that by talking to people. I really don't think there is any substitute for walking around, meeting with different groups, talking to individuals and asking them what they think about the place. I ask them questions to get to know how they feel.

A lot of it comes down to mission. Why are they there? What is their vision for the organization? What drives them to come to work every day and continue to struggle with others to try to be successful individually and for the organization?

There is also the issue of values. Values can serve as a guidepost for behavior. This is one area where you can go about making change. By instilling and applying a set of values within the organization, you can begin to change the culture. Talking to people, understanding what they think about the organization, finding out why they are there and what guides them in the way they approach their jobs every day, provides a good sense of the culture of the organization.

Moderator: Al, as I listened to what Dave just said, there's the idea of how the individual employee's beliefs and cultures impact an organization. Employees, of course, spend time outside of work with their families, in their own communities. They come from different cultures. It's inevitable that they bring some of their beliefs and values to the workplace with them. Every hospital that I've ever visited has a culture distinctive in itself. It's driven by mission, religious affiliation, among other things. How do you take a diverse group of people that come from different cultural backgrounds, with their own families and their own personal situations, and try to create a culture that can be distinct when they are inside your walls?

Al Stubblefield (Baptist Health Care): Dave's use of the terms mission, vision and values was right on.

I learned about culture as we started on our journey toward service excellence. Going into the process, I didn't realize that what we were really doing was creating a culture of service excellence and focusing on our employees.

We, at the senior management level, said we weren't going to sell out on service. We placed service at the top of our list. It was non-negotiable. We won't allow any excuses for poor service. We began to live out service excellence, driving it deep into our culture, into the everyday life of the organization. You have to find ways to do that. It's not easy making it part of the organization. You can't just make a plaque and place it on your wall. You can't just say that it is your mission. You have to live it every day.

The dynamic is interesting. The employees learn the organization's expectations pretty quickly. They pick up on your ideals. If you are consistent with your message, if you don't waver, they will follow suit. But you have to ingrain it into the culture, set the tone, provide direction and make it non-negotiable. You have to let your employees know that it is up to them whether they want to be a part of the new culture. They have to decide whether they want to work in that environment. If not, then you find a way for them not to be a part of it.

Part of it is leadership development. You find ways to involve your workforce and help them achieve. You give your leaders the tools they need to keep the issue at the forefront and never let it fall to the wayside.

Investing in leadership development is something that you have to start if you are going to make this happen. And then you never, ever back away from it, even when your CFO tells you that you need to make some cuts. During our budget process, that always comes up. It seems like an easy cut. But you have to stick with it. You have to maintain focus.
Kurt Metzner (Mississippi Baptist Health System): Yes, but I guess the other word that comes to mind is foundation. At our organization, which of course has a Christian affiliation, the foundation is human

ministry. Having a solid foundation in place makes it easier from the get-go. In other words, starting out with that foundation helps build the mission, values and vision and so forth. Of course, everyone doesn't have to subscribe to the Baptist theology. But it does create a solid foundation from which to build the culture of the organization.

When I first arrived at Mississippi Baptist, the organization was just starting a service excellence vision. The purpose wasn't to build a different culture as much as it was to create differentiation from our competitors. We are all in the same business. We are all competitors. We are all going after the same population pool of potential employees. We all have the same opportunities.

We decided that service excellence was going to differentiate us. Certainly making the patient experience a very positive one would make a difference in terms of our competitive position.

Our goal wasn't simply to become competitive as much as it was an initiative to get back to the foundation that was created back when the organization first started.
Bruce Lawrence (Integris Health): I agree with what everyone has said so far. It's important that there is a level of expectation set for everyone in the organization. Of course, expectations have to be set for the leadership down to the front-line workers.

As was stated earlier, every hospital has a unique culture and there are multiple cultures within an organization. What I have seen through the years is that basically every department has its own culture and every shift has its own culture in that department. Even in a multiple hospital system, you will see different cultures among all of the different organizations. You are going to see that from major medical centers to the smaller rural facilities. So if you think about it, there are hundreds of sub-cultures in any organization.

I don't know who said this originally, but it's true that culture trumps strategy every time. It is hard to be on point with your strategic initiatives if you don't have a positive culture. It gets down to individual leaders. The supervisor of the lab on the 11 p.m. to 7 a.m. shift has to be supportive of the overall mission, vision, and values of the organization. He or she has to find ways to put that into action with the employees on that particular shift.

We spend a lot of time on the development side talking about the culture that has to be there.

[1]Excerpted from *Hospitals & Health Networks*, Vol. 80, No. 10, by permission, October 2006, Copyright 2006, American Hospital Publishing, Inc.

natural forces (Gove, 1971). To the Algonquin, everything that could not be comprehended was attributed to *manitou.* Similarly, the very modern concept of organizational culture has been described as a mystical, magical (Atchison, 1990; Deal & Kennedy, 1982; Morgan, 1986), and invisible (Kilmann, 1984) power that can appear to influence organizations in supernatural ways. Many of the apparently inexplicable and irrational acts that occur in organizations can be attributed in large part to the concept of organizational culture (Schein, 1985). Much like the concept of *manitou,* culture feels illusory; nevertheless, it is a very real phenomenon governing the beliefs and behaviors in organizations. For this reason, an understanding of culture is *essential* for health care managers. If ignored, not adequately considered, or poorly understood and managed, it can work quite like a supernatural force controlling health care organizational behavior.

Because many different meanings and connotations have been attributed to culture (Schein, 1985), the term tends to be especially confusing. For example, microbiologists grow bacterial cultures. Anthropologists analyze ethnic cultures. Others refer to highly civilized societies as being cultured and more primitive ones as being uncultured. In this latter regard, European societies are often thought of as being more highly refined than American culture, especially in areas such as the arts, literature, music, architecture, and fashion. This view of culture, as measured disparities in level of social refinement, although still commonly used, is old-fashioned and should not be confused with contemporary notions of organizational culture in any way.

What then is corporate or organizational culture? Innumerable definitions have been advanced in the literature, but an exclusive definition of the concept

does not exist (Ott, 1989). Cryptic explanations such as "the glue that holds organizations together," "the lubrication that makes the gears mesh," or "the way we do things around here," while conveying the fundamental essence of what is meant by the term, are not nearly complete enough to be useful on their own (Duncan, 1989b). However, the reader will see that these abbreviated descriptions become more meaningful as the concept becomes better understood.

Perhaps the best place to begin gaining a true understanding of organizational culture is to examine Schein's (1985) definition and three-level model. Schein (1985) defines culture as the:

> pattern of basic assumptions—invented, discovered, or developed by a group as it learns to cope with its problems of external adaptation and internal integration—that has worked well enough to be considered valid and, therefore, to be taught to new members as the correct way to perceive, think, and feel in relation to these problems. (p. 9)

In addition, culture exists in three interacting, hierarchical levels called (1) **artifacts,** (2) beliefs and values, and (3) **basic underlying assumptions** (Schein, 1985).

Artifacts

Artifacts represent the most visible and objective aspect of organizational culture (Duncan, 1989b). Anything in an organization's physical, social, and emotional environment potentially can be a cultural artifact. Examples of artifacts include group member dress and deportment, facility layout and decor, furnishings and equipment, written documents, spoken words, and work outputs.

Artifacts serve as the highly visible manifestation or outgrowth of culture, and are thus relatively easy to examine and describe. For this reason, many writers have tended to view artifacts *as the culture* (Nystrom, 1993). Anthropologists who examine fragments of pottery, jewelry, and tools excavated from an archeological site are examining artifacts of a culture. The difficult task is to infer the content of the culture based on those artifacts. Likewise, when one views the immense Margaret Mead Hall of Pacific Peoples in New York's American Museum of Natural History, one is not observing a complete culture—only artifacts of that culture. Thus, although cultural artifacts are easily observed, they tend to be difficult to decode without the benefit of the information contained in the two levels beneath them (Sathe, 1985b). Specific categories of artifacts include symbols; language; ceremonies and **rituals;** stories, myths, and legends; and heroes and heroines.

Symbols

Symbols are physical representations of shared values that can be used to fortify a culture by evoking in workers a profound sense of self-esteem and pride. Symbols can be almost anything—a sculpture, building, picture, expression, flag, logo, or award.

Language

Language is such an important element that a culture cannot remain intact without it. The significance of language derives from its ability to influence how people think, behave, and perceive. In the Navajo language, for example, corresponding words for *boss, subordinate,* or *hierarchy* do not exist (Ott, 1989). As such, members of this culture cannot be expected to assimilate easily into formal bureaucratic structures without changing the language and attenuating their culture.

Language contains expressions, phrases, jargon, and acronyms that cultural outsiders may not be able to interpret. The vernacular of the health administration subculture is replete with representative jargon (e.g., matrix structure, strategic business units, corporate culture, informatics) and an alphabet soup of acronyms (e.g., HMO, CMS, DRG, HIPAA, RHIO). Likewise, the language of interns and residents is central to the physician socialization

process. Konner's (1987) "Glossary of House Officer Slang" (pp. 379–390) provides more than 200 expressions and acronyms used by American interns and residents. These types of expressions are indispensable to members of the culture, but are virtually incomprehensible to people from the outside. To genuinely comprehend and influence a culture, one must learn to speak its language.

Ceremonies and Rituals

While ceremonies refer to the occasional events when a culture's values and assumptions are deliberately showcased (Deal, 1985), rituals refer to the habitual and customary approaches to work that convey and sustain culture. Organizational activities such as meetings, strategic planning, and the process of budgeting can become ritualized approaches to work from which "people learn, celebrate, and reshape core values" (Deal, 1985, p. 310). A classic example is the scrubbing and gowning process of surgical culture (Deal, 1985). Konner (1987) describes this mechanical and protracted hand washing as being

> so exceedingly thorough, that it [is] like a ritual confirmation of the germ theory, a self-reteaching of that theory, every day. The gowning and gloving [are] equally ritualistic but more dramatic, since they [involve] nurses attending the surgeon . . . like priestesses who . . . [are] responsible for the purity of the ritual and who [will] pounce mercilessly on a technical blemish. (p. 37)

Stories, Myths, and Legends

Accounts of previous incidents in an organization's history are known as stories. Stories impart the ideal standard suggestive of a culture's favored values, behaviors, and outlooks by delivering "their core messages implicitly, metaphorically, and usually symbolically. They tend to have a greater impact on attitudes than most other forms of verbal communication" (Ott, 1989, p. 32). As such, members of the culture better retain the central ideas communicated in stories than through other types of communiques that may be more to the point, but much less intense. As time progresses, some stories may become less factually accurate by being embellished and accentuated. These types of stories are known as *myths* and *legends*. Organizational members are aware that the truth may be slightly misrepresented, but a myth or legend still serves the same function as the more factually correct story.

Heroes and Heroines

All organizational stories contain characters known a *heroes* and *heroines*. These key individuals epitomize the core cultural elements that the organization wishes to preserve or bolster. Heroes and heroines are role models (Deal, 1985) who render testimony to the significance and vitality of the values underlying the culture.

The illustrations below are powerful examples of genuine cultural stories in use at Miami Children's Hospital and New Orleans' Ochsner Health System.

⚜ Once Upon a Culture²

On Christmas Eve 1928, a baby was abandoned in Pittsburgh's Sheridan Square Theater. "Please take care of my baby," a note pleaded. "Her name is Catherine. I can no longer care for her. I have eight others. My husband is out of work. I have always heard of the goodness of show business people, and I pray you will look after my little girl."

The theater's manager found Catherine and took her to members of the Variety Club, who were meeting in the building that evening. The chapter's 11 members took in the infant as their own. And so, the story goes, because of Catherine and those Variety Club folks, needy kids became the special interest of show business pros.

The story is told as part of the history of Miami Children's Hospital. Never mind that it took place 22 years before the hospital was founded. Never mind that it happened in the industrial Northeast, more than a thousand miles from Miami. It doesn't matter. You see, Miami Children's was founded as Variety Children's Hospital by another chapter of Variety Clubs International.

Why tell a story like this? The answer goes well beyond spinning a feel-good tale. The story succinctly communicates the goals and culture of Miami Children's. It shows people stretching beyond what is required of them to care for a child in need. It connects people to organizational roots. It makes intuitive sense—ways that no statement of values can.

Stories are the single most powerful form of human communication. A truth the world over for thousands of years, it remains just as true in today's organizations, writes Peg C. Neuhauser in *Corporate Legends and Lore: The Power of Storytelling As a Management Tool* (1993). If you want people to remember information and believe it, your best strategy in almost every case is to give that information in the form of a story.

Neuhauser puts stories into six categories: hero, survivor, steam valve, aren't we great, we know the ropes, and kick-in-the-pants. Each type can be told at the appropriate time to have a positive effect. That doesn't mean every story is positive. Hospital ER stories often describe "the big night," when wave after wave of patients arrived, taxing the physical and emotional limits of the staff. These survivor stories, though full of negative events, have a strong positive: They communicate perseverance and dedication to mission in the face of adversity.

Other stories floating through organizations have both negative content and outcome. They range from those about the loyal employee who got the shaft to stories depicting the CEO as out of touch. You can't stop watercooler negativism, but you can give your staff an arsenal of stories to tell. The trick is to incorporate storytelling into your management style. Use stories to illustrate major goals. Use them to motivate. Mostly, tell them again and again, so that your employees learn them and pass them on.

²This illustration is from Solovy, A. (1999). Once upon a culture. *Hospitals & Health Networks, 73*(5): 26.

🪷 Building a culture of "yes"[3]

Ochsner Health System in New Orleans, Louisiana, is a national leader in the delivery of health care services in the United States and the largest multispecialty group practice in the Gulf South. In addition to over 600 employed physicians in over 70 medical sub-specialties practicing in 24 sites, Ochsner operates seven hospitals totalling over 1,550 licensed beds, a home health agency, and a full-service hotel, as well multiple fitness centers.

With over 7,500 employees, Ochsner's biggest strength is its people. Ochsner recently achieved Magnet Nursing Status and was named the Employer of Choice in a national survey of hospitals. Likewise, Ochsner received the 2005 VHA Leadership Award for Performance Management and Leadership Development and was named Best Place to Work in New Orleans in 2006 by City Business Magazine. Ochsner was also a finalist for Fortune Magazine's 100 Best Companies to Work For.

Ochsner was moving toward a shift in its culture, even prior to the Hurricane Katrina experience. Immediately prior to Katrina, the 60 top physician leaders and the executive leadership of the organization held a two-day, off-site meeting to discuss the culture of the organization and the organization's future direction. At this meeting, the physician leadership discussed the need to move more toward a "Culture of Yes" where the needs of the patient, their physician partners, and the organization come first. There was a defined need to hold each other, as physician leaders, accountable to one another and to move away from a culture of "No" to a culture of "Yes."

Roughly three days after Hurricane Katrina struck New Orleans, when Ochsner had over 400 patients in-house and a total of 2,000 people in the facility, bright green signs with the lone word "YES" began appearing throughout the facility. These signs were put up by the Chairman of the Department of Hematology and Oncology—one of the physician leaders present at the meeting just days before.

During this difficult period, the answer was always "Yes." The employees, physicians, and leaders at Ochsner, faced with challenges never before anticipated, fully embraced this Culture of Yes. Several years later, every new employee is trained in orientation on the Culture of Yes and their role and responsibility of living and promoting this culture—daily.

Another story that continues to be told at Ochsner several years after Katrina shows the value of every employee and the realization of the level playing field upon which great cultures are built. One area where Ochsner was short-staffed immediately post-Katrina was in Food Services. With over 400 patients in-house and over 2,000 total people living at the main campus hospital, meal service proved very challenging. Roughly four days after Katrina, before air conditioning was restored in the cafeteria, an ophthalmologist, a vascular surgeon, an orthopedic surgeon, and a cardiovascular surgeon relieved four of the food service workers and served lunch to all the employees and family members staying at the facility. This example of physician leadership and support for the role each employee plays at Ochsner is only one of the examples that evolved from Katrina and showed the tremendous importance of every employee's role and the value of a culture of service to one another.

[3]These illustrations courtesy of Mr. Michael Hulefeld, Senior Vice President and Chief Operating Officer, Ochsner Clinic Foundation.

Beliefs and Values

Knowledge of the second level of culture—beliefs and values—can offer insights into how individuals explicitly interpret, account for, and uphold their actions as organizational members (Sathe, 1985b).

Values, perhaps better referred to at this level as *espoused values,* refer to the *conscious* outcomes that are considered desirable or meaningful to organizations (Beyer, 1981). An organization's espoused values are relatively easy for the membership to voice and on which to agree. Typically, they are expressed in documents such as mission or philosophy statements (Gibson, Newton, & Cochran, 1990).

Beliefs, although similar to espoused values, are less of an aspiration and more of a conscious understanding of what is believed to be *real* and *true* in an organization. Whereas "beliefs provide cognitive justification for organizational action patterns, . . . values provide the emotional energy or motivation to act on them" (Ott, 1989, p. 40). "Whether they are aware of the values they are expressing or not, your employees reflect a certain set of core values in the service they provide" (Stubblefield, 2005, p. 24).

Basic Underlying Assumptions

The level that comes closest to characterizing a culture is that of basic underlying assumptions (Ott, 1989; Sathe, 1985b; Schein, 1985). The assumptions operating at this level, although unstated and unrecognized, strongly regulate behavior (Kilmann, 1984) by showing members which actions are regarded indisputably as appropriate or inappropriate to the group.

Espoused values can often be detected by asking people about them directly or by reading about them in organizational literature. Underlying assumptions, however, are "the out-of-conscious system of beliefs, perceptions, and values" (Ott, 1989, p. 42). They are much more difficult to uncover because they have dropped from awareness and exist only in the subliminal backwaters of the mind.

Espoused values are normative statements of desired outcomes or conditions that an organization believes ought to exist. However, espoused values do not become basic underlying assumptions automatically unless they work effectively and repetitively over time. To the degree that espoused values, or any other ways of behaving or perceiving, *work* over time, they will inevitably fall from the organization's consciousness and become collectively and implicitly acceptable. When this occurs, they will not be questioned, challenged, or even talked about, thus making it extremely difficult for even organizational members to articulate them. However, because they represent the intrinsic "way we do things around here," they will be earnestly adhered to. It is this level of basic underlying assumptions that comes closest to giving meaning to the idea of culture.

An example of a basic underlying assumption operating in modern American culture is that we respect and honor our elderly parents and grandparents. The idea that they should be left to die unattended when they become too old, frail, and burdensome is repulsive to us. Rarely is this assumption talked about explicitly. However, if someone were to challenge it seriously, such as when former Colorado Governor Richard Lamm publicly stated, "the old should die and get out of the way," the tacit assumption—that it is very wrong to hurry the deaths of the elderly because they may be a burden to others—became explicit (i.e., surfaced) in the public reaction that followed.

We can contrast this implicit value with pre-twentieth century arctic Inuit culture, in which it was believed proper to abandon the elderly by leaving them to freeze to death or to be eaten by wild animals when they became unable to contribute to tribal survival adequately (Salloway, 1982). In that particular culture, the notion that the elderly "should die and get out of the way" was not challenged nor debated vigorously. In fact, the elderly themselves often indicated when their time had come. Jack London's (1981) short story "The Law of Life" recounts how an old man left to die did not complain about his treatment, rather he affirmed that it "was the way of life, and it was just" (p. 280). Because this practice effectively and consistently allowed Inuit families and tribes to survive in an inordinately harsh physical environment, as time progressed, the practice fell from conscious consideration and became a basic underlying assumption (i.e., "the way we do things around here").

It is also important to recognize that consciously espoused values do not always correspond with deeper underlying assumptions. For example, a new hospital administrator who has not had the opportunity to explore the organization's culture fully may be at a loss to explain the very strong resistance to the hospital's publicly stated values of: (1) patients are the reason we exist; (2) all employees will be treated fairly, equitably, and with dignity; and (3) employees are encouraged to participate in the management process. By taking the time to examine the culture carefully, it would become apparent that it is not a supernatural force bringing about this resistance, but espoused values that are at odds with the basic underlying assumptions that maintain that: (1) patients are the problem; (2) women and minorities are second-class citizens; and (3) employees cannot be trusted to be empowered with managerial responsibilities.

In sum, all health care organizations possess specific and identifiable cultures (Deal, 1990) that are characterized by a pattern of beliefs, behaviors, and unspoken underlying assumptions that are conveyed to, and shared by, all members (Conner, 1990). An organization's culture can be analyzed in terms of artifacts and/or espoused **values and beliefs,** but the surest (and most difficult) way to grasp it is to understand its basic underlying assumptions.

CULTURAL STRENGTH

Organizational cultures can be characterized as being strong or weak. In **strong cultures,** a dominant and unified set of shared assumptions is adhered to consistently by members throughout the organization (Rakich, et al., 1992). Sathe (1985b) specifies three attributes that contribute to a culture's strength: (1) thickness, which represents the number of underlying assumptions in use by members; (2) extent of sharing, which denotes the degree to which assumptions are shared throughout the organization; and (3) clarity of ordering, which refers to how evident it is that some assumptions are more prominent than others. Strong cultures tend to be thick, widely shared, and ordered more clearly than **weak cultures.**

A health care organization can benefit from a strong and widely shared culture in a variety of ways. First, it can provide employees with a clear sense of direction, meaning, and guidance (Atchison, 1990), which can obviate the need for extensive or restrictive systems of bureaucratic control (Ott, 1989). Second, strong cultures can allow health care organizations and their employees to achieve valued outcomes. In a strong culture, employees are able to identify better with the organization and consequently tend to demonstrate greater commitment, cooperation, loyalty (Martin, et al., 1983), satisfaction, morale, pride (Atchison, 1990), and sense of purpose (Studer, 2003). Third, a strong culture is imperative for the establishment and perpetuation of high technical and consumer-perceived service quality (Albert, 1989; O'Connor & Bowers, 1990; Stubblefield, 2005). Last, strong and widely shared cultures are also likely to improve decision making and communication (Sathe, 1985a), as well as to facilitate succession planning (Schein, 1985). For these reasons, health care organizations that feature strong cultures are frequently viewed as superior performers (Nystrom, 1993).

Alternatively, weak cultures are splintered and lack consensus on, and commitment to, the overarching values, beliefs, and assumptions that characterize the dominant culture. In other words, they are cultures in disarray (Rakich, et al., 1992). They emerge from the existence of splinter groups, conflicting subcultures, and a general lack of *shared,* organization-wide values and assumptions.

The lack of connectedness and *esprit de corps* brought about by weak cultures can result in situations in which animosity, conflict, and divisiveness run rampant and even the most minor problems become overblown. Absent a collective focus, employees find themselves "compelled to use their own values as a basis for making decisions, they are inclined to say, 'You haven't given me anything to believe in, so I'm going to make decisions in my own best interest' " (Atchison, 1990, p. 130).

Weak cultures usually are viewed unfavorably because they frequently create a less gratifying work experience, and consequently employees who are reluctant to work very hard on behalf of the organization. Additionally, weak cultures can have a negative impact on an organization's bottom line by insidiously contributing to erosion in profitability, productivity, and market share (Atchison, 1990).

Subcultures

Unfortunately, the cultures of many health care organizations tend to be weak and in disarray (Bice, 1984). This is due largely to the fact that they harbor numerous and diverse subcultures that must be fused together to achieve organizational objectives (Lombardi, 1992). Although some of these subcultures are supportive and advance the values of the principal culture, others conflict by maintaining distinct and rival value systems.

Subcultures can be categorized into three groups called: (1) enhancing, (2) orthogonal, and (3) **counterculture** (Siehl & Martin, 1984). As the name suggests, the **enhancing subculture** is supportive and very much in harmony with the principal culture. An example might be a hospital's sponsoring religious congregation. The **orthogonal subculture** partially overlaps the principal culture by sharing some of the same values, but also simultaneously adheres to others that are different. An example of an orthogonal subculture might be a radiology group organized as an independent professional corporation that contracts exclusively with a specific hospital. *Countercultures* are confederate subcultures that are inimical to the value structure of the overall organizational culture. Because trade unions can be conceived as counterorganizations that often are at ideological odds with the main organization, they exemplify the archetypal counterculture (Morgan, 1986).

In health care organizations, subcultures can emerge almost *anywhere a group can be identified,* such as on nursing units, in service-line programs, and in ancillary departments, as well as among governing bodies. However, the presence of numerous and assorted professional subcultures such as nursing, administration, medicine, and other health-related occupations is probably most responsible for the observation that health care organizations are culturally weak. Different professions arise from distinctive theoretical paradigms and professional socialization processes that leave their imprint in the form of unique frames of reference that serve to shape priorities and guide organizational activity differentially. Thus, for example, although physicians are considered essential to the functioning of most health care organizations, their distinctive and strong professional subculture frequently clashes with the dominant culture (Myer & Tucker, 1992; Raelin, 1986), as well as the administrative subculture (O'Connor & Shewchuk, 1993; Shortell, 1991).

Most complex health care work places possess weak cultures due to their highly differentiated and professionalized nature, which contributes to the formation of orthogonal and countercultural subcultures. Indeed, the need to bring order to this chaos can be quite daunting. Nevertheless, the obligation for doing so rests squarely with the chief executive officer (CEO) (Stevens, 1991; Zuckerman, 1989), who must clarify purposes and values as well as convey them continuously through as many vehicles as possible (Filerman, 1989). Accordingly, the CEO must act as (1) a role model, and (2) a skilled storyteller (Atchison, 1990).

As the leading behavioral role model, the CEO can do much to facilitate a desired culture. Because "actions speak louder than words," a leader's behavioral conduct conveys more convincing messages than oral and written exhortations. The aphorism, "Walk your talk" (Nystrom, 1993, p. 47) is especially valuable in this regard.

In addition to playing the proper roles, the CEO must develop skills in orchestrating artifactual expressions—symbols; language; ceremonies and rituals; stories, myths, and legends; and heroes and heroines—that furnish insights into the main culture (Deal, 1985; Sathe, 1985b).

A Cautionary Caveat

Although strong cultures are considered generally desirable, it is important to note that they do not *always* enhance performance. Inappropriate values and beliefs, particularly when widely shared and strongly adhered to, may cause organizations to march in the wrong direction and to resist change efforts.

The content of culture, as described by specific types of values and beliefs is, therefore, equally critical in influencing organizational performance (Sathe, 1985a). Environmental conditions may make some types of cultures more appropriate than others. In high-tech, research-driven environments, hospitals whose cultures stress values such as innovation and risk-taking may be more successful than hospitals that share risk aversion and traditionalism as values. In stable environments, however, the opposite may be true. Cultures emphasizing efficiency and tradition may outperform those that place a high priority on constant and unnecessary change. Furthermore, as the environment has placed increased emphasis on quality, patient safety, and medical errors, health care organizations characterized as strong individual and competitive cultures find that "adverse event reporting systems with root-cause analysis tend not to work" (Wilson, 2001, p. 82). Thus, in this "who's to blame" winner-or-loser culture, people will not readily report involvement in an adverse event. As such, the strong culture serves as a powerful barrier to improving quality and patient safety efforts.

Accordingly, in rapidly changing environments such as health care, even strong and appropriate cultures may not always improve performance. As environmental opportunities and threats change, values and norms that have worked well in the past may no longer suffice. Organizations have to discard old values and beliefs and adopt new ones. In such cases, adaptive cultures are called for (Kotter & Heskett, 1992). Organizations whose cultures promote flexibility and adaptability in values and norms are more likely to survive and to succeed in turbulent environments.

Health care administrators seeking to manage culture for superior performance need to understand the relationship between the two concepts. How does organizational culture influence performance? It is believed that culture affects performance through other organizational practices (Sathe, 1985a). The following sections address the interaction of culture with two such practices—strategic management and human resources management.

ORGANIZATIONAL CULTURE AND CORPORATE STRATEGY

Organizational culture affects and is affected by the strategic context of the firm. It influences the various steps of the strategic management process, from environmental analysis and goal setting to strategy formulation, implementation, and control. It influences the kinds of strategies selected by an organization, and it determines the effectiveness with which the selected strategies are implemented. The strategies adopted by an organization also affect its culture. Every strategy has a unique configuration of structure, management systems, and organizational processes that it imposes on an organization. This unique configuration is likely to affect the existing culture of the organization (Joyce & Slocum, 1990).

Managers' perceptions of cultural values in the organization affect the manner in which they monitor, interpret, and evaluate environmental issues. Issues such as pay-for-performance initiatives may be interpreted as a threat by administrators of hospitals with traditional, risk-averse cultures. The same issues may be perceived as an opportunity in hospitals with innovative, risk-taking cultures. An organization's culture may also determine the aspects of the environment to which it gives higher priority. Hospitals with innovative, research-oriented cultures may pay more attention to the technological aspects of the environment. Religious hospitals with charity-oriented cultures may be more concerned about the social aspects of the environment.

An organization's culture is also reflected in its mission and objectives. Hospitals with a mission to provide "high-tech" care are often characterized by innovative cultures, whereas those with missions to provide "high-touch" care have patient-focused cultures. The former will have objectives in the areas of medical research and technology acquisition, and the latter will have objectives in the area of patient satisfaction.

Strategy formulation is ideally an analytical decision-making process based on economic realities. In practice, however, this process is often biased by political and cultural realities within the organization (Bower & Doz, 1979). Incomplete financial information often forces managers to use value-based judgments in evaluating strategic alternatives and making strategic choices. Often, strategies that make the best economic sense are discarded because they run afoul of the values of powerful subcultures within the hospital. Cost containment strategies may have to be pared down in the face of quality-related values. Cultural values also provide a framework that facilitates the interpretation of large amounts of information that would otherwise overwhelm the decision maker.

Strategy implementation is facilitated when organization members' values are incorporated in business strategies. Strong cultures ensure that values and beliefs are shared by both managers and employees and improve the chances that employees' values are represented in the strategies selected by management. As a consequence, employees are committed to strategy adopted by the organization and motivated to implement this strategy more effectively. If physicians and managers share the belief that costs can be cut without sacrificing quality, then it will much easier to implement a cost-containment strategy. Managers could promote effective implementation by incorporating physician values (in the form of quality safeguards) in the cost-containment practices.

It has been widely recommended that organizations find a fit between their strategies and their cultures (Deshpande & Parasuraman, 1986;

Schwartz & Davis, 1981; Shrivastava, 1984). Organizations whose strategies match their cultures are likely to perform better than organizations whose cultures clash with their strategies (Bourgeois & Jemison, 1982). Strategy-culture congruence results in the formulation of better strategies and superior implementation. Lack of congruity, however, results in conflicts of interest, confusion, and resistance to implementation.

CULTURAL FORMATION, MAINTENANCE, AND CHANGE

The association between human resources management practices and organizational culture is best understood in the context of the formation, maintenance, and change of culture. Selection, socialization, compensation, reward systems, and removal are some commonly suggested means for the propagation of culture (Sathe, 1985a). In order to understand the relationship between human resources strategies and the culture of an organization, we have to look at culture formation from a behavioral point of view.

The Behavioral Aspect of Culture

Thompson and Luthans (1990) describe culture as socially learned values and norms that help organization members cope with their experiences. What are the implications of this statement? First, it implies that culture formation involves learning through social interaction. Culture is a system of values that have been learned during a period of time as a result of past experiences, both successful and unsuccessful. Second, it implies that behavior is connected to the development of culture. Organization members modify their behaviors by observing others and learning which behaviors are rewarded and which ones are disciplined (Kerr & Slocum, 2005; O'Reilly, 1989; Thompson & Luthans, 1990).

The learning and behavioral aspects of culture are fundamental to its formation and transmission.

According to social learning theory (Bandura, 1977), learning occurs either through direct experience or through vicarious processes. Direct learning follows the notion that behavior is a function of its consequences (Skinner, 1938). Individuals learn which behaviors are expected and which ones are not by recognizing the connection between their various behaviors and the consequences of such behaviors. Accordingly, they modify their behaviors, repeating those that result in favorable consequences and reducing the frequency of those that produce unpleasant reactions.

Management can aid this learning process by providing feedback to the employee. Positive feedback reinforces the behavior and negative feedback deters its occurrence. This interaction between management and employees facilitates the learning process and leads to the formation of culture. The same holds true for interactions between employees and their peers, mentors, or subordinates. By learning to associate behaviors with consequences, employees learn to cope with experiences in the organization. The feedback they receive enables them to articulate the behavioral norms in the organization, and as they accumulate this knowledge, they develop an understanding of the organization's culture. Management propagates the culture by providing the feedback and reinforcement.

The behavior–consequence association can also be learned vicariously. Employees learn by observing what happens to other employees or by hearing about the experiences of others through formal (e.g., memos, meetings) or informal (e.g., newsletters, grapevine) channels of communication. The direct and indirect learning of the connection between behaviors and consequences leads to a modification of behaviors to maximize favorable outcomes. As these behaviors are internalized into norms and values, culture is formed. The formal and informal communications can be used by management as transmitters of culture.

Thompson and Luthans (1990) also suggest that employees learn by recognizing the appropriate antecedents for a particular behavior. A behavior that is appropriate in some situations may not be tolerated in others. Organizations that place a higher value on autonomy in certain administrative tasks may demand absolute adherence to rules in certain clinical procedures. Once again, the learning process here occurs through direct experiences as well as through vicarious means. As employees develop a knowledge of the antecedents-behaviors links in the organization, they improve their perception of the organizational culture.

The preceding discussion can be summarized by stating that direct and vicarious social interactions allow members to interpret the relationships among antecedents, behaviors, and consequences in an organization. This facilitates individual assimilation of behavioral norms and values within the organization. As more employees are exposed to a common set of experiences, there is a shared perception of the values and beliefs in the organization, and a strong culture develops.

The extent to which management can influence the formation, transmission, and change of culture depends on its ability to dictate the antecedents and consequences of behavior in the organization. Human resources management practices and policies constitute an important avenue available to management for this purpose.

The Role of Human Resources Practices in Culture Transmission

Human resources management strategies such as selection, socialization and development, and rewards systems and performance evaluation can be used to set the antecedents and consequences in the organization. They can also reinforce those behaviors that management wants internalized in the form of organizational culture.

Selection

In addition to the interactions within the organization, employee perceptions of organizational culture are influenced by predispositions formed outside of the organization. The society from which an organization draws its human resources inculcates certain norms and values in its members.

In the course of a lifetime of social interaction with family, friends, and institutions (e.g., schools, churches, work organizations), individuals go through a continuous process of matching antecedents–behaviors–consequences to form a host of behavioral norms and values.

These extra-organizational norms and values influence an individual's perception of the organizational culture when he or she joins the organization. They also may influence an individual's image of the organization before joining it. Organizations may be variously perceived as having task-oriented or people-oriented cultures (Sheridan, 1992). Some hospitals may be viewed as having highly stressful but high-paying work environments. Others may be seen as lower-paying organizations but with pleasant, low-stress environments. Perceptions of an organization will determine the kind of individuals who seek employment in it. Applicants who thrive on competition and who place a relatively high value on compensation may be attracted to high-pay, high-stress organizations. Those who value cooperation and pleasant working conditions are likely to be willing to sacrifice pay for low-stress work environments.

Societal predispositions require management to review the values and expectations of potential employees carefully. Selection and recruitment practices should ensure that applicants whose values are compatible with those of the organization will be hired and that applicants whose values are incompatible will be screened out (Chatman, 1991). In addition to job-related criteria such as skills, knowledge, intelligence, and ability, selection processes should also include criteria measuring the fit of values between the applicant and the organization.

Organizations are recognizing that the formation, maintenance, and change of culture is facilitated by hiring individuals whose values and expectations match the profile desired by the organizational culture. Conversely, the selection of individuals with values that are inconsistent with or contrary to the culture make the management of organizational culture even more difficult (Trice & Beyer, 1993). Organizations are finding it useful to provide applicants with information about the organization through realistic job previews. If candidates perceive a mismatch between their values and those of the organization, they can withdraw from the recruitment process.

Organizations are trying to learn as much as they can about applicants by spending time with them prior to hiring. The pre-hiring stage has become an important part of the recruitment process. Potential employees are invited to spend time with different members of the organization. Applicants whose values match those of successful members of an organization have a better chance of being selected (Rothstein & Jackson, 1981). Traditional recruitment practices have given way to psychological testing, structured interviews, and behavioral interviews.

Socialization and Development

Human resources managers can use selection practices to match the external experiences of applicants to the organization's culture. In a similar fashion, they can use socialization to direct the internal experiences of employees toward the formation and assimilation of organizational culture. **Organizational socialization** is a process by which individuals learn the values and behavioral norms that contribute to the culture. Learning occurs through a variety of activities that facilitate social interaction.

Mentor programs are a commonly used form of socializing new employees. New recruits are encouraged to form relationships with senior organizational personnel. The senior member serves as a source of cultural information for new recruits who want to learn the antecedent-behavior-consequence links in the organization. New employees can use the values and norms of their mentors to guide their own behaviors (Terborg, Castore, & DeNinno, 1976).

For employees who have been in the organization for some time, socialization serves to foster maintenance or even change of culture. Training and development is a form of socialization often used for this purpose (Van Maanen, 1977). Employees go through intensive training programs aimed at reinforcing existing values and norms, or in the case of change, replacing existing values and norms with new ones. Existing perceptions of culture are very difficult to change. Change will come only in incremental form unless concerted efforts are made through comprehensive organizational development programs.

Effective socialization techniques also may include the use of clear career paths and management role models to exemplify strong, visible values. Employees who perceive their organizations as having intensive socialization and support programs are more committed to the organization. This indicates that socialization promotes the direct, as well as vicarious, learning of norms and values, thus helping in the creation, maintenance, and change of organizational culture.

Reward Systems and Performance Evaluation

Reward systems represent a powerful tool for influencing an organization's culture (Kerr & Slocum, 2005). One of the lessons from the behavioral perspective of culture is that organizations can facilitate the learning of behavioral norms by providing a range of reinforcements through a variety of reinforcing agents. **Motivation theory** stipulates that individuals will gravitate toward behaviors associated with positive reinforcement and away from behaviors that produce negative reinforcement. Hence, rewards and penalties play an important role in the learning process and its outcomes.

Individuals qualify for rewards according to their ability to meet a variety of needs and wants. Extrinsic rewards such as salary increases, bonuses, promotions, stock awards, and other perquisites may be preferable to some employees. Intrinsic rewards, such as the provision of a sense of achievement, responsibility, and competence, may provide a more positive reinforcement for others.

In addition to rewards, performance evaluation processes also influence organization culture. Evaluation protocols specify what is expected from employees. They communicate the values and norms that the organization expects its employees

to conform to and they set out the consequences that individuals can expect to face as a result of their behaviors and performance. They represent another way by which organizational members learn the antecedents-behavior-consequence linkage. Kerr and Slocum (2005) described how two combinations of rewards and evaluation systems, which they termed as the **hierarchy-based system** and the **performance-based system,** produced two different types of cultures in organizations.

In the hierarchy-based system, superiors evaluated performance of employees largely through subjective criteria based on interdepartmental cooperation, interactions with consumers, interpersonal relationships, and teamwork. Rewards were largely in the form of salary, with increases according to formal salary plans or perks based on rank and tenure. Bonuses constituted a very small percentage of the total compensation and were based on team, rather than individual, performance. Promotion was largely from within. These rewards and evaluation criteria emphasized the importance of long-term commitment, cooperation, teamwork, and the dependence of subordinates on superiors. The cultures of organizations that adopted a hierarchy-based reward system were characterized by values and norms that emphasized fraternal relationships, loyalty to the organization, sense of tradition, pride in organizational membership, and conformity to the common good rather than to individual wants.

The performance-based system evaluated employees solely on objective and measurable performance criteria. Quantitative outcomes such as return on assets, pre-tax profits, and sales and production figures were used as evaluation criteria. Rewards were directly based on performance and results, not on the methods by which results were achieved. Rewards were largely in the form of bonuses and stock awards and were based on individual, rather than on team, performance. Hiring from outside was more common than promotion from inside, and perks based on tenure were rare. These rewards and evaluation protocols emphasized individual initiative and performance, short-term commitment, and independence from peers.

The culture of organizations with performance-based reward systems were found to include values and norms that emphasize contractual relationships, loyalty to self, limited interaction with other organizational members, and priority of individual needs over organizational needs.

Organizations do not only differ in types of reinforcements; they also have different types of reinforcing agents. Management, professional associations, peers, subordinates, and superiors are some of the sources that individuals rely on for reinforcement of behavior. In new organizations that are preoccupied with stabilizing work norms, work groups develop that become additional sources of reinforcement. These groups may often encourage norms and values different from or opposite to the ones supported by management, which leads to the development of subcultures and countercultures (Siehl & Martin, 1983). The transmission or change of culture through rewards is thus not entirely under the control of management. The influence of professional and peer groups may have to be taken into account when designing incentive systems.

Assessing Culture

Any attempt to create, change, or reinforce a given health care organizational culture requires that some method be available for its assessment. However, because culture is multitiered and ill-defined, it is not surprising that issues surrounding its measurement have been hotly debated. The heart of this controversy centers on the relative merits of quantitative versus qualitative methods of cultural assessment.

Quantitative methods, which utilize techniques such as standardized questionnaires and interview formats, quasi-experimental designs, and multivariate statistical analyses, have been criticized for their unsuitability (Deal & Kennedy, 1983) and apparent lack of success in providing penetrating insights into organizational cultures (Van Maanen, Dabbs, & Faulkner, 1982). As a result, the state of organizational culture research and assessment is increasingly turning to qualitative methods such as participant observation, interactive probing, and ethnography.

It is important to remain flexible on this issue (Duncan, 1989a) because the most appropriate method may depend on the level of culture we wish to assess (Rousseau, 1990). Although qualitative techniques, such as interactive probing, may be the only ones compatible with surfacing basic underlying assumptions, quantitative survey methods may be better suited for eliciting organizational values, norms, and beliefs.

Rousseau (1990) provides an excellent overview of the qualitative-versus-quantitative debate and makes the strong case for using a variety of methods when assessing organizational culture. In addition, she provides a comparison of several widely known culture assessment tools that are likely to be of value to health care management practitioners and researchers. Several of these and others are included in the following list of instruments for assessing organizational culture:

1. Kilmann-Saxton Culture-Gap Survey (Kilmann & Saxton, 1983)

2. Organizational Value Congruence Scale (Enz, 1986)

3. Organizational Culture Profile (O'Reilly, et al., 1991)

4. Critical Incident Technique (Mallak, et al., 2003)

5. Medical Group Practice Culture Questionnaire (Kralewski, et al., 2005)

SUMMARY

Culture is an ethereal concept that is one of the more mysterious and magical elements operating in health care organizations. Given its supernatural aura and assessment difficulties, some health administrators readily attribute all facets of organizational life to it, and others just ignore it. The point remains, however, that all health care organizations maintain specific and distinct cultures that can serve to influence performance positively or negatively. Thus, it behooves the health care manager to attempt to understand the organization's culture and to set in motion appropriate interventions when necessary.

MANAGERIAL GUIDELINES

1. *Know your culture.* Because organizational- and individual-level performance is related to culture, understanding the culture can provide baseline information for future performance improvements. Knowing your culture means more than being familiar with norms, beliefs, and the espoused values articulated in documents such as the mission statement; it means being cognizant of basic underlying assumptions as well.

2. *Create a strong, appropriate, and flexible culture.* Strong cultures are generally preferred to weak ones because of the clear sense of meaning and guidance they offer employees. However, given the high rate of change and turbulence associated with the health care environment, strong and appropriate cultures can become strong and *inappropriate* ones quickly. For this reason, cultural flexibility is paramount. Senior-level managers play a key role in correcting inappropriate cultures and reinforcing appropriate ones. In addition, careful attention to human resources management practices (e.g., selection, socialization and development, reward systems and performance evaluations, dismissal) is necessary.

3. *Match organizational strategy to organizational culture.* Strategies that incorporate the values of managers as well as other organizational members generally tend to be implemented more effectively. Managers in charge of strategy formulation should perform a cultural audit of their organization before they generate and evaluate strategic alternatives. One of the evaluation criteria should be the fit between the behaviors demanded by the strategy and the behaviors stemming from the organizational culture values.

4. *Employ value congruence as one of the selection criteria in the hiring process.* Candidates whose values are congruent with the values of the organization will be more committed to the organization. They will also be more satisfied and will remain longer in the organization. Hiring practices should include structured interviews aimed at identifying the value fit between applicants and the organization. Key organizational personnel should spend time with candidates to convey the value systems of the organization.

5. *Tailor evaluation and compensation systems to reward culturally correct values and behaviors.* Employees will engage in behaviors that produce positive evaluations and rewards. Organizational monitoring and reward systems should be designed so as to provide reinforcement of those behaviors considered desirable by the organizational culture. Continuous reinforcement of such behaviors will internalize them as norms and values.

6. *Use socialization to propagate, maintain, or change culture.* Use mentor programs, pre-hiring seminars, and orientation programs as socialization techniques to inculcate organizational culture into new recruits. Management development seminars, employee training programs, retreats, social gatherings, and ceremonies can be used to maintain or change cultural values and beliefs among existing employees.

DISCUSSION QUESTIONS

1. Is it possible for a strong health care organizational culture to be an ineffective one? Explain.
2. What kinds of cultural changes will hospitals have to make in order to adapt to the changing health care environment? How can these changes be achieved most efficiently?

3. What are the cultural implications of the quality and patient safety movement in the health care industry? Can culture provide a solution to the cost-versus-quality debate?
4. "Any culture becomes dysfunctional over time." Explain.
5. What steps are required to change a dysfunctional culture?

CASE: THE RECALCITRANT MEDICAL STAFF

St. Vincent's Hospital is a 200-bed hospital in a northeastern city. The institution was established in 1908 by the Sisters of Charity, a Roman Catholic religious order. The hospital has been known for providing humane patient care in a Christian environment.

In 1999, the hospital joined a nonprofit, Catholic, multiunit system based in the Northeast called Health Care Services, Inc. The reasons for the merger were to achieve economies of scale and lower purchasing costs and to obtain greater managerial expertise in certain areas.

Recently, however, St. Vincent's has been receiving pressure from the home office to reduce patient lengths of stay and total costs per case, both of which are above the average for the city. Sister Elizabeth, the administrator of the hospital, has spoken with Dr. Thurston, president of the medical staff, about the problem. His response was that he would discuss the issue, but was "reluctant to push too hard" because it might be viewed as "infringing on the physician's right to practice good medicine."

After meeting with the medical staff, Dr. Thurston reported strong resistance to "any type of controls on the practice of medicine." The staff also asked him to express disappointment that Sister Elizabeth would even raise the issue. In their view, each case is unique, and only the attending physician can determine what length of stay or total expenditure is reasonable. The staff also stated that bureaucratic standards on averages for large numbers of dissimilar cases are irrelevant and that Christian institutions, above all others, should support the principle that patient care comes first.

Several months went by, and the performance level of the facility did not improve. As occupancy rates declined, the hospital began to develop deficits. Pressure on Sister Elizabeth increased, and she knew she had to do something. Although she sympathizes with the medical staff in terms of their concern for patient care, she is also disturbed by their unwillingness to curb their use of resources and their support of one another.

CASE DISCUSSION QUESTIONS

1. What is the major problem? How did it develop?
2. What alternatives does Sister Elizabeth have? What are the advantages and disadvantages of each?
3. What solution would you propose? Why? Provide a step-by-step plan for implementation of your proposal.
4. How could such a problem be avoided in the future?

REFERENCES

Albert, M. (1989). Developing a service-oriented culture. *Hospital & Health Services Administration, 34*(2): 167–183.

Alexander, M. (1978). Organizational Norms Opinionnaire. In J.W. Pfeiffer & J.E. Jones (eds.) *The 1978 Annual Handbook of Group Facilitators* (pp. 81–88). La Jolla, CA: University Associates.

Archison, T.A. (1990). *Turning Health Care Leadership Around: Cultivating Inspired, Empowered, and Loyal Followers.* San Francisco, CA: Jossey-Bass.

Bandura, A. (1977). *Social Learning Theory.* Englewood Cliffs, NJ: Prentice Hall.

Baraga, F. (1850). *A Theoretical and Practical Grammar of the Otchipwe Language, the Language Spoken by the Chippewa Indians; which is also Spoken by the Algonquin, Otawa and Potawatami Indians, with Little Difference. For the Use of Missionaries and*

Other Persons Living Among the Indians of the Above Mentioned Tribes. Detroit, MI: Jabez Fox.

Bice, M.O. (1984). "Corporate culture and business strategy: A health management company perspective." *Hospital & Health Service Administration, 29*(4): 64–78.

Bourgeois, L., & Jemison, D. (1982). "Analyzing corporate culture in its strategic context." *Exchange: The Organizational Behavior Teaching Journal, 7*(3): 37–41.

Bower, J.L., & Doz, Y. (1979). Strategy Formulation: A Social and Political Process. In D.E. Schendel & C.W. Hofer (eds.) *Strategic Management: A New View of Business Policy and Planning* (pp. 52–166). Boston: Little, Brown.

Chatman, J.A. (1991). Matching people and organizations: Selection and socialization in public accounting firms. *Administrative Science Quarterly, 36*: 459–484.

Conner, D. (1990). Corporate culture: Healthcare's change master. *Healthcare Executive, 5*(2): 28–29.

Deal, T.E. (1985). *Cultural Change: Opportunity, Silent Killer, or Metamorphosis.* In R.H. Kilmann, M.J. Saxton, R. Serpta, & Associates (eds.) *Gaining Control of the Corporate Culture.* San Francisco, CA: Jossey-Bass.

Deal, T.E. (1990). "Healthcare executives as symbolic leaders." *Healthcare Executive, 5*(2): 24–27.

Deal, T.E., & Kennedy, A.A. (1982). *Corporate Cultures.* Reading, MA: Addison-Wesley.

Deal, T.E., & Kennedy, A.A. (1983). Culture: A new look through old lenses. *Journal of Applied Behavioral Sciences, 19*: 498–505.

Deshpande, R., & Parasuraman, A. (1986). Linking corporate culture to strategic planning. *Business Horizons, 29*: 28–37.

Duncan, W.J. (1989a). *Great Ideas in Management: Lessons from the Founders and Foundations of Management Practice.* San Francisco, CA: Jossey-Bass.

Duncan, W.J. (1989b). Organizational culture: "Getting a fix" on an elusive concept. *The Academy of Management Executive, 3*(3): 229–236.

Enz., C. (1986). *Power and Shared Values in the Corporate Culture.* Ann Arbor, MI: UMI.

Filerman, G.L. (1989). Toward a future of consequence: The education of a health service administrator. In G.L. Filerman (ed.) *A Future of Consequence: The Manager's Role in Health Services* (pp. 3–28). Arlington, VA: Princeton University Press.

Gibson, C.K., Newton, D.J., & Cochran, D.S. (1990). An empirical investigation of the nature of hospital mission statements. *Health Care Management Review, 15*(3): 35–45.

Glaser, R. (1983). *The Corporate Culture Survey.* Bryn Mawr, PA: Organizational Design and Development.

Gove, P.B. (1971). *Webster's Third New International Dictionary, Unabridged.* Springfield, MA: G. & C. Merriam Co.

Joyce, W.F., & Slocum, J.W. (1990). Strategic context and organizational climate. In B. Schneider (ed.) *Organizational Climate and Culture* (pp. 130–150). San Francisco: Jossey-Bass.

Kerr, J., & Slocum, J.W. (2005). Managing corporate culture through reward systems. *Academy of Management Executive, 19*(4): 130–138.

Kilmann, R.H. (1984). *Beyond the Quick Fix: Managing Five Tracks to Organizational Success.* San Francisco: Jossey-Bass.

Kilmann, R.H., & Saxton, M.J. (1983). *The Kilmann-Saxton Culture-Gap Survey.* Pittsburgh: Organizational Design Consultants.

Konner, M. (1987). *Becoming a Doctor: A Journey of Initiation in Medical School.* New York: Penguin Books.

Kopelman, R.E., Brief, A.P., & Guzzo, R.A. (1990). The role of climate and culture in productivity. In B. Schneider (ed.), *Organizational Climate and Culture* (pp. 282–319). San Francisco: Jossey-Bass.

Kotter, J.P., & Heskett, J.L. (1992). *Corporate Culture and Performance.* New York: Free Press.

Kralewski, J., Dowd, B.E., Kaissi, A., Curoe, A., & Rockwood, T. (2005). Measuring the culture of medical group practices. *Health Care Management Review, 30*(3): 184–193.

Lombardi, D.N. (1992). *Progressive Health Care Management Strategies.* Chicago: American Hospital Publishing.

London, J. (1981). The Law of Life. In L. Teacher & R.E. Nicholls (eds.) *The Unabridged Jack London* (pp. 279–284). Philadelphia: Running Press.

Mallak, L.A., Lyth, D.M., Olson, S.D., Ulshafer, S.M., & Sardone, F.J. (2003). Diagnosing culture in health-care organizations using critical incidents. *International Journal of Health Care Quality Assurance, 16*(4/5): 180–190.

Martin, J., Feldman, M., Hatch, M., & Sitkin, S. (1983). The uniqueness paradox in organizational stories. *Administrative Science Quarterly, 28*: 438–453.

McLean, L.D. (2005). Organizational culture's influence on creativity and innovation: A review of the literature and implications for human resources development. *Advances in Developing Human Resources, 7*(2): 226–246.

Mirvis, P., & Sales, A. (1990). Feeling the elephant: Culture consequences of a corporate acquisition and buy-back. In B. Schneider (ed.) *Organizational Climate and Culture* (pp. 345–382). San Francisco: Jossey-Bass.

Morgan, G. (1986). *Images of Organizations.* Newbury Park, CA: Sage Publications.

Myer, P.G., & Tucker, S.L. (1992). Incorporating an understanding of independent practice physician culture into hospital structure and operations. *Hospital & Health Services Administration, 37*(4): 465–476.

Nystrom, P.C. (1993). Organizational cultures, strategies, and commitments in health care organizations. *Health Care Management Review, 18*(1): 43–49.

O'Connor, S.J., & Bowers, M.R. (1990). An integrative overview of the quality dimension: Marketing implications for the consumer-oriented health care organization. *Medical Care Review, 47*(2): 193–219.

O'Connor, S.J., & Shewchuk, R.M. (1993). Enhancing administrator-clinician relationships: The role of psychological type. *Health Care Management Review, 18*(2): 57–65.

O'Reilly, C.A. (1989). Corporations, culture, and commitment: Motivation and social control in organizations. *California Management Review, 31*(4): 9–24.

O'Reilly, C.A., Chatman, J., & Caldwell, D.F. (1991). People and organizational culture: A profile comparison approach to assessing person-organization fit. *Academy of Management Journal, 34*(3): 487–516.

Ott, J.S. (1989). *The Organizational Culture Perspective.* Chicago: Dorsey Press.

Pascale, R., & Athos, A. (1981). *The Art of Japanese Management.* New York: Simon & Schuster.

Peters, T., & Waterman, R. (1982). *In Search of Excellence.* New York: Harper & Row.

Pettigrew, A. (1979). On studying organizational cultures. *Administrative Science Quarterly, 24*(4): 570–581.

Raelin, J.A. (1986). *The Clash of Cultures: Managers and Professionals.* Boston: Harvard Business School Press.

Rakich, J.S., Longest, B.B., & Darr, K. (1992). *Managing Health Services Organizations* (3rd ed). Baltimore: Health Professions Press.

Rothstein, M., & Jackson, D. (1981). Decision-making in the employment interview: An experimental approach. *Journal of Applied Psychology, 65*: 271–283.

Rousseau, D.M. (1990). Assessing Organizational Culture: The Case for Multiple Methods. In B. Schneider (ed.) *Organizational Climate and Culture* (pp. 153–192). San Francisco: Jossey-Bass.

Runy, L.A. (2007). Creating a culture of patient safety. *Hospitals & Health Networks, 81*(5): 51–55.

Salisbury, N. (1982). *Manitou and Providence: Indians, Europeans, and the Making of New England, 1500–1643.* New York: Oxford University Press.

Salloway, J.C. (1982). *Health Care Delivery Systems.* New York: Westview Press.

Sathe, V. (1985a). *Culture and Related Corporate Realities.* Homewood, IL: Irwin.

Sathe, V. (1985b). How to Decipher and Change Corporate Culture. In R.H. Kilmann, M.J. Saxton, R. Serpta, & Associates (eds.) *Gaining Control of the Corporate Culture* (pp. 230–261). San Francisco: Jossey-Bass.

Schein, E.H. (1985). *Organizational Culture and Leadership: A Dynamic View.* San Francisco: Jossey-Bass.

Schwartz, H., & Davis, S. (1981). Matching corporate culture and business strategy. *Organizational Dynamics, 10*: 30–48.

Sherer, J.L. (1994). Corporate cultures: Turning "us versus them" into "we." *Hospitals & Health Networks, 68*(9): 20–22, 24, 26–27.

Sheridan, J.E. (1992). The relationship between organizational culture and employee retention. *The Academy of Management Journal, 35*(5): 1035–1056.

Shortell, S.M. (1991). *Effective Hospital-Physician Relationships.* Ann Arbor, MI: Health Administration Press.

Shrivastava, P. (1984). Integrating strategy formulation with organization culture. *The Journal of Business Strategy,* Winter: 103–111.

Siehl, C., & Martin, J. (1984). The Role of Symbolic Management: How Can Managers Effectively Transmit Organizational Culture? In J.G. Hunt, D.M. Hoskig, C.A. Schriesheim, & R. Stewart (eds.) *Leaders and Managers: International Perspectives on Managerial Behavior* (pp. 227–269). New York: Pergamon Press.

Siehl, C., & Martin, J. (1990). Organizational culture: A key to financial performance. In B. Schneider (Ed.), *Organizational Climate and Culture*. San Francisco: Jossey-Bass.

Silverzweig, S., & Allen, R.E. (1976). Changing corporate culture. *Sloan Management Review, 17*(3): 33–49.

Skinner, B.F. (1938). *The Behavior of Organisms*. East Norwalk, CT: Appleton & Lange.

Solovy, A. (1999). Once upon a culture. *Hospitals & Health Networks, 73*(5): 26.

Solovy, A. (2005). Good hire, good fire. *Hospitals & Health Networks, 79*(9): 42.

Stevens, R.A. (1991). The hospital as a social institution, new fashioned for the 1990s. *Hospital & Health Services Administration, 36*(2): 163–173.

Stubblefield, A. (2005). *The Baptist Health Care Journey to Excellence: Creating a culture that WOWs!* Hoboken, NJ: John Wiley & Sons.

Studer, Q. (2003). *Hardwiring excellence: Purpose, worthwhile work, making a difference*. Gulf Breeze, FL: Fire Starter Publishing.

Terborg, J., Castore, C., & DeNinno, J. (1976). A longitudinal field investigation of the impact of group composition on group performance and cohesion. *Journal of Personality and Social Psychology, 34*: 782–790.

Thompson, K., & Luthans, F. (1990). Organizational Culture: A Behavioral Perspective. In B. Schneider (ed.) *Organizational Climate and Culture* (pp. 314–344). San Francisco: Jossey-Bass.

Trice, H.M., & Beyer, J.M. (1993). *The Cultures of Work Organizations*. Englewood Cliffs, NJ: Prentice Hall.

Van Maanen, J. (1977). Toward a Theory of the Career. In J. Van Maanen (Ed.), *Organizational Careers: Some New Perspectives* (pp. 67–130). New York: Wiley.

Van Maanen, J., Dabbs, J.M., & Faulkner, R.R. (eds.) (1982). *Varieties of Qualitative Research*. Beverly Hills: Sage Publications.

Wade, R. (2006). Creating a learning culture for quality and leadership. *Hospitals & Health Networks, 80*(10): 78–87.

Weinstock, M. (2007). Can your nurses stop a surgeon? *Hospitals & Health Networks, 81*(9): 38–41, 42, 44–45.

Wilkins, A. (1983). The culture audit: A tool for understanding organizations. *Organizational Dynamics, 12*(2): 24–38.

Wilson, N.J. (2001). Creatures of culture. *Hospitals & Health Networks, 75*(5): 82.

Zuckerman, H.S. (1989). Redefining the role of the CEO: Challenges and conflicts. *Hospital & Health Services Administration, 34*(1): 25–28.

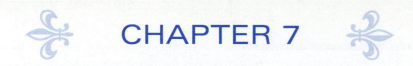

CHAPTER 7

Managing a Diverse Health Services Workforce

Richard M. Shewchuk, PhD and Windsor Westbrook Sherrill, PhD, MBA, MHA

LEARNING OBJECTIVES

Upon completing this chapter, the reader will be able to:

1. Describe the demographic trends that are changing the nature of the health services workforce and patient populations.
2. Offer a definition of "cultural diversity" as it relates to management of health services organizations.
3. Identify different organizational approaches for managing cultural diversity and delineate the characteristic values or assumptions underlying each approach.
4. Describe specific diversity management strategies associated with health services organizations.
5. Identify and describe characteristics and assumptions of multicultural organizations.

KEY TERMS

Americans with Disabilities Act (ADA)

Affirmative Action

Cultural Competence

Diversity

Diversity Management

Equal Employment Opportunity Commission (EEOC)

Equal Employment Opportunity (EEO) Laws

Golden Rule Approach

Monolithic Organization

Multicultural Approach

Multicultural Organization

Plural Organization

Workplace Diversity

INTRODUCTION

The environment in which health care organizations operate is characterized by constant change and upheaval. In recent years, hospitals and other health care organizations have had to keep pace with significant technological developments, confront a challenging array of new regulatory and reimbursement mechanisms, and meet increasing demands of patients and third party payers. A diverse workforce and diverse patient populations add to the volatility of the health services industry. Organizational viability is likely to depend on how well and how quickly leaders can respond and adapt to changing environmental conditions, including the needs of an increasingly diverse population.

One of the most critical elements of the changing health care environment concerns the demographic and cultural profile of the workforce emerging in the United States. Until recently, the workforce employed in most organizations could be described as being "monolithic" with respect to its demographic and cultural characteristics. In general, the typical employee conformed to a "homogeneous ideal" that was found in most corporate settings. In 1991, Loden and Rosener noted that the ideal or successful employee embodied several specific attributes; "he" was between the ages of 35 and 49 and was married with children, college educated, heterosexual, in good physical condition, Protestant or Jewish, and competitive. However, it also must be recognized that, to some degree, the concept of the typical employee traditionally has been influenced by the specific occupational roles found in a particular organizational setting. In health care organizations, for example, nurses and allied health personnel have been fairly homogeneous with respect to gender. Similarly, the demographic profile of hospital administrators, especially those who have attained upper management positions, also has tended to conform to fairly well-defined characteristics. The concept of the "homogeneous ideal" and the historically close correspondence between occupational roles and the demographic profiles of the employees who have occupied those roles have helped to define a management dynamic in which assimilation and conformity were dominant strategies for developing a productive workforce. In organizations in which the majority of employees conformed to an "ideal type," a management approach based on relatively narrowly defined norms, values, and expectations of a homogeneous workforce, although perhaps somewhat constrictive, was, nonetheless, probably functional.

As the growth rate of the workforce slows in general and as the traditional pool of potential employees shrinks, the concept of the "homogeneous ideal" has become increasingly obsolete. Additionally, as organizations have faced competition for entry-level and skilled workers, they have incorporated nontraditional entrants in the workforce. Therefore, the current health care workforce is characterized by its **diversity.** Consequently, management practices that seemed to be appropriate when most employees were thought to be similar (and when those who were different were encouraged to adapt to the norm) have become less effective, and even dysfunctional, in work places where there are many different individuals, each of whom requires understanding and respect (Jamieson & O'Mara, 1991). To survive in this new environment, health services organizations must develop a new workforce management paradigm.

It is important to recognize that diversity can exert both positive and negative effects on organizational performance. To leverage the potential benefits of a diverse workforce while avoiding its negative consequences, management must understand the complex nature of diversity and how it should be managed within different contexts and under different conditions. In this chapter, we first define the concept of diversity as it relates to human resource management. We then explore several environmental realities that impact **diversity management** issues. Next, we describe several different approaches that organizations have adopted in dealing with diversity. Finally, we conclude by outlining specific strategies that have been used by various organizations to manage the impact of a diverse workforce effectively.

DEFINING DIVERSITY

Diversity is best defined broadly, because it comprises all the similarities and differences that make individuals unique. Traditionally, human resources diversity has been focused on "numbers" of people, largely connected to the initiation of **affirmative action.** Organizations that employed individuals from minority groups claimed to be "diverse" to avoid the perceptions of being discriminatory. Loden and Rosener originally (1991) defined diversity as "otherness," or those human qualities that are different from our own and outside the groups to which we belong, yet present in other individuals and groups. The meaning of diversity has evolved as the concept increasingly encompasses those who are different in terms of race, age, religion, disability, marital status, ethnicity, ancestry, gender, physical abilities/qualities, sexual orientation, educational background, geographic location, income, military experience, parental status, and work experience.

The change in the racial and ethnic composition of the United States perhaps provides the most powerful illustration of the challenges and opportunities that arise with increasing demographic heterogeneity and shifting personal beliefs about diversity. The cornerstone of strategic diversity management is **cultural competence,** which embraces the "information value of diversity" and the importance of "celebrating our differences" (Dreachslin, 2007).

Cultural competence is defined by the Office of Minority Health as "a set of congruent behaviors, attitudes, and policies that come together in a system, agency, or among professionals that enables effective work in cross-cultural situations" (Beal, 2006). It is a critical component to the provision of quality health care because beliefs shape the way people define health problems, seek assistance, and

adhere to medical regimens (Aries, 2004). According to Sondra Thiederman, an author specializing in **workplace diversity** and communications issues:

> Growing diversity affects everyone who works in the healthcare industry, and introduces new imperatives that healthcare organizations did not face before. Chief among these imperatives is the need to ensure effective interaction among physicians, staff, and patients whose cultural values, language, and points of view may be different. (1996, p. 72)

Managing Diversity to Maximize Institutional Effectiveness

Diversity management differs from affirmative action when management maximizes the ability of all employees to contribute to organizational goals. Affirmative action emphasizes legal requirements and social responsibility; managing diversity emphasizes business maximization. To address diversity issues, health care organizations need to consider several challenges:

- Are there practices, policies and paradigms in the organization that have differential or unintended impact on different groups?
- Are there organizational changes that can enable diverse work groups in the institution to be more productive?

Increased workforce productivity directly contributes to organizational viability. Organizations must be aware of the changing needs of a diverse workforce as a key in establishing a successful business model. Organizational leaders have a critical role in transforming the organizational culture so that it more closely reflects the values of a diverse workforce. Some of the skills needed are

- an understanding and acceptance of managing diversity
- recognition that diversity is a component of all aspects of management

- self-awareness within the organization of organizational culture, identity, biases, prejudices, and stereotypes that exist within the organization
- willingness to challenge and change institutional practices that present barriers to different groups and to the development of a diverse workforce

Managing diversity means acknowledging people's differences and recognizing these differences as valuable; it enhances good management practices by preventing discrimination and promoting inclusiveness, but it also provides for business maximization within the organization.

Demographic Factors

Several demographic forces are altering the workforce available to health services organizations. Data from the U.S. Census projects that by 2030, four of every ten Americans will identify themselves as a member of a racial or ethnic minority group (Dreachslin, 2007; Shin & Bruno, 2003). African Americans, Hispanic Americans, and Native Americans compose nearly 34% of the total U.S. population, yet only account for 6% of the nation's physicians, 9% of its nurses, and 5% of its dentists (Maxwell, 2005). As many as 20 languages may be encountered among the staff and patients in a single health care facility (Thiederman, 1996). Furthermore, studies by the American College of Healthcare Executives (ACHE) indicate that women earn approximately 20% less than men, yet women and minorities make up at least 62% of the health care workforce (Warden, 1999). In the section that follows, we examine some of the primary factors that are changing the workforce. We also briefly discuss some of the implications that a changing workforce has for health services organizations.

The Generational Workforce

The "aging of America" is potentially the single most significant demographic force that will influence management strategies of health services organizations in the foreseeable future. According to the U.S. Bureau of Labor Statistics, studies indicate that as many as 40% of the nursing workforce are considering retirement. Furthermore, fewer qualified graduates are available to take the place of the aging "Baby Boomer," thus leading to a knowledge and skills gap, along with a generational gap and a substantial gap in number of workers available compared to those that are needed (D'Aurizio, 2007). A generation is defined by demographics and key life events that contribute to the shaping of generational characteristics (Bell & Narz, 2007). There is slight disagreement among sources on exact birthdates, but the general consensus is that there are four generations working side by side in today's workforce. These generations, as defined by Bell and Narz (2007), are

- The Traditionalist Generation—those employees over 60. These employees can be credited with the "typical" work environment. They tend to work from 8:00 a.m. to 5:00 p.m. with frequent evening and weekend hours during the tax season. Traditionalists are frugal, hardworking conformists who respect authority and put duty before pleasure.

- The Baby Boomers—those employees in their mid-40s to 60s. These employees, being raised by Traditionalist parents, entered the workforce with a strong work ethic. Baby Boomers value personal growth, hard work, individuality, and equality of the sexes.

- Generation X—those employees in their late 20s to early 40s. Generation Xers are children of the Baby Boomers, so they witnessed the sacrifice of both parents working in order to "have it all." They are a relatively small generation and are self-reliant, optimistic, and confident. Generation Xers value education, independence, and parenting above work.

- Generation Y—the new generation entering the workforce; those employees in their early 20s or younger. This generation constitutes the largest generation since the Baby Boomers, and they are sometimes referred to as the "Echo Boomers." Generation Yers were exposed to diverse lifestyles and cultures at an early age and tend to respect different races, ethnic groups, and sexual orientations. Approximately one-third of this generation are members of a minority group. They are accustomed to computer technology, immediacy, and multitasking. As Generation Y enters the workforce, organizational culture change will be a necessity.

There are at least two realities that accompany an aging and slowly growing workforce. The first, which is likely to be a boon to health services organizations, is that there will be a large pool of workers 55 years and older who are well-educated, highly skilled, and eager to retire. Less fortuitous will be the task of juggling the demands of work with personal life for Generation Xers and Generation Yers, who will be less flexible with respect to training or relocation (Bell & Narz, 2007). Furthermore, the limited ability to hire a supply of younger and lower-paid workers will make it more difficult for organizations to diversify rapidly or to expand operations in response to changing environmental conditions.

Women in the Workforce

The continuing influx of women into the workforce is another dominant demographic trend that holds far-reaching implications for health services organizations. During the last three decades, employment patterns have been altered dramatically as increasing numbers of women entered the workforce. In 1950, 34% of women worked in paying jobs outside of the home and made up about 30% of the workforce. In 1990, 57.5% of women working in jobs outside of the home made up approximately 46% of the U.S. workforce (Fernandez, 1991). Currently, representation of women in the overall workforce is almost equal to that of men. According to ACHE's survey from the year 2000, women with the same education and experience as their male counterparts earned, on average, $19,400 less per year (ACHE, 2000). Studies by the American College of Healthcare Executives indicate that less than 2% of top health care positions are filled by minorities and that women earn 20% less than men. However, women and minorities make up 62% of the health care workforce (Warden, 1999). Researchers have found that gender tends to work

with race and ethnicity to exacerbate disparities in career attainment (Dreachslin, 2007).

Many of the women who enter the workforce are married mothers of young children. In fact, Hoffman (1989) has observed that 71% of mothers in two-parent families have full-time employment outside of the home and, as a group, represent one of the most rapidly growing segments of the workforce. There is considerable evidence that supports the notion that most women, including mothers of young children, work primarily because of economic need. Higgins, Duxbury, and Johnson (2000) observe that most professional working women with children prefer part-time jobs with flexible hours or jobs that would permit them to work at home.

As the feminization of health services organizations further evolves, new management approaches will be required to fully capture the potential of this large pool of workers. In particular, attention must be focused on further development of family-friendly benefits and human resources policies and practices that allow women to balance their career and home responsibilities effectively. It is possible that in addition to appearing more attractive to potential employees, health services organizations that provide assistance with childcare arrangements and institute policies that allow flexible work options (e.g., job sharing, voluntary reduced time, flex-time, compressed work week, work-at-home options) could prevent or help resolve much of the family-work conflict that can undermine women's productivity (Jamieson & O'Mara, 1991). Organizations that actively offer such benefits to all employees rather than focusing on one group such as women also reduce potential conflict among workgroups.

Organizations must also do more to develop professional opportunities and employment functions for women. Many jobs for women are clustered in "female" occupations that pay poorly. Many institutions are making an effort to promote and educate women about opportunities so that women may achieve higher-paying jobs and leadership roles. If health services organizations are to benefit optimally from a feminized workforce, they must resolve several lingering management practices that discriminate against women. It is especially important to remove the many barriers that deny women access to upper management levels (Morrison, 1992). The issue of differential salaries is another gender bias issue that should be addressed by organizations hoping to attract and retain qualified women. Undergirding these and other changes that must occur are educational and training initiatives and "a thoroughgoing reform of the institutions and policies that govern the workplace, to insure that women can participate fully."

Minority and Immigrant Workers

According to a study by the executive search firm Witt/Kieffer, women in general have achieved a greater breakthrough in health care senior leadership ranks than minorities (1999). The increasing rate at which people of color born in the United States and new immigrants to this country enter the workforce is a third dominant demographic trend that has a profound influence on health services organizations. It is estimated that native-born people of color, primarily African Americans, Latinos, and Asians, make up only slightly less than one-third (29%) of the new workforce entrants. Approximately 600,000 people who immigrate to this country each year (most from Latin America and Asia) make up another 14% of the new entrants to the workforce. As a result of their rapid entry into the workforce, minority and immigrant workers will occupy 26% of all jobs nationwide (Fernandez, 1991; Jamieson & O'Mara, 1991). Hispanics have surpassed African Americans as the largest minority group in the United States (U.S. Bureau of the Census).

The overall impact of this changing demographic profile will be significant. According to some sources, the concept of "minority" will assume a different meaning in some regions of the country, where much of the population will consist of people of color. Of particular significance to health services organizations is the fact that many of these new workers are being raised in poverty

with many of its attendant disadvantages, especially being "ill-served by the nation's school system" (Offermann & Gowing, 1990, p. 97). Johnston and Packer suggest that the lack of adequate education and training could place minority workers at a distinct disadvantage as increasing numbers of jobs are created in which more education and higher skill levels are required.

In light of the impending shortage of qualified workers, it seems clear that health services organizations would be well-served if they were to commit educational and training resources to those segments of minority and immigrant populations that are in need of such assistance. However, effective management of a culturally diverse workforce will entail more than helping nontraditional employees gain entry into the workforce. If health services organizations are to integrate people of various cultural, ethnic, and racial backgrounds into the workplace successfully, they also must implement programs that foster a recognition and appreciation of the meaningful differences that employees manifest.

Other Dimensions of Diversity

Another population segment that traditionally has been underrepresented in the workforce, but one that is expected to participate more extensively in the future, consists of people with disabilities and various chronic diseases. Although a majority of persons with disabilities express a desire to work, for several reasons, only approximately one-third of the working-age members of this population have found their way permanently into the workforce (Jamieson & O'Mara, 1991, p. 25). Employment policies should take into account a personalized assessment of disability to account for the various personal and environmental factors which lead people to achieve employment in spite of disability, or what researchers call the "capability approach" to disability (Mitra, 2006). In the past, many disabled persons confronted significant social and physical barriers that made it difficult to obtain employment. The **Americans with Disabilities Act (ADA)** includes provisions that "prohibit discrimination in employment against individuals who, with reasonable accommodation, can perform the essential functions of a job."

It can be reasonably expected that health services organizations may wish to help offset the developing workforce shortage by integrating qualified workers from the large population of disabled persons and a growing number of persons with chronic disease into the work place. Effective strategies for enhancing the productivity of the many elements of this population demand innovative and flexible work approaches that accommodate workers' limitations. Also called for are educational efforts that are directed at enhancing all employees' levels of tolerance and understanding of this dimension of otherness, thereby helping to remove the attitudinal barriers that interfere with cooperative work place efforts.

Equal employment opportunity (EEO) laws make it illegal for employers to discriminate against an employee or potential employee in certain workplaces. The **Equal Employment Opportunity Commission (EEOC),** which was created by the Civil Rights Act of 1964, is the federal agency that has the responsibility to handle discrimination complaints. Concurrent with the very observable workforce changes that are already occurring, health services organizations are likely to encounter workers who possess diverse attitudes, motivations, and values that may seem to be at odds with those that were held by the traditional workforce. Although perhaps less obvious, these psychologically oriented dimensions of diversity are very salient for workers and can have an important influence on productivity levels. Characteristic of the value orientation of the emerging workforce is an "increased desire for autonomy, self-development . . . more meaningful work experiences, as well as more involvement in decisions pertaining to themselves" (Offermann & Gowing, 1990, p. 98). One would expect that health services organizations would gain some advantage over competitors in terms of being able to attract and retain qualified workers in productive roles by acknowledging the validity of each employee's values and attitudes. Although this is an area that requires additional

research, Jamieson and O'Mara (1991) suggest that value-sensitive management policies are those that link reward and recognition mechanisms with employee values, allow a large measure of worker autonomy and self-management, and seek and consider employee input concerning decisions that affect the quality of life in the work place.

The evolving workforce of today's health services organizations reflects, to a large degree, the major demographic transitions that are occurring within society at large. Accumulating evidence suggests that the rate of workforce growth is slowing and that, unlike the traditional, predominantly white male workforce of the past, this new workforce will be older and have more women, minority, immigrant, and disabled workers. Furthermore, it is likely that employees will express values and attitudes that are unfamiliar to most managers. Taken together, these transitions pose a significant challenge for health services organizations. In the section that follows, we examine several approaches organizations have adopted in dealing with issues of diversity.

Multiculturalism offers tremendous competitive benefits to an organization (Lim, Winter, & Chan, 2006). The nation's most successful firms are already adept at using diversity and cultural differences as a tool rather than an obstacle (Vallario, 2006). Employing a diverse workforce will be advantageous because workers bring multiple perspectives to a problem and thus will create more creative solutions, especially to the needs of a diverse customer base (Aries, 2004). In addition, according to Cynthia Waller Vallario, in *Financial Executive,* "The human capital, namely the competence and capabilities of the employees, is broadened and deepened with increased diversity and by cultural development and talent investment strategies" (2006, p. 51).

Diversity in the workplace is not only a human resources issue but also a business strategy: "It is a mix of people skills and cultures that enables a range of viewpoints to challenge traditional thinking" (Vallario, 2006). The changing nature of workforce demography will result in a shift in people's values, attitudes, and beliefs, which will affect the importance placed on a variety of work aspects (Lim, et al., 2006). Workplace diversity will be a tool for success in the ever-changing environment of the future (Lawrence, 2005).

Diversity policies need to be solidly integrated throughout the organization, with executive leadership, and in ongoing training and support (Vallario, 2006). A strategic plan for diversity that sets goals, assesses the environment, and evaluates the organization's strengths and weaknesses must come into play in order for diversity to work (Warden, 1999). The concept of building a diverse organization must become integrated throughout the organization; time should be taken to educate and train management in diversity and to enhance the human resources support systems to make diversity possible in leadership (Warden, 1999). The active participation of managers will be critical in creating a culturally competent and cohesive workforce (Aries, 2004).

Cultural competence throughout the health care industry begins in the interview process. Interviews are used in recruitment, selection, promotion, identifying training needs, and performance reviews. Career development professionals must understand the potential impact of discrimination that might be caused by cultural incompetence rather than blatant discrimination (Lim, et al., 2006). The success of an organization is heavily dependent on its human and intellectual capital. As such, human resource professionals and managers need to be aware of the cultural forces involved during an interview. In order to reinforce the importance of cultural competence, training policies need to focus on raising cultural awareness and improving cross-cultural communication, so interviewers will be able to differentiate between skills, personality, and culturally based behaviors (Lim, et al., 2006).

The incorporation of diversity into the health care organization will ultimately lie in changing the organizational culture. The scope of being diverse needs to go beyond a focus of recruiting more people from minority groups (Lawrence, 2005). The restructure of the organization will be a result of organizational leaders listening to new perspectives

(Lawrence, 2005). As attitudes of inclusion improve, employees with different opinions who work in an open and honest environment will lead to a better product—or in the case of the health care industry, better service with a higher level of customer satisfaction (Maxwell, 2005).

The views of all staff should shape the way an organization is run, and all employees must have access to development and promotion opportunities if they are to reach their full potential (Lawrence, 2005). The competence and capabilities of employees is broadened and deepened with increased diversity (Vallario, 2006).

Health care organizations must view diversity as a long-term approach to organizational culture change. Success in reaching meaningful diversity goals will require at least a five-year plan, with practical and measurable goals (Maxwell, 2005). To promote a new organizational culture of diversity, the plan must offer frequent and visible communication and support. Acceptance of the diversity initiative will be the key to a successful initiative (Maxwell, 2005).

DIFFERENT APPROACHES TO DIVERSITY: ORGANIZATIONAL TYPOLOGIES

Ignoring diversity or failing to manage it effectively will most certainly undermine organizational performance. Increased conflict, complaints, and legal actions related to diversity issues decrease productivity. Resultant tensions or conflict among workers can reduce the institution's ability to recruit and retain diverse work groups and to maintain a positive work environment, impacting the effectiveness of the organization.

Just as definitions of diversity have varied, so have typologies that describe organizational approaches to handling diversity. Morrison (1992) described five organizational approaches to diversity, including: (1) the **golden rule approach,** (2) assimilation, (3) righting the wrongs, (4) the culture-specific approach, and (5) the **multicultural approach** (see Table 7.1). Some organizations have encouraged employees and managers to focus on incorporating "the golden rule" philosophy in human resources management dealing with co-workers; the maxim states that one should treat others as one would want to be treated. Organizations adopting this approach rely on individual integrity and morality to make diversity work. Yet differences among employees based on characteristics such as age, gender, race, and ethnicity are not recognized explicitly by organizations that ascribe to the golden rule approach. The implicit assumption in the golden rule approach is that how one individual wants to be treated is how others want to be treated. As they expand beyond this approach, organizations increasingly recognize that respect may not be the same for everyone. Individuals may share similar values, such as respect or need for recognition, but how we show those values through behavior may be different for different cultures or groups. Another maxim is to "treat others as *they* want to be treated." In this approach, the frame of reference moves from an ethnocentric view ("our way is the best way") to a culturally relative perspective ("let's take the best of a variety

of ways") and facilitates management in a diverse work environment.

Assimilation relates to shaping people to the style already dominant in an organization. Organizations that adopt this approach expect individuals to suppress their differences and to accommodate the notion of the "homogeneous ideal." This relates to the idea of approaching fairness in human resource management as "treating everyone the same," but this is not always effective among a diverse staff. One example is when employees have limited reading proficiency. Providing important information through detailed memos might not be an effective mode of communication, even though it might constitute same treatment. A staff member who missed out on essential information might feel that the communication process was "unfair." A process that takes account of the diverse levels of English language and reading proficiency among the staff might include taking extra time to be sure that information in an important memorandum is understood. Efforts on the part of supervisors and managers should be supported and rewarded as good management practices for working with a diverse staff. The third approach, righting the wrongs, targets groups who have suffered past

Table 7.1. Organizational Approaches to Diversity

Stage	Morrison (1992)	Thomas (1991)	Cox (1991)	Adler (2002)
Do nothing/denial of differences or impacts of diversity	Golden rule			Parochial
Acknowledge differences; avoid problems by avoiding diversity	Assimilation		Monolithic	Ethnocentric
Acknowledge differences; take action only if legally mandated	Rights the wrongs	Affirmative action	Plural	
Acknowledge differences; minimize inevitable dysfunctional impacts by fostering understanding and acceptance	Culture-specific	Valuing cultural differences		
Full recognition of differences, problems, and benefits; productively encourage and manage diversity	Multicultural	Managing cultural diversity	Multicultural	Synergistic

discrimination and attempts to compensate for past injustices. Organizations that favor this approach rely primarily on legal mandates for guidance in handling diverse employees, and these approaches only serve the organization in a limited fashion.

The multicultural approach "involves increasing the consciousness and appreciation of differences associated with the heritage, characteristics, and values of many different groups, as well as respecting the uniqueness of each individual" (Morrison, 1992, p. 7). Organizations that embrace this approach consciously acknowledge differences among employees along a number of dimensions and promote understanding and respect of such differences.

A similar typology, reflecting an organization's strategy for dealing with cultural diversity, was offered by Thomas (1991). He notes that organizations can use a strategy of: (1) complying through affirmative action, (2) simply valuing cultural differences, or (3) proactively managing cultural diversity. The goals of the first approach are to provide opportunities for upward mobility for minorities and women and to comply with legal and social responsibilities. However, the affirmative action approach, as a single strategy for dealing with diversity, has significant disadvantages. Although such an approach may succeed in increasing numbers of women and minorities in key positions, little is done to change negative attitudes toward these individuals. Indeed, in many cases, a "backlash" of negative attitudes may occur, resulting in charges of reverse discrimination and feelings that all minorities and women achieve key positions through quotas rather than qualifications.

The goals of the second approach, valuing diversity, are to establish quality interpersonal relationships; to reduce conflict; and to minimize overt expressions of racism, ethnocentrism, and sexism. Essentially, such an approach is aimed toward eliminating or minimizing the negative impact of a culturally diverse workforce. The focus of this strategy is on avoiding trouble rather than on maximizing benefits.

According to Thomas (1991), "acceptance, tolerance, and understanding of diversity are not by themselves enough to create an empowered workforce. To empower a diverse group of employees to reach their full potential, managing diversity is needed" (p. 25). Thus, organizations adopting the third strategy of proactively managing diversity view cultural differences as offering specific advantages. Organizations adopting this strategy recognize and confront the realities of today (e.g., changing demographics of the U.S. workforce, increased competition, external pressure for quality products and services) and believe that they will achieve a competitive advantage only by fully integrating and utilizing a culturally diverse workforce.

Cox (1991) presented a typology describing three organizational prototypes that differ according to six factors: (1) mode of acculturating diverse employees, (2) methods and degree of structural integration of diverse employees, (3) methods and degree of informal integration of diverse employees, (4) degree of cultural bias within the organization, (5) identification (e.g., loyalty, commitment) of employees, and (6) degree of intergroup conflict among diverse employees. He viewed these prototypes as representing different stages of development in an organization's ability to deal effectively with diversity.

The first type of organization, which Cox labeled as *monolithic*, is characterized by assimilation of diverse employees (i.e., expecting them to conform to a homogeneous norm), minimal structural and informal integration of diverse others, presence of prejudice and discrimination against diverse employees, large gaps in the degree of organizational commitment of diverse versus dominant employees, and low intergroup conflict due to high homogeneity. Thus, the **monolithic organization** reflects the first, or least effective, stage of development in managing cultural diversity.

The **plural organization** reflects "middle ground" on the six factors identified by Cox (1991) and is the second stage of development. This organization also is characterized by assimilation of diverse others, but has greater structural and informal integration of diverse employees, less prejudice and discrimination, and smaller gaps in employee identification than the monolithic organization.

However, intergroup conflict may be higher in a plural organization because although heterogeneity is greater, prejudice and discrimination still exist.

The organization that handles diversity most effectively, according to Cox (1991), is the **multicultural organization.** This organization incorporates diverse employees into its workforce by recognizing differences and valuing heterogeneity. Diverse employees are fully integrated into the organization, both structurally and informally, resulting in little intergroup conflict. Prejudice and discrimination are minimal, as are gaps in the level of employee commitment among groups.

Adler (1991) offered yet another typology of organizations, based on their recognition of the potential impact, both positive and negative, of cultural diversity. She stated that "the extent to which managers recognize cultural diversity and its potential advantages and disadvantages defines the organization's approach to managing that diversity" (p. 104). According to Adler, the most common organizational approach is to ignore the impact of diversity (i.e., to assume that differences among people are irrelevant). Adler (1991) maintains that managers in such organizations confuse judgment with recognition; she stated:

> Recognition occurs when a manager realizes that people from different cultural groups behave differently and that that difference affects their relationship to the organization. People from one ethnic group are not inherently any better or worse (judgment) than those from another group; they are simply different. To ignore cultural differences is unproductive . . . . Judging cultural differences as good or bad can lead to inappropriate, offensive, racist, sexist, ethnocentric attitudes and behaviors. Recognizing differences does not. Choosing not to see cultural diversity limits our ability to manage it. (p. 97)

Organizations in which managers ignore the potential impact of cultural diversity are labeled "parochial" by Adler (2002). Parochial organizations neither benefit from employee diversity nor resolve problems associated with such differences.

A second type of organization, labeled "ethnocentric" by Adler (2002), assumes that cultural diversity among employees has clear disadvantages, but no advantages. Such organizations seek to minimize the source and impact of cultural diversity by selecting a monocultural workforce and by forcing diverse others to assimilate to the values, attitudes, and behaviors of the predominant group. Obviously, ethnocentric organizations fail to benefit from the diversity that exists among the workforce.

In contrast, the "synergistic" organization, according to Adler (2002), recognizes the potential advantages and problems associated with a culturally diverse workforce. Such organizations, which Adler believes are uncommon, directly address potential problems (e.g., miscommunication, lack of consensus regarding appropriate behaviors) while simultaneously embracing the benefits offered by diversity among its employees (e.g., greater creativity and flexibility).

Summary of Typologies

The various typologies discussed above are summarized and compared in Table 7.1. Basically, organizations might be viewed along a diversity continuum, ranging from passive denial to proactive management of the impact of a diverse workforce. Stage 1 organizations deny the importance of cultural differences, assuming that *equal* treatment for all will naturally prevail and will result in perceived equity and productivity. Morrison's (1992) golden rule organizations and Adler's (2002) parochial organizations adopt this approach.

At Stage 2, organizations acknowledge that differences exist, assume that they are counterproductive, and seek to minimize problems by consciously avoiding diversity in their workforce. Such organizations may avoid diversity through the selection process or through assimilation of the limited number of "others" who do enter the workforce. Morrison's (1992) assimilation, Cox's (1991) monolithic, and Adler's (2002) ethnocentric organizations are at Stage 2 of the diversity continuum.

Stage 3 organizations, like those at Stage 2, acknowledge that differences among people exist and view them as generally dysfunctional. Organizations at this stage, however, actively seek to expand the diversity of the workforce, but only within the boundaries mandated by law. Diversity is seen by such organizations as a necessary evil. Organizations labeled by Morrison (1991) as "righting the wrongs" and by Thomas (1991) as "affirmative action" are representative of this stage.

At Stage 4, organizations recognize that diversity is a way of life and realize that benefits may accrue to the organization if greater understanding and acceptance can be fostered among employees. Thus, educational efforts may be undertaken by such organizations to enhance understanding of cultural differences and to minimize problems related to communication or conflict. Stage 4 organizations, however, still fail to achieve maximum benefit from the diversity of employees because their efforts are directed only toward minimizing problems, not toward developing strengths. Organizations fitting this description are labeled by Morrison (1991) as "culture-specific" and by Thomas (1991) as "valuing cultural differences." Cox's (1991) plural organization combines elements of Stages 3 and 4 (i.e., complying with legal mandates and making some efforts to minimally integrate diverse employees and to lessen dysfunctional effects of diversity).

Stage 5 organizations clearly understand both the problems and the benefits associated with employee diversity. They view the management of a diverse workforce as an ongoing activity that necessitates fundamental changes in the values and assumptions that define the organization's culture. Cultural differences are recognized fully, and efforts are made to develop an organizational culture that supports differences, develops individual strengths, and benefits from the range of experiences, values, and skills offered by its diverse others. Multicultural organizations (Cox, 1991; Morrison, 1992), organizations that manage cultural diversity (Thomas, 1991), and synergistic organizations (Adler, 2002) are organizational types described as operating at Stage 5.

Although these five stages seem to reflect the range of philosophies and actions that might be found in different organizations, it should be noted that the categories are not mutually exclusive.

Morrison (1992), for example, concludes that "perhaps the most promising approach to diversity is one that combines the premises and practices of several of the approaches . . . particularly the goals of the multicultural approach and the affirmative action types of practices in the approach of righting the wrongs" (p. 8). Likewise, Thomas (1991) stated that effective managers cannot rely exclusively on any of the three strategies that he described, but "will want to use all three" (p. 26) to achieve maximum productivity.

As organizations move through the continuum to the latter stages, it is likely that they retain characteristics of earlier stage organizations. Thus, the process might be viewed as cumulative or additive; organizations retain some practices (e.g., affirmative action) while adding new ones (e.g., training and education). As organizations advance toward Stage 5, they do not reject worthwhile policies or practices of the past; rather, they refine beneficial policies, discontinue policies or practices that are detrimental, and extend efforts to include new and innovative approaches to managing employee diversity.

CHARACTERISTICS AND ASSUMPTIONS OF MULTICULTURAL COMPANIES

Loden and Rosener (1991) surveyed 50 organizations, both public and private, that are innovators in managing diverse employees. Their goal was to identify the underlying values or assumptions that are shared by such organizations. Labeled "leading-edge organizations," they were described as "those with a declared commitment to the value of diversity that are actively engaged in a variety of efforts aimed at institutionalizing this philosophy" (p. 160). Loden and Rosener (1991) found three common characteristics among the 50 organizations: (1) support and involvement of top management; (2) operating philosophy of different but equal; and (3) expanded, more flexible definitions of effective performance. Loden and Rosener (1991) stated that within leading-edge institutions, senior-level managers have "become visibly and philosophically identified with efforts to promote a culture of diversity" (p. 161). Senior-level managers serve as critical role models for other employees and act as protagonists in efforts to change underlying cultural values. They also emphasized that managers in leading-edge organizations recognize the distinction between equality and sameness. Because they understand true differences among diverse employees (e.g., communication styles), these managers adapt their styles to accommodate varying needs. Finally, leading-edge organizations tend to be more flexible in their definitions of effective performance. Loden and Rosener (1991) stressed that organizations need not sacrifice performance standards; rather, they recognize that high levels of performance can be attained in different ways. For example, traditional approaches to identifying employees with management potential have tended to be gender-biased (e.g., emphasizing the value of competitive, combative behavior, rather than supportive behavior). Loden and Rosener (1991) stated that performance assessment tools "need to be modified to reflect the diverse communication styles of the multicultural workforce" (p. 164).

Furthermore, Loden and Rosener (1991) delineated three common assumptions among leading-edge organizations. First, such companies assume that employee diversity is a competitive advantage, rather than a disadvantage. They recognize that a culturally diverse workforce can serve as a "means of enhancing their recruitment, marketing, and customer service effectiveness" (Loden & Rosener, 1991, p. 164). Second, leading-edge companies assume that the organization is in transition; they recognize the need for continuous monitoring and alteration of the organization's culture, policies, and practices. Finally, leading-edge companies assume that they must change the organizational culture, rather than the people. They have abandoned the practice of assimilation (i.e., forcing diverse others to "fit" their organization) and have embraced the idea that the organization's culture must change to support a variety of diverse others.

STRATEGIES FOR MANAGING A DIVERSE WORKFORCE

Morrison (1992) reported the results of in-depth interviews of managers in 16 organizations that were considered to be "role models in developing diversity in management" (p. 271). She reported that organizations used many different strategies for dealing with workforce diversity; however, she also observed much overlap in strategies. The seven practices that ranked highest were: (1) top management intervention and influence; (2) targeted recruitment of women and persons of color for entry-level, nonmanagerial jobs; (3) internal advocacy groups; (4) reliance on equal employment opportunity statistics and employee profiles; (5) incorporation of diversity into the performance review process; (6) targeting of women and people of color in the management succession process; and (7) revision of promotion criteria to include diversity goals.

Morrison noted that the 16 organizations in her study engaged in 52 different practices related to diversity, and that a majority of the organizations used numerous different (at least 20) practices as part of their diversity efforts. Further examination of these 52 practices suggested that they comprised three broad categories: (1) accountability practices, (2) development practices, and (3) recruitment practices.

Accountability practices included such things as the use of internal advocacy groups; inclusion of diversity in performance evaluation, promotion decisions, management compensation, and management succession planning; policies against racism or sexism; inclusion of diversity in the mission statement; and internal audits or surveys regarding cultural diversity.

Among those initiatives that were development related were practices such as diversity training programs, formal mentoring programs, support groups, job rotation, career planning, and targeted job assignments for diverse employees. Recruitment practices were also cited, including targeted recruitment of diverse employees for nonmanagerial and/or managerial positions, recruitment incentives for diverse persons, partnerships with nontraditional organizations or groups, and creation of a corporate image of supportiveness for diverse individuals.

Morrison (1992) also provided guidance for organizations considering the implementation of diversity-related strategies. Specifically, she recommended that organizations: (1) match practices to the organization's problems and culture, (2) select practices that provide for sustained leadership development within the organization, (3) choose practices that will reach as many employees as possible, (4) provide the necessary education and training to support each practice and to ensure its successful implementation, and (5) be reasonable— narrow the list of problems and strategies to a few immediate priorities.

Several steps are recommended for organizations to follow if they are interested in developing effective programs for managing cultural diversity. The first step is discovery of problems and issues. Organizations hold rich information related to existing problems; such information may be captured by asking employees about their knowledge, perceptions, or attitudes (e.g., through focus groups or survey instruments) or by utilizing existing personnel data. Both objective and perceptual data are important during the discovery phase.

Second, organizations must strengthen top management's commitment to the process. Top management must recognize that the process represents a long-term effort and must endorse it through words and actions. Third, organizations must choose a balanced strategy. Specific practices should reflect all three overarching strategies (i.e., accountability, development, and recruitment), and they should support both short-term and long-term goals.

Fourth, organizations should identify ways to evaluate the results of their diversity-related efforts to determine whether they are achieving desired goals. If not, they should reexamine both goals and practices. Morrison (1992) stated that "the degree of emphasis that organizations place on results may separate those that succeed in their diversity efforts from the field of hopefuls" (p. 226). Morrison (1992) recommended that organizations "plan beyond the short-term impact of diversity practices" (p. 251). Initial plans should include both short-term and long-term goals; continuous evaluation and revision must take place to ensure that momentum is maintained.

Finally, it is crucial for managers to comprehend the complex relationship that exists between diversity and organizational performance and how this can be moderated by situational context and culture. Diversity can enhance innovation and exploration of new ideas and opportunities. However, diversity often can undermine efforts to implement or execute programs and policies (Mannix & Neale, 2005). To benefit from diversity it is crucial to understand how groups function and to appropriately modulate conditions within the organization (Bachmann, 2006).

SUMMARY

In summary, effective human resources managers must recognize the increasing demographic and cultural diversity in the United States and its workforce, and they must understand the significant challenges that such changes will present to organizations. Human resources managers must assume the responsibility for developing plans and strategies that are designed specifically to help them compete for an increasingly limited pool of knowledgeable and skilled employees. A key element of their success will be the degree to which they understand and appreciate meaningful differences among employees; such understanding must provide the underpinning for human resources policies and practices that will optimize the organization's ability to attract, retain, and utilize fully qualified employees. Finally, effective human resources managers must become familiar with the wide array of strategies available to them in their efforts to manage and benefit from an increasingly diverse workforce. They should evaluate strategies in light of their own organization's goals and culture. They must select strategies with great care and consideration in order to preserve what is valuable within their organization, while simultaneously changing goals or cultural values that are unlikely to be effective in the context of the rapidly emerging, nontraditional workforce.

MANAGERIAL GUIDELINES

1. *Recognize the critical need for diversity-friendly employment policies.* The changing health care work environment reflects the increasingly more diverse cultural profile of the workforce emerging in the United States.

2. *Leverage potential benefits to the organization's benefit.* Managers should understand how diversity is complex and how it should be managed in different contexts and under different conditions. Programs that foster recognition and appreciation of meaningful differences in diverse groups of employees should be implemented and integrated throughout the organization.

3. *Develop a diversity skill set.* Managers should understand and accept the management of diversity. They need to recognize that it is a management component, and should be aware of organizational culture, identity, biases, prejudices, and stereotypes. They should challenge and change policies that prohibit development of diversity.

4. *Tailor HR policies to be more female/family-friendly.* Managers should allow women to balance career and home responsibilities

effectively. They should assist with childcare and institute flexible work options. Doing so may enhance female employee productivity and reduce potential conflict among workgroups. Practices that discriminate against women should be eliminated.

5. *Develop professional opportunities and employment functions for women and people of color.* Managers should promote and educate them, where appropriate, to leadership and higher positions, and commit educational and training resources to segments of minority and immigrant populations in need of such assistance. Training policies should raise cultural awareness and improve cross-cultural communication.

6. *Strike a wise balance between skills, personality, and culturally-based behavior.* Managers need to understand that discrimination can result from cultural incompetence, and should be aware of cultural forces during interviews and employee interaction.

7. *Institutionalize one's diversity philosophy.* Top management must be involved and supportive. Managers should operate under the philosophy of "different but equal," and continuously expand to include flexible definitions of effective performance in performance review processes. Managers should aim to change the organizational culture, not the people.

DISCUSSION QUESTIONS

1. Discuss the management implications of the demographic changes that are occurring in today's workforce.

2. Compare and contrast different organizational typologies for managing a diverse workforce. Address underlying values, assumptions, strategies, policies, and practices.

3. List and discuss practices related to diversity management in the areas of (1) accountability, (2) development, and (3) recruitment.

REFERENCES

Adler, N.J. (2002). *International Dimensions of Organizational Behavior* (4th ed.). Cincinnati: South Western: Thompson Learning.

American College of Healthcare Executives. (2000). *A Comparison of the Career Attainment of Men and Women Healthcare Executives.* Chicago: ACHE.

Aries, N. (2004). Managing diversity: the differing perceptions of managers, line workers, and patients. [Electronic Version]. *Healthcare Management Review, 29*(3): 172–180.

Bachmann, A.S. (2006). Melting pot or tossed salad? Implication for designing effective multicultural workgroups. *Management International Review, 46*: 721–747.

Bell, N.S., & Narz, M. (2007). Meeting the challenges of age diversity in the workplace. [Electronic Version]. *The CPA Journal, 77*(2): 56–60.

D'Aurizio, P. (2007). Onboarding: delivering the promise. [Electronic Version] *Nursing Economics, 25*(4): 228–230.

Dreachslin, J. (2007). Diversity management and cultural competence: research, practice, and the business case. [Electronic Version]. *Journal of Healthcare Management, 52*(2): 79–86.

Fernandez, J.P. (1991). *Managing a Diverse Work Force: Regaining the Competitive Edge.* Lexington, MA: D.C. Heath.

Fyock, C.D. (1990). *America's work Force is Coming of Age.* Lexington, MA: DC Heath.

Higgins, C., Duxbury, L., & Johnson, K.L. (2000). Part-time work for women—does it really help balance work and family. *Human Resource Management, Spring, 39*(1): 17–32, John Wiley and Sons.

Hoffman, L.W. (1989). Effects of maternal employment in the two-parent family. *American Psychologist, 44*: 283–292.

Jamieson, D., & O'Mara, J. (1991). *Managing Workforce 2000: Gaining the Diversity Advantage.* San Francisco: Jossey-Bass.

Lawrence, T. (2005). Why diversity matters. [Electronic Version]. *The Scientist, 19*(21): 20–21.

Lim, C., Winter, R., & Chan, C.(2006). Cross-cultural interviewing in the hiring process: challenges and strategies. [Electronic Version]. *Career Development Quarterly, 54*(3): 265–268.

Loden, M., & Rosener, J.B. (1991). *Workforce America! Managing Employee Diversity as a Vital Resource.* Homewood, IL: Business One Irwin.

Mannix, E., & Neale, M.A. (2005). What differences make a difference? *Psychological Science in the Public Interest, 6*(2): 31–55.

Maxwell, M. (2005). It's not just black and white: how diverse is your workforce? [Electronic Version] *Nursing Economics, 23*(3): 139–140.

Mitra, S. (2000). The capability approach and disability. *Journal of Disability and Policy Studies, Spring, 16*(4): 236–247.

Morrison, A.M. (1992). *The New Leaders: Guidelines on Leadership Diversity in America.* San Francisco: Jossey-Bass.

Offermann, L.R., & Gowing, M.K. (1990). Organizations of the future: Changes and challenges. *American Psychologist, 45*(2): 95–108.

Shin, H.B., and Bruno, R. (2003). *Language Use and English-Speaking Ability: 2000.* Washington, DC: U.S. Census Bureau.

Thiederman, S. (1996). Improving communication in a diverse healthcare environment. [Electronic Version] *Healthcare Financial Management, 50*(11): 72–74.

Thomas, R.R. (1991). *Beyond Race and Gender: Unleashing the Power of Your Total Work Force by Managing Diversity.* New York: AMACOM.

Towers Perrin & Hudson Institute. (1990). *Workforce 2000: Competing in a Seller's Market.* Valhalla, NY: Towers Perrin.

Vallario, C.W. (2006). Creating an environment for global diversity: global diversity in the workplace is not just a human resources issue, but also a business strategy that embraces many elements. [Electronic Version]. *Financial Executive, 22*(3): 50–52.

Warden, G. (1999) Leadership Diversity. *Journal of Healthcare Management, 44*(6): 421–423.

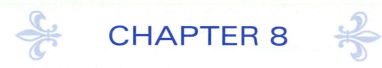

CHAPTER 8

Leadership Development, Succession Planning, and Mentoring

Amy Yarbrough Landry, PhD and Lee W. Bewley, PhD, FACHE

LEARNING OBJECTIVES

Upon completing this chapter, the reader will be able to:

1. Describe the different approaches to developing leaders in organizations.
2. Discuss a model of leadership development and its application in health care organizations.
3. Define succession planning and discuss the two general approaches.
4. Describe the way succession planning is used in health care organizations.
5. Define mentoring.
6. Describe the multi-dimensional aspects of mentoring and how each dimension may be applied in leadership development.
7. Describe different ways that mentoring is used in health care.

KEY TERMS

360-Degree Feedback

Action Learning

Career Sponsoring

Challenging Job Assignment

Classroom Instruction

Coaching

Developmental Relationships

Job Coaching

Leadership

Leadership Development

Mentoring

Personal Development

Skill-Based Training

Succession Planning

Team Training

INTRODUCTION

Strong **leadership** is essential to the strategic management of organizations in any industry. Good leaders facilitate planning and coordination, and they direct employees to behave in a manner that is in the best interests of the organization (Drucker, 2002; Mintzberg, 2004). Most importantly, top level leadership represents an organization's mission, vision, and values. The decisions that leaders make determine the implementation of strategic initiatives that can lead to either the success or failure of the organization (Hambrick & Mason, 1984). Leadership is particularly important in health care organizations, where managerial decisions can directly influence patient outcomes.

Health care organizations are among the most complex entities to manage (Burke & Scalzi, 1988). Typically, they employ a variety of occupational groups, including different levels of clinical and administrative staff. They are subject to rigorous regulatory scrutiny at both the state and federal levels, and often these organizations provide services for which they are either underpaid or not reimbursed. Internal processes among clinical and administrative staff are difficult to coordinate, and the environment in which these organizations operate is uncertain and complicated (Begun & Kaissi, 2004). These complexities surrounding the industry underscore the need for qualified leadership in health care organizations.

Although many organizations have institutionalized **leadership development** activities, including training courses and **succession planning,** health care has not kept pace with businesses in other industries in this regard. Scarce time and resources are one possible reason for the lack of participation in such activities. Health care organizations are constantly under pressure to reduce costs while increasing the quality of care provided. Reallocating resources to leadership development likely does not fit with the priority scheme present in many such organizations. Further complicating the issue,

the competencies and experience required to adequately fill top management roles at such institutions have not been firmly established. Leadership development might not be viewed as a good investment given such ambiguity.

Despite a need for strong leadership, a shortage of qualified health care executives is looming (Dye, 2005; Thrall, 2001). While much attention is given to the deficit of clinical personnel, including registered nurses, the lack of managerial talent in health care has gone largely unnoticed. One possible solution to this dilemma is an increased emphasis on leadership development in health care organizations.

Leadership Development

Although organizational leaders are often employed in formal management positions, the terms "leader" and "manager" are not interchangeable. A topic of much debate, the fundamental difference between leaders and managers is simple. Managers are those individuals who simply control organizational processes, while leaders are those individuals who set an organization's strategic direction (Kotterman, 2006). Leaders may have some management responsibility consistent with their job roles, but their main purpose is to lead the organization in the direction of success. Leading an organization refers to an individual's ability to galvanize resources and motivate employees to work collectively to further organizational goals, which goes beyond simply controlling day-to-day operations (Day, 2001).

With the distinction between leaders and managers clarified, leadership development can be defined as any activity that improves the ability of an individual to lead, including both formal and informal methods (Hernez-Broome & Hughes, 2004). While some overlap exists among the activities of both management and leadership development, the overall spirit of leadership development is the preparation of a leader for unanticipated circumstances and challenges (Day, 2001). A formal leadership development activity is one that is specifically designed to facilitate leadership. For example, if a hospital offers a course on leadership skills to its managers, this is a formal activity. If a leader learns a lesson through the everyday performance of his or her job, this in an informal leadership development activity.

Several different approaches to leadership development exist. The focus might be on the development of an individual leader (Conger & Benjamin, 1999). In such a case, an organization might finance the continuing education of an employee. For example, a health insurance company might pay for a nurse leader to pursue a master's degree. While this additional education will benefit the organization indirectly through the nurse's application of knowledge gained at school, the primary benefit of this type of development goes to the nurse leader. The beneficiary of the education can take this degree with them if they choose to leave the organization. In contrast, activities might focus on developing leaders in a manner that specifically facilitates the fulfillment of the organization's mission, vision, and values (Conger & Benjamin, 1999). This approach involves leadership development activities that are designed to increase a leader's ability to achieve a particular organizational goal. For example, a hospital might desire to improve its patient satisfaction scores, in which case the organization might offer a leadership course that teaches techniques for improving patient satisfaction. The beneficiary of this type of activity would be the hospital.

The tactical approaches to leadership development vary among organizations, but include the following activities: (1) **classroom instruction,** (2) **skill-based training,** (3) **challenging job assignment,** (4) **team training,** (5) **action learning,** (6) **360-degree feedback,** and (7) **developmental relationships** (Bewley, 2005; McAlearney, 2006).

Classroom Instruction

The classroom instruction approach to leadership development typically refers to didactic learning that is either internal or external to the organization. External classroom instruction encompasses both degree-seeking academic programs, such as a Master's in Business Administration or a Master's in Health Administration, or continuing education administered through a third party such as a professional association or foundation. For example, a hospital might choose to send its executive team to a leadership development seminar sponsored by the American College of Healthcare Executives or send its nurse leaders to a program hosted by the American Association of Nurse Executives.

An internal approach to leadership development involves some type of classroom instruction created or hosted by a particular organization for its employees. Organizations in other industries have long practiced this approach to leadership development. For example, General Electric's corporate university at Crotonville has a long history of internally educating future organizational leaders (Grenier, 2002). While internal leadership development programs certainly exist within the health care industry, these organizations have adopted this approach to leadership development at a slower rate than other industries (McAlearney, 2006).

Skill-Based Training

Skill-based training involves initiatives targeted at the development of specific skills required for effective leadership. The competencies required to be an effective health care leader have not been empirically verified, and probably vary depending on the job role of the individual leader. However, studies of hospital CEOs and various other health care executives identify several skill areas that future leaders need to master. Skills in strategy formulation, negotiation, interpersonal, financial management, human resource management, marketing, and information technology are all thought to be useful for future health care leaders (Parsons, et al., 1997; Sievking & Wood 1992; Waldman, et al., 2006). Development activities targeted at these skill areas are the most beneficial for health care organizations. However, these are very broad skill areas, so specific training activities might be difficult to define.

Challenging Job Assignment

Challenging job assignment is an applied method of leadership development that involves assigning challenging jobs consisting of diverse tasks and levels of responsibility and rigor that progress with the individual as leadership is demonstrated (Bass, 1981; Hernez-Broome & Hughes, 2004). For example, a student might enter a managed care organization as an intern. As he or she demonstrates leadership abilities, he or she is reassigned to an entry-level staff position and eventually a managerial role. Based on individual job performance, promotion to more challenging roles occurs. This method of leadership development is widely used in organizations of all types, and it has proven to assist employees in team building, strategic thinking, and interpersonal skills (Day, 2001).

Team Training

Team training is a form of leadership development that occurs when members of a team interact, bringing various experiences, skills, and knowledge to the team processes (Hernez-Broome & Hughes, 2004). Many health care organizations utilize multidisciplinary groups in problem solving, so team training is a frequently used informal method of leadership development. For example, in a nursing home, a committee consisting of a registered nurse, a dietician, a pharmacist, and a physical therapist might be assembled to generate ideas that increase the quality of care in the facility. Through their interaction, all team members may derive skills that will help them develop into effective leaders.

Action Learning

Similar to team training, action learning is a form of leadership development that occurs when groups of employees are assembled to solve a specific problem. This process is thought to promote collaborative leadership through requiring participants to apply familiar problem-solving approaches to unique or unfamiliar contexts (Raelin, 2006). Formal approaches to action learning might involve focused strategic initiatives that are undertaken with the goal of developing leaders while simultaneously solving an organizational problem. For example, an organization might host a planning retreat that involves both administrative and clinical leadership with the goal of creating a strategic plan and developing leadership skills. The advantage of this approach to leadership development is the ability of an organization to conduct business while simultaneously developing leaders (Hernez-Broome & Hughes, 2004). Informally, action learning probably occurs whenever a group or committee meets to solve a problem within an organization.

360-Degree Feedback

One leadership development technique that provides multisource information is 360-degree feedback. The process of 360-degree feedback involves administering a survey about a particular leader's strengths and weaknesses to his or her supervisors, peers, and subordinates. The survey results are then aggregated by a third party and returned to the leader that is the subject of the survey. This allows for a confidential, honest review of leadership ability and identifies areas to target for improvement. The review is also comprehensive, as job performance or perception of performance vary depending on the context (Day, 2001). For example, a manager might receive a positive annual performance review from his or her superiors. However, his or her subordinates might think the manager is performing poorly. The 360-degree feedback technique provides information on positive and negative aspects of individual performance from all vantage points.

While the 360-degree feedback technique is widely employed, it is not used as often in health care organizations as in other industries. One reason for the lack of use in health care may be the absence of an instrument specifically designed for leaders in health care organizations. A secondary reason might include the costliness of performing such an assessment (Garman, Tyler, & Darnall, 2004). The usefulness of the process also varies among individuals. Although the technique provides valuable multisource feedback to a specific individual, research suggests that the way in which the leader in question chooses to use the information determines the usefulness of the process. If a manager or leader chooses to ignore the negative feedback or opportunities for improvement he or she receives from the surveys, no performance improvement or leadership growth will occur (Day, 2001).

Developmental Relationships

Leadership development often occurs in the form of developmental relationships such as **mentoring** and **coaching.** A mentoring relationship involves two individuals: a mentor and a protégé. A mentor is often a more senior executive or member of an organization's staff, while the protégé or student is typically in a more junior position. The crux of the relationship involves the mentor guiding the protégé to success relative to his or her career (Kram, 1983). The relationship can be formal or informal in nature, and the mentor and protégé do not necessarily have to belong to the same organization. Mentoring will be explored more thoroughly later in this chapter.

Coaching (sometimes called executive coaching) refers to the practice of establishing a relationship between two individuals with the hope of developing one individual's career, improving his or her performance, or working through a specific challenge or issue (Day, 2001; Katz & Miller, 1996). Organizations may choose to hire an external consultant to fill the role of coach for a particular employee, or they may select an internal coach, though this occurs less commonly. Although multiple models of coaching exist, the process basically consists of problem definition and individual assessment, development of a plan, and implementation and support of such a plan (Day, 2001; Saporito,

1996). The employment of external consultants in a coaching capacity can be very expensive. Therefore, health care organizations often choose mentoring relationships for leadership development.

A MODEL OF LEADERSHIP DEVELOPMENT

The tactical approaches to leadership development fall into three broad categories that have some overlap: training and education, interpersonal interaction, and job performance. All classroom-based instruction or training, both within the organization and outside the organization, fall into the training and education category. Interpersonal interaction includes all activities that involve communication among people, such as developmental relationships and 360-degree feedback. Activities that are conducted within the scope of an individual's job, such as action learning, challenging job assignments, and team training fall into the job-performance category (Bewley, 2005).

Bewley's graphical depiction of this model (Figure 8.1) demonstrates the overlap that occurs between categories. For example, an individual

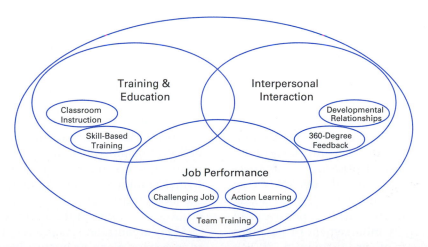

Figure 8.1. A Model of Leadership Development Encompassing Three Broad Clusters of Leadership Development and Seven Tactical Approaches (Bewley, 2005).

involved in a developmental relationship such as mentoring is likely to be assigned a challenging job through his or her mentor. Additionally, a mentor might tap a protégé to participate in a formalized leadership course that falls into the training and education category. Though leadership development activities are distinct enough to fall into separate clusters, the categories are related enough that they probably cannot be considered totally independent.

LEADERSHIP DEVELOPMENT IN HEALTH CARE

Leadership development activities have been treated as a source of competitive advantage in many industries (Day, 2001). The cultivation of human capital within organizations is often viewed to be as important as the development of products or services. However, the utilization of leadership development techniques in health care has lagged behind other industries, and this lag can be attributed to several reasons.

First, numerous interests and projects compete for time and money in health care organizations. The adoption of electronic medical records and other types of information technology have received increased attention in recent years as a way to improve the quality of health care and reduce medical errors. Implementing such systems can be extremely expensive and time consuming for health care organizations (McAlearney, 2006). Secondly, operating margins in health care organizations can be extremely slim, limiting the amount of extra resources such entities have to devote to leadership development activities. Health care organizations are under constant pressure to cut costs while simultaneously increasing the quality of care provided. Unlike organizations in other industries, health care facilities often provide expensive care and receive either no reimbursement or payment that is below the cost of care (Gapenski, 2003). Finally, the organizational structures of health care

organizations are extremely complex. Both clinical and administrative executives have leadership roles in such organizations, and, often, clinical leaders are not direct employees. For example, most physicians serving on the medical staff of a hospital are not directly employed by the organization. Therefore, it makes coordinating leadership development activities extremely difficult. The cultural differences that exist between administrative and clinical leaders also contribute to challenges with regard to leadership development (McAlearney, 2006). For example, a chief medical officer might place a higher priority on competencies related to quality of care, while a chief financial officer might prioritize financial management skills as more important. Designing a program to develop leadership competencies can be extremely difficult if organizational leaders cannot agree on what competencies are of most importance.

Despite these challenges, leadership development is extremely important in health care organizations. Research suggests that these activities are effective in cultivating organizational leaders (Burke & Day, 1986; Collins & Holton, 2004), indicating that leadership development deserves a high prioritization in light of the pending shortage of leadership in health care organizations.

Next, we will discuss a potential solution to the leadership deficit in health care organizations: succession planning.

SUCCESSION PLANNING

Succession planning is one strategy that health care organizations may use in addressing the future deficit of qualified health care leaders. Succession planning refers to any leadership development activities employed by an organization that lead to the identification of a replacement for existent executives in advance of their turnover.

Many organizations take a very narrow approach to succession planning by focusing activities around specific positions, typically limited to those at the executive level, including the chief executive officer (CEO). However, some organizations maximize succession-planning activities to create an internal talent pool. This broad approach involves the training and development of managers and employees at all organizational levels with the goal of enhancing and identifying the skills, attributes, and experiences employees need to fill various positions as they become vacant (Berchelman, 2005).

Selection of an Heir Apparent

The identification of a specific successor or "heir apparent" for a particular position is the activity most often associated with the idea of succession planning. For example, a hospital executive with a plan for retirement might collaborate with the board of directors and the hospital's management team to select an appropriate successor for his or her position. Once this individual is selected, he or she will begin preparing to take on the future role of CEO by participating in different training and leadership development activities. Additionally, the current executive can groom his or her successor for the position through mentoring and other coaching activities. This process can provide time for a successor or new management candidate to prepare to meet future organizational needs in his or her new role. Such training can reduce disruption that might surround a management transition (Harris & Helfat, 1997; Zhang & Rajagopalan, 2004) and make the organization's employees and various stakeholders more comfortable with the new executive.

While this is the most common type of succession planning, the selection of an heir apparent can alienate other leadership talent present in the organization. If the successor for an upper management position is identified in advance, other managers with growth potential might look outside the organization for job opportunities. Additionally, this approach is probably not very effective if the organization seeks a new type of leader to move the organization in a different strategic direction. When a successor for an executive position is identified by sitting executives, the organization risks "executive cloning," or the development of a leader

that is similar to the incumbent leader. Current organizational leadership will likely select a successor that fits well with the current organization, and this type of individual will not be a champion for change (Karaevli & Hall, 2003). Despite these disadvantages to this approach to succession planning, the presence of an heir apparent is beneficial to organizations because it prepares an organization to face the reality of a management turnover event, whether it is planned or unexpected.

Developing a Talent Pool

Some organizations take a broad approach to succession planning. In lieu of identifying one heir apparent for a specific position, these businesses create and develop an internal pool of managerial talent. This form of succession planning produces a group of employees with high potential for management that are prepared to move into a variety of positions as needed.

The identification of key positions is the first step in designing an organization-wide succession-planning initiative. Executives and key stakeholders must decide what leadership roles are pivotal to the organization's functioning and have the potential to cause the most disruption in the event of a resignation or turnover event (Karaevli & Hall, 2002). Continuing our hospital example, the executive leadership team and the board of directors might decide that the chief executive officer, chief nursing officer, and chief financial officer are the positions that most need succession planning. In thinking about those positions, the job roles that prepare management candidates for these key positions also must be considered. Therefore, the director of nursing, director of finance, and director of operations might be included in this initiative.

Once the key positions in an organization are identified, employees with the leadership potential to eventually fill these roles are identified. Tools such as performance appraisals, 360-degree feedback, and competency assessments can indicate the potential leadership ability of employees. Additionally, any interaction between existing leadership and potential future leaders can also indicate aptitude for upper management. The selection of employees for leadership development can occur through either a group or individual process. For example, the hospital used in our example might formally identify high-potential employees for leadership development each year. The executive team might meet once a year and discuss the candidates for the program. However, another approach might involve each executive identifying a certain number of employees with leadership potential in their areas.

After their identification, employees with high potential are notified and leadership development activities begin (Karaevli & Hall, 2002). As mentioned in the previous section of this chapter, different approaches to leadership development exist. Organizations can choose to focus on developing the organization-specific skills and knowledge that employees need to excel or they can focus more on the personal development of the employee. Regardless of the approach, when organizations dedicate resources to developing an internal pool of management talent, succession problems are minimized and leadership transitions are easier.

The creation of a talent pool grants organizations more flexibility in selecting leaders than the identification of an heir apparent. Organizations can place these employees with high leadership potential into transitional roles to further evaluate their abilities to assume an executive-level role. This type of transitional on-the-job training also allows the organization to assess what area of leadership provides the best fit for a particular employee. With a cadre of trained leaders internally available, the organization has several choices when selecting the appropriate candidate for a vacancy in a key position. Depending on the specific needs of the organization and the skills and knowledge necessary to fill a particular role at a particular time, the type of leader desired will vary.

Succession Planning in Health Care

Research suggests that organizations with succession plans in place perform better financially than organizations without such plans (Zajac, 1990).

Despite these findings, many organizations do not plan for management succession (Zhang & Rajagopalan, 2004), and health care organizations are even less likely to plan for succession than companies in other sectors of the economy (Garman, et al., 2004). This failure to plan for leadership succession among health care organizations is disappointing. Aside from the looming shortage of available health care executives, health care organizations exist in a volatile, complex environment (Begun & Kaissi, 2004). Research indicates that organizations that function in highly dynamic industries benefit more from succession planning with regard to performance than businesses in other industries (Zhang & Rajagopalan, 2004).

Health care executives need skills in finance, marketing, negotiating, planning, and information systems (Parsons, et al., 1997, Sieveking & Wood, 1992). While many organizations employ mid-level managers with skills in one of these areas, leadership development and education is often necessary to prepare these individuals to advance to the executive level. Succession planning offers organizations a way of cultivating an internal group of employees that are trained and ready to ascend the ladder to upper management.

MENTORING

The concept of mentoring, a major component of leadership development, is thought to be partially inspired by Homer's ancient epic poem, *The Odyssey*. Ulysses, the central character, entrusts his son, Telemachus, with Mentor while he leaves his homeland to rescue the princess, Helen, from the kingdom of Troy. In Ulysses' absence, Mentor assumes the paternal role of raising Telemachus and preparing him for his future role as the leader (Homer, 1961). Modern academic scholars have generally adopted this character to label the concept of mentoring without necessarily accepting the entire portfolio of responsibilities assumed by Mentor as the definition of mentoring. Clearly, Ulysses valued leadership development as a critical element of succession planning in ancient Ithaca.

Views of mentoring have evolved over the past quarter-century. The traditional perspective of mentoring generally holds that a seasoned senior executive will guide and sponsor a young protégé over the course of his or her career (Kram, 1985; Levinson, et al., 1978). For example, a health care executive might hire an administrative fellow into his or her organization. The fellow would work directly with the executive, completing assigned projects and learning how the organization functions. In this mentoring relationship, the executive would fill the mentor role while the fellow would be the protégé.

Modern views of mentoring incorporate a more refined, dynamic personal-development relationship perspective. This new perspective generally holds that mentoring is a developmental relationship that is mutually maintained by two people for professional, social, or other benefit. Furthermore, this relationship may include peers and may range from an episodic period to a lifelong commitment to development. Finally, a mentoring relationship may exist within the context of a network of multiple mentoring relationships (Higgens & Kram, 2001; Kram, 1985).

The mentor–protégé relationship has evolved with changes occurring in the workplace. Arrangements such as "free agent" employee–employer contracts, dramatic changes in communication technology, organizational structure evolutions, and the ever-increasing diversity of the workplace environment have dictated a reciprocal evolution in the traditional mentor–protégé relationship. Accordingly, developmental networks of multiple mentors with varying relationship strengths and opportunities for mentors and protégés will likely become more prevalent (Higgins & Kram, 2001).

While many definitions of mentoring exist, scholars often describe a mentor as an influential individual that provides counsel, instruction, and support in the development of a person (Levinson, 1978). When such an individual offers psychosocial support and sponsorship, this is an indication that a mentor relationship exists (Kram, 1985). The United States Army defines mentoring as "the proactive development of each subordinate through observing, assessing, coaching, teaching, developmental counseling, and evaluating that results in people being treated with fairness and equal opportunity" (United States Army, 1999). What is common in these and other definitions of mentoring is that no consistent definition exists; however, recurring functions or traits generally emerge in broad definitions that describe a dyadic relationship between someone who is relatively advanced in position, experience, and/or knowledge and another individual who seeks to enhance their standing by association with that person.

Another key aspect of mentoring is the multidimensional form in which it may be applied in leadership development. While there are a number of specific mentoring processes or techniques such as counseling or exposing protégés to higher strata of management decision-making, clearly defined dimensions of mentoring have emerged in research and practice (Bewley, 2005; Dreher & Ash, 1990; Kram, 1986; Steinberg & Foley, 1999; Turban & Dougherty, 1994). These broad areas of mentoring include **personal development, career sponsoring,** and **job coaching.**

Personal Development

Personal development in mentoring is generally achieved by processes associated with positively shaping a protégé's attitude about the context or environment. These mentoring activities are focused on emphasizing values, esprit de corps, and camaraderie in the working environment so that an individual becomes more fully invested or committed to the organization and/or the mentor and associated leaders. Examples of these type of activities include social and family-oriented events or celebrations of individual or group achievement.

Career Sponsoring

Career sponsoring is an aspect of mentoring that focuses on the process of enabling a protégé to pursue or assume advanced levels of responsibility and authority in an organization or in the working environment. The prime function of mentoring in this context is for the mentor to directly or indirectly influence the environment or provide counsel to a protégé so that a position, assignment, or some developmental opportunity is made available to the protégé. For example, an executive who serves as a mentor to a junior manager in a health care organization might advocate for his or her protégé to be hired into a director-level position over other qualified candidates.

Job Coaching

Job coaching is the dimension of mentoring that enhances the ability or competence level of the protégé. Mentors performing job coaching activities will focus on process and content elements of a job or working environment to enhance the ability of a protégé to make a contribution to the firm. Activities such as training, development, observation, practice, and modeling are all aligned with enabling a protégé to be able to perform general work requirements or tasks in a proficient manner.

While each of the dimensions of the mentoring process are clearly interconnected and important to the leadership development of protégés, research indicates that each of these dimensions may have varying levels of importance to protégés depending upon the career-life stage of the protégé. For instance, a young careerist would likely find the job coaching aspect of mentoring most valuable, while a competent mid-careerist would seek career-sponsoring mentoring to facilitate advancement in the organizational hierarchy. Similarly, a seasoned senior executive who is clearly competent and has achieved wide success in attaining higher levels of authority and responsibility would seek personal development from his or her mentor to provide validation to his or her continued contributions in the field (Bewley, 2005).

Mentoring in Health Care

The multidimensional model of mentoring provides a framework for describing how it is utilized

in the health care market. Job coaching, career sponsoring, and personal development are perpetually being utilized as mechanisms for leadership development. These processes of leadership development also provide a substantial basis for organizational processes aligned with near-term and future succession planning. Figure 8.2 provides a graphical depiction of how health care organizations, including health systems, hospitals, group practices, and other firms in the market, utilize mentoring to develop leaders and facilitate succession planning.

Nominating, coordinating, or public recognition for cumulative service in a field or firm such as "life-time achievement" or "emerging star" are often utilized in the health care field as a form of mentoring by providing opportunities for *personal development* to an individual. Similarly, enabling an individual to be recognized as a fellow in an organization or to awarding him or her more senior rank or status—for example, associate professor or chief resident—provide mentoring that strengthens the personal ties and dedication of the individual to the organization and the mentor who is responsible for providing that recognition.

Hiring and promotion or activities associated with shaping the environment leading to an advancement of a protégé in a firm or the field are the most common mechanisms for mentoring via *career sponsoring* in the health care market. References or personal associations provide the most direct mechanism for mentoring to individuals. Hires or promotions can be largely based on the personal recommendations of a mentor, which moderates or eliminates competence and ability unknowns that a potential supervisor or employer may have regarding a protégé relative to other applicants.

The health care field abounds with examples of mentoring in the form of *job coaching.* Graduate medical education, training programs, and first-line service activities constantly operate in the context of on-the-job training, continuous process improvement, and observation learning. Practically every major field of the health care landscape has fellowships, residencies, internships, or technical training relationships where mentors and protégés are

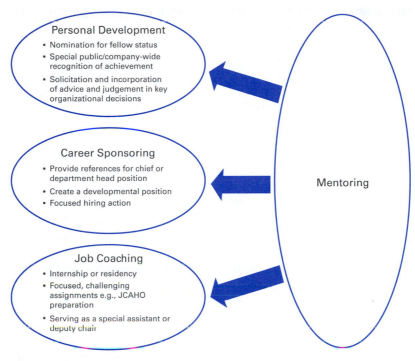

Figure 8.2. A Multidimensional Model of Mentoring Examples in the Health Care Field.

perpetually interacting to facilitate leadership development via enhanced competency levels in job performance.

SUMMARY

The United States Army in the 20th century provides a remarkable example of how organizations may properly integrate mentoring, leadership development, and succession planning into strategic human resource management. General of the Army John J. "Blackjack" Pershing personally selected and developed a precocious, earnest young lieutenant colonel during World War I who later became chief of staff of the army during World War II and who is credited with the leadership development and mentoring of no less than one hundred general officers, including general of the army and future president, Dwight D. Eisenhower. General George C. Marshall served as the capstone of a leadership development cycle between multiple organizational periods spanning Pershing and Eisenhower that achieved victory in two world-wide conflicts and ensured a positive, seamless transition of Army leadership.

Modern health care organizations are not required to win wars nor maintain national security, but the battles that exist in the market for health services require quality leadership and management at the most senior levels in order to ensure that respective organizations do not become casualties of the marketplace. Leadership development processes that incorporate multidimensional mentoring can enhance the human resource stock of an organization and contribute to succession planning for senior organizational positions.

MANAGERIAL GUIDELINES

1. *Dedicate resources to leadership development.* Developing leaders is a good investment. Organizations that use leadership development tools such as mentoring and succession planning outperform their counterparts who do not make the investment. It is worth the time and money to implement a leadership development program in your organization.

2. *Choose an approach to leadership development that is appropriate for your organization.* The resources (both financial and human) available in your organization for leadership development might be scarce or ample. If you have scarce resources, using external resources to develop individuals might be the best approach to leadership development. In contrast, if you have ample resources, developing a leadership development program that is tailored to your organizational strategy might be beneficial.

3. *Consider developing a talent pool.* Selecting and developing a pool of employees with high leadership potential is a proactive approach to planning for leadership succession events. Not only will your organization be prepared for leadership turnover events, the employees selected will become more invested in your organization's future.

4. *Facilitate mentoring in your organization.* No better way of developing leaders exists than mentoring. Encourage senior level leaders to take on more junior employees and guide them as they navigate their careers. This will not only benefit the employees (both mentor and protégé) but it will also benefit your organization by helping retain leadership talent.

DISCUSSION QUESTIONS

1. What are the prime goals of leadership development?
2. How might a health care organization organize a leadership development program?
3. Who should lead succession-planning processes?
4. How can effective mentoring, succession planning, and successful current operations be simultaneously achieved?
5. What are some successful examples in contemporary management and health administration of mentoring? succession planning? leadership development?

CASE

The board of directors of Breckinridge Community Hospital (BCH), a large, acute-care hospital with extensive community outreach services including primary care, rehabilitation, and long-term care has been facing a recurring problem in retaining hospital leadership. This problem is present most notably at the chief executive officer (CEO) position, but also at mid and lower levels of health care management. BCH is located in a rural southern county near a military base and more than 50 miles from a major metropolitan area; consequently, it is the prime source of health care for most patients in the area. While the quality and cost of living in the area is very competitive, the hospital has experienced significant turnover in all levels of management, despite offering compensation consistent with health care facilities within the state and region. Management turnover is beginning to significantly decrement operational outcomes within the hospital. The prime reason that health care managers cite as to why they left BCH is that there is no plan or promise for management development or upward progression within the facility. Currently, the hospital is operating with a temporary CEO provided by a staffing agency, but it is seeking to find an executive that can develop and implement a plan to solve the systematic health care management problem at BCH.

CASE DISCUSSION QUESTIONS

1. What should the Board expect to hear as a sound plan for addressing the problems at BCH?

REFERENCES

Begun, J.W., & Kaissi, A. (2004). Definition and scope of health services administration. *Journal of Health Administration Education, 21*(2): 227–239.

Berchelman, D.K. (2005). Succession planning. *The Journal for Quality and Participation, 28*(3): 11–12.

Bewley, L. (2005). Seasons of Leadership Development: An Analysis of a Multi-Dimensional Model of Mentoring Among Career Groups of United States Army Officers. Doctoral dissertation, University of Alabama at Birmingham: Alabama.

Burke, M., & Day, R. (1981). *Stodgill's Handbook of Leadership: A Survey of Theory and Research.* New York: The Free Press.

Burke, C., & Scalzi, C. (1988). Role stress in hospital executives and nursing executives. *Healthcare Management Review, 13*(3): 67–72.

Collins, D., & Holton, E. (2004). The effectiveness of managerial leadership development programs: A meta-analysis of studies from 1982–2001. *Human Resources Development Quarterly, 15*(2): 217–248.

Conger, J., & Benjamin, B. (1999). *Building Leaders: How Successful Companies Develop the Next Generation.* San Francisco: Jossey-Bass.

Day, D. (2001). Leadership development: A review in context. *Leadership Quarterly, 11*(4): 581–613.

Dreher, G., & Ash, R. (1990). A comparative study of mentoring among men and women in managerial, professional, and technical positions. *Journal of Applied Psychology, 75*(5): 539–546.

Drucker, P. (2002). *Managing the Next Society.* New York: St. Martin's Press.

Dye, C. (2005). Is Anyone Next in Line? *Healthcare Financial Management, 59*(2): 64–67.

Garman, A., Tyler, L., & Darnall, J. (2004). Development and validation of a 360-degree-feedback instrument for healthcare administrators. *Journal of Healthcare Management, 49*(5): 309–322.

Gapenski, L. (2003). *Understanding Healthcare Financial Management: Fourth Edition.* Chicago: Health Administration Press.

Grenier, L. (2002). Steve Kerr and his years with Jack Welch at GE. *Journal of Management, 11*(4): 343–350.

Hambrick, D., & Mason, P. (1984). Upper Echelons: The Organization as a Reflection of Its Top Managers. *Academy of Management Review, Vol. 9*(2): 193–206.

Harris, D., & Helfat, C. (1998). CEO duality, succession, capabilities and agency theory: Commentary and research agenda. *Strategic Management Journal, 19*(9): 901–904.

Haworth, M. (2005). Tips for better succession planning. *The Journal for Quality and Participation, 28*(3): 13.

Hernez-Broome, G., & Hughes, R. (2004). Leadership development: Past, present, and future. *Human Resource Planning, 27*(1): 24–32.

Higgens, M., & Kram, K. (2001). Reconceptualizing mentoring at work: A developmental network perspective. *Academy of Management Review, 26*(2): 264–289.

Homer. (1961). *The Iliad.* Translated by T. Murray. Cambridge, MA: Harvard University Press.

Karaevli, A., & Hall, D.T. (2003). Growing leaders for turbulent times: Is succession planning up to the challenge? *Organizational Dynamics, 32*(1): 62–79.

Katz, J., & Miller, F. (1996). Coaching leaders through culture change. *Consulting Psychology Journal: Practice and Research, 48*: 104–114.

Kotterman, J. (2006). Leadership versus management: What's the difference? *The Journal for Quality and Participation, 29*(2): 13–17.

Kram, K. (1983). Phases of the mentor relationship. *Academy of Management Journal, 26*(4): 608–625.

Kram, K., & Isabella, L. (1985). Mentoring alternatives: The role of peer relationships in career development. *The Academy of Management Journal, 26*(1): 110–132.

Kram, K. (1985). *Mentoring at Work: Developmental Relationships in Organizational Life*. Glenview, IL: Scott, Foresman, and Company.

Kram, K., & Hall, D. (1996). Mentoring in a context of diversity and turbulence. In Kossek & Lobel (eds.), *Management Diversity: Human Resource Strategies for Transforming Organizations* (pp. 108–136). Oxford: Blackwell Publishers.

Levinson, D., Darrow, C., Klein, E., Levinson, M., & McKee, B. (1978). *Seasons of a Man's Life*. New York: Knopf.

Levinson, D. (1986). A conception of adult development. *American Psychologist, 41*(1): 3–13.

McAlearney, A. (2006). Leadership development in healthcare: A qualitative study. *Journal of Organizational Behavior, 27:* 967–982.

Mintzberg, H. (2004). *Managers Not MBAs: A Hard Look at the Soft Practice of Managing and Management Development*. San Francisco: Berret-Koehler.

Parsons, R.J.., Gustafson, G., Murray, B.P., Dwore, R.B., Smith, P.M., & L.H. Vorderer. (1997). Hospital administrators' career paths: Which way to the top? *Health Care Management Review, 22*(4): 82–96.

Raelin, J. (2006). Does action learning promote collaborative leadership? *Academy of Management Learning & Education, 5*(2): 152–168.

Saporito, P. (1996). Business-linked executive development: Coaching senior executives. *Consulting Psychology Journal: Practice and Research, 48:* 96–103.

Sieveking, N., & Wood, D. (1992). Hospital CEOs view their careers: Implications for selection, training, and placement. *Health Care Management Review, 37*(2): 167–179.

Steinberg, A., & Foley, D. (1999). Mentoring in the army: From buzzword to practice. *Military Psychology, 11*(4): 365–379.

Thrall, T. (2001). A leadership vacuum. *Hospitals and Health Networks, 75*(9): 44–47.

Turban, D., & Dougherty, T. (1994). Role of protégé personality in receipt of mentoring and career success. *The Academy of Management Journal, 37*(3): 688–702.

United States Army. (1999). *FM 22-100: Army Leadership*. New York: McGraw-Hill.

Waldman, J.D., Smith, H., Hood, J., & Pappelbaum, S. (2006). Healthcare CEOs and physicians: Reaching common ground. *Journal of Healthcare Management, 51*(3): 171–184.

Zajac, E. (1990). CEO Selection, Succession, Compensation and Firm Performance: A Theoretical Integration and Empirical Analysis. *Strategic Management Journal, 11:* 217–230.

Zhang, Y., & Rajagopalan, N. (2004). When the Known Devil Is Better than an Unknown God: An Empirical Study of the Antecedents and Consequences of Relay CEO Successions. *Academy of Management Journal, 47*(4): 483–500.

THREE

Human Resources Processes

CHAPTER 9

Job Analysis

Barbara A. Wech, PhD and Anantachai Panjamapirom, MS, MBA

LEARNING OBJECTIVES

Upon completing this chapter, the reader will be able to:

1. Determine the benefits of job analysis on all human resource activities.
2. Identify the classifications of job analysis methods.
3. Identify the steps in conducting a job analysis.
4. Discuss the necessities of job analysis in relation to the qualification requirements specified by major health care accrediting entities.
5. Address the significance of job analysis in the changing health care environment and its impacts on health care organizations.
6. Identify the legal aspects of job analysis.

KEY TERMS

Accreditation

Cognitive Task Analysis (CTA)

Critical Incident Technique

Functional Job Analysis

Job Analysis

Job Specification

Position Analysis Questionnaire (PAQ)

Protected Groups

Time-and-Motion Studies

Work-Oriented Methods

Worker-Oriented Methods

INTRODUCTION

A crucial foundation of strategic human resources management is **job analysis.** Job analysis is the process by which we systematically and thoroughly describe jobs in an organization. These descriptions include identifying and evaluating the job tasks, responsibilities, and the context or environment associated with a particular job. Job analysis

> may be viewed as the hub of virtually all human resources administration and management activities necessary for the functioning of organizations. Hardly a program of interest to human resource specialists and other practitioners whose work pertains to organizational personnel does not depend on or cannot benefit from job analysis results. (Gael, 1988, p. xv)

Information obtained from a job analysis impacts all human resource activities including, but not limited to, planning, recruiting, selection, performance appraisal, training, and compensation. The resulting job description is important to human resources planning in deciding what jobs and employee skills will be needed in the future. In recruiting and selection, job analysis information can be used to find the best qualified applicants and communicate with them the job expectations. In identifying the specifications of the job, job analysis is an integral part of the performance appraisal process aiding the organization and the employee in understanding the performance standards and facilitating the comparison of actual performance to the standards. Training is guided by the job analysis in identifying the knowledge, skills, and abilities necessary to successfully perform a job. In the area of compensation, job analysis provides invaluable information about all the jobs in an organization, making it possible to determine each job's worth to the company through assessing the skills, knowledge, responsibilities, and the work environment.

In addition to its role in all aspects of human resources management, the court system has also contributed to the importance of job analysis. Two major court cases have lead to job analysis being critical in discrimination cases. In *Griggs v. Duke Power Company* (1971) the Supreme Court noted that a selection device should measure the person for the job, not the person in the abstract. It focused attention on the importance of conducting an analysis of a job for which a selection procedure has been developed. A few years later, the Supreme Court reinforced the idea that selection tests should be designed with supporting job analysis data (*Albemarle v. Moody*, 1975).

In this chapter, we discuss job analysis methods and the steps used to conduct a job analysis, including the outcomes produced that are of crucial use in other aspects of human resources. We also highlight the legal importance of job analysis to organizations and the role job analysis plays in the health care industry with respect to **accreditation.**

JOB ANALYSIS METHODS

The methods of job analysis available can be classified as work oriented or worker oriented (Brannick, Levine, & Morgeson, 2007). **Work-oriented methods** focus attention on tasks the worker performs, machines used, and the job context. As its name implies, worker-oriented approaches identify what the person needs to successfully perform the job, such as the knowledge, skills, abilities, licensure requirements, and so on. Some of the more common methods are highlighted below.

Work-Oriented Methods

Time-and-Motion Studies

Time-and-motion studies are aimed at making jobs more efficient. Time studies focus on the time it takes to complete various job aspects, while motion studies examine the sequence of steps performed to complete a job. The health care industry has used time-and-motion studies in a variety of jobs to make job functioning more effective and efficient.

Functional Job Analysis

A **functional job analysis** is oriented toward what gets accomplished in a particular job. It currently uses seven scales to describe what workers deal with in their jobs: (1) things, (2) data, (3) people, (4) worker instructions, (5) reasoning, (6) math, and (7) language. Each of the seven scales has several levels, using behavioral statements and illustrative tasks as anchors to assist job analysts in their role.

Critical Incident Technique

Critical incident technique identifies behaviors that differentiate good job performers from poor ones. The job analyst interviews incumbents and/or other job experts to compile the critical behavioral incidents. Incidents are examined by determining what led to the employee's behavior, the behavior itself, and the consequences of the employee's actions. This information provides future job holders with thorough details about critical job behaviors.

Worker-Oriented Methods

Position Analysis Questionnaire

The **Position Analysis Questionnaire (PAQ)** is a 300-item questionnaire that consists of worker-oriented items focused on generalized job activities (e.g., analyzing data or information). It looks at the extent to which certain tasks are involved in the performance of the analyzed job.

Cognitive Task Analysis

Cognitive task analysis (CTA) is the most recently developed method and was created out of the recognition that when jobs involve tasks that are complex, assessing behavior will not be sufficient. CTA focuses on the mental processes that lead to

behaviors. The technique describes the cognitive processes and skills necessary to perform a job.

JOB ANALYSIS PROCESS

Conducting a job analysis involves several steps. While the exact steps may differ somewhat from organization to organization, the following is a general guide (Bratton & Gold, 2000): (1) Familiarize yourself with the organization and the type of work performed within it; (2) Identify the jobs to be analyzed; (3) Collect pertinent job information; (4) Write job description; (5) Detail the **job specifications;** (6) Identify the performance standard.

Be Familiar with the Organization and Its Jobs

Jobs are impacted by the strategy and direction of the organization, as well as the industry it is in. The health care industry has confronted various significant changes, such as more rigid regulations, increasing demand, and decreasing supply. Therefore, it is important to recognize the current and future needs within the organization in relation to these environmental changes, so that it can effectively conduct job analyses that will benefit the current circumstances as well as its future goals and objectives.

Identify the Jobs to Be Analyzed

Job identification entails ascertaining the jobs to be analyzed. This identification can be accomplished through examining previous job analyses, interviewing upper management about the strategic objectives of the organization and trends in the health care industry, and having discussions with employees and lower level managers. Also, organization charts can be helpful in identifying jobs currently in the organization or jobs that have been in place in the past.

Collect Pertinent Job Information

The most common method is through the use of a questionnaire. Questionnaires can be completed either using paper and pencil or via the Internet using a survey-generating Web site. The questionnaire is developed in such a way as to gather information about a specific job's tasks, duties, responsibilities, required abilities of the employee who fills the job, and performance standards associated with the job. The advantages associated with using a questionnaire include employee involvement and input. The questionnaire allows input from a large number of people for the inputs to be gathered fairly quickly. Moreover, from a cost standpoint, it is more reasonable than other methods. However, the information gathered is only as good as the questions asked and as accurate as the employees can recall or want the analyst to know.

There are other ways to collect job analysis information. Employees can write job diaries detailing the tasks and activities associated with their job. The job analyst can conduct face-to-face interviews with job incumbents. This may be the best way to collect information because it allows for two-way communication in order to gain as much useful information as possible; however, it is very time consuming. Job analysts can also conduct direct observations, noting for themselves the duties and activities associated with a particular job. A job analyst may identify and document duties that the job incumbent views as unimportant and consequently would not have noted in his or her job analysis. This is also a very time-consuming method. For many jobs, prior information is usually available and should be used, such as previous job descriptions, policies and procedures related to the job being analyzed, training manuals and other documents, and performance appraisals. Information on jobs can also be obtained from other employers and/or professional and trade organizations. In addition, the U.S. Department of Labor's O*NET is a free and useful source of occupational information available at www.onetcenter.org. The O*NET database contains updated information on hundreds of occupations using job-oriented, worker-oriented, and occupation-oriented data. The Department of Labor also allows the free use of its job analysis method.

There are many sources of job information available other than the incumbent employee and job analyst. Supervisors and managers are another excellent source of job information. Experts who have recent knowledge of the job being analyzed can provide useful additional job information. Experts can include such people as previous job holders, customers, and consultants.

Discrepancies in viewpoint between individuals that provide job information are not unusual. Managers may not be close enough to a job to know all that it encompasses, for example. You can call a meeting of those who provided data and discuss the job details. Failure to support the results of a job analysis is often a result of lack of commitment. Thus, everyone on the team should come to agreement and sign off on the job analysis, so that there is commitment to it.

Write a Job Description

Once the information for the job analysis is compiled, a job description summarizes the results in a document that is useful to human resources and management. Appendix 9.1 is an example of a job description for a registered nurse at St. Vincent's Hospital in Birmingham, Alabama. It is a very thorough description that includes qualifications, work environment description, physical demands, and detailed job duties. The developmental inventory includes other important and expected activities that accompany the registered nurse job. It is important to verify the job description with those involved in the job analysis process to ensure that the information is complete and accurate.

Detail the Job Specifications

Another important outcome of the job analysis is a job specification. A job specification focuses on the human attributes identified as important to the successful performance of the job. These characteristics can include such factors as knowledge, skills, abilities, license requirements, physical and mental demands, and experiences. Depending on the organization, job specifications can be a separate document from the job description or part of it. As can be seen in Appendix 9.1, job specifications are included in this job description example.

Identify the Performance Standard

Lastly, job analysis can identify the performance standard for a given job. The performance standard is the minimum acceptable level of performance. As can be seen in Appendix 9.1, the performance standard is noted, starting with the key result areas (KRA) description. It is made clear to the employee performing the job and the individual assessing performance what is expected.

JOB ANALYSIS AND THE HEALTH CARE INDUSTRY

There are specific issues in health care that are related directly and indirectly to job analysis. In particular, we will address job analysis and its relation to various accreditation requirements and future health care industry trends.

Accreditation

There are numerous accrediting bodies in health care. The principal accrediting body is the Joint Commission (JC). It accredits approximately 15,000 health care organizations and programs in the United States. The JC has numerous standards that impact the human resources function. In particular, health care organizations should provide an adequate number and mix of employees and have a competent staff whose qualifications are consistent with their responsibilities. The organization should provide an orientation

program that provides initial job training and information. All employees should be capable of describing or demonstrating their safety roles and responsibilities in terms of their job duties or responsibilities. The organization is responsible for providing continuous education and training to its employees. Furthermore, it should assess, maintain, and improve the competence of its employees and perform performance evaluations. Each of these activities is crucially and directly tied to job analysis. A job analysis provides all the information necessary for an organization to meet the JC accrediting requirements.

The Healthcare Quality Association on Accreditation (HQAA) accredits organizations in the durable medical equipment industry. A portion of their accrediting requirements focuses on the human resources function. They require their suppliers to specify the qualifications, training, experience, and continuing education requirements of their employees. Their technical staff must be able to deliver and set up equipment and items as well as train customers in the operation of the equipment. Professional employees are required to be appropriately licensed, certified, or registered and to perform consistently within those requirements. Again, job analysis is crucial in establishing the job qualifications, education, and licensing required for each position.

The Accreditation Commission for Health Care, Inc. (ACHC), the first health care accrediting organization to achieve ISO 9001: 2000 certification, accredits health care organizations in the following areas: Specialty Pharmacy, Women's Post-Breast Surgery Fitter Services, Respiratory Nebulizer Medication Programs, Medical Supply Provider Services, and Rehabilitation Technology Supplier Services. To become accredited by ACHC, firms must have job descriptions for each position, have an orientation plan, assess the competency of their staff, and provide a continuing education plan for all staff. Importantly, all employees needing licenses or certification must have and maintain such. Similar to the accreditation requirements above, job analysis is a critical foundation in the accreditation requirements of ACHC.

Lastly, the Magnet Recognition Program, developed by the American Nurses Credentialing Center, grants Magnet status to health care organizations providing nursing excellence. In relation to job analysis, Standard VIII covers performance appraisal. The standard has a number of requirements, including regular scheduled performance appraisals that comprise an assessment of strengths and development needs and a focus in assisting the achievement of goals. As already noted in the introduction, job analysis is a key component of the performance appraisal process, providing the information, usually in the form of a job description, that allows for performance to be assessed according to the requirements of the position and creates information crucial to goal formation.

Future Trends

There are a few health care industry forecasts that will directly impact job analysis. As in other industries, technology is ever- and quickly changing in health care. Such technology makes new procedures and treatments possible (Bureau of Labor Statistics, 2005). These new treatments and procedures provide a solution that meets medical needs for a number of patients, which leads to an increasing survival rate and the rising life expectancy of the nation as a whole (National Center for Health Statistics, 2006). In order to safely and effectively utilize this innovative technology, employees are required to have and develop skills to perform the tasks. This changing technology must be anticipated by health care administrators, and job analysis plays a critical role in identifying skills and knowledge requirements for a myriad of health care employees.

There is a growing consensus that over the next 15 years, the United States will experience a shortage of physicians because demand will exceed supply (U.S. Department of Health and Social Services, 2006). In particular, projections are that an imbalance in demand and supply will be especially noticeable in specialties that serve the geriatric population. We will see the average age of the U.S. population to continue increasing through 2020 (He, et al., 2005). This demographic change will be driven by the aging of the "baby boomers." By 2020, most baby boomers will have reached 65 years of age, and we will see a large portion of the U.S. population at age 55 and older. This population change will have a strategic impact on the health care industry. Clearly, as we age, we have higher needs of health care. As a result, job analysis will play a large role in identifying the changing skill and knowledge needs among health care professionals of the future.

We will see a similar trend in the supply of nurses. The shortage of nurses is expected to continue as baby boomer nurses retire, leaving many open nursing positions. With the demand for quality health care increasing by an aging population demanding more health care services, the nursing shortage will be an important strategic human resource issue in the health care industry. Job analysis will play a role similar to that noted above in the physician shortage.

Given the changing nature of the health care industry, the idea of strategic job analysis surely will become a major focus as health care organizations try to strategically anticipate and plan for future needs. Strategic job analysis is the identification and specification of future job tasks and responsibilities and the knowledge, skills, and abilities needed to perform those jobs that currently do not exist but that are anticipated to be needed in order to address future organizational needs (Schneider & Konz, 1989). Important to this analysis is the anticipation of the future changes in terms of laws and regulations, employee demographics, profession shortages, technology, information technology, and other possible changes. Experts in these various areas will play a vital role in proactively anticipating changes so that the health care organization can plan accordingly. Knowing which jobs and their associated tasks will be needed in the future, along with identifying the knowledge, skills, abilities, and other requirements needed to perform such jobs, will be a potential advantage for health care organizations desiring to effectively compete into the future.

JOB ANALYSIS AND THE LEGAL ENVIRONMENT

The legal system does not require organizations to conduct job analyses. However, conducting thorough job analyses increases the likelihood that employment decisions are based on job-related criteria, resulting in a reduction in the organization's exposure to employment-related lawsuits.

Job analysis can assist organizations in avoiding lawsuits in connection with several laws. The Fair Labor Standards Act (FLSA) (1938) delineates the difference between exempt and nonexempt employees; essentially, nonexempt employees must be paid overtime for work performed outside of usual work hours. Job analysis provides indispensable information that is used in the determination of which jobs are classified in each particular category. The Civil Rights Act of 1964 made it illegal to discriminate in employment practices based on race, color, sex, religion, or national origin. So, if an employment practice disproportionately and negatively affects any of these **protected groups,** it is discrimination unless it is job related. As a result, job analysis is a large factor in determining the job relatedness of various employment requirements. Moreover, the Equal Pay Act of 1963 states that men and women must be paid equally for the same job. Job descriptions are crucial to demonstrate the existence of substantive differences between jobs.

The Americans with Disabilities Act (1990) prohibits discrimination against those with disabilities. In terms of employment, a person with a disability is someone who is qualified for the job and who, with or without a reasonable accommodation, can perform the essential functions of the job. Job analysis is a critical technique used to define the essential functions of a job and in defining a reasonable accommodation.

The Equal Employment Opportunity Commission (EEOC) and the Office of Federal Contract Compliance Programs (OFCCP) are responsible for the enforcement of equal employment opportunity laws in the U.S. In 1978, the EEOC published the Uniform Guidelines on Employee Selection Procedure. It states that a thorough job analysis is a necessary support for a selection procedure. A selection procedure should be validated and the validation process includes a job analysis. It also notes that:

> There should be a job analysis, which includes an analysis of the important work behavior(s) required for successful performance and their relative importance, if the behavior results in work product(s), and an analysis of the work product(s). Any job analysis should focus on the work behavior(s) and the tasks associated with them. If work behavior(s) are not observable, the job analysis should identify and analyze those aspects of the behavior(s) that can be observed and the observed work products. The work behavior(s) selected for measurement should be critical work behavior(s) and/or important work behavior(s) constituting most of the job. (Equal Opportunity Employment Commission, 1978)

SUMMARY

Job analysis is the systematic process through which job descriptions, job specifications, and performance standards are produced. Job descriptions identify task requirements, responsibilities, qualifications, and physical work environment, whereas job specifications explicitly state the individual attributes required to achieve the tasks. These results from the analysis lay a foundation for all human resources management activities.

Even though various methods are available for conducting a job analysis, these methods are classified into two major categories: work-oriented and worker-oriented. Work-oriented techniques encompass different components related to the job context, including the tasks, sequence of steps toward completing the tasks, and machines or tools used in the operation. Some of the common work-oriented methods are time-and-motion studies, functional job analysis, and critical incident technique. Conversely, worker-oriented methods focus on individual specifications and qualifications needed to accomplish the tasks. These attributes may include, but are not limited to, knowledge, skills, abilities, licensure requirements, and experiences. Some of the worker-oriented approaches are position analysis questionnaires and cognitive task analysis.

A general guideline for conducting a job analysis provides six steps: (1) Familiarize yourself with the organization and the type of work performed within it; (2) Identify the jobs to be analyzed; (3) Collect pertinent job information; (4) Write a job description; (5) Detail the job specifications; (6) Identify the performance standard. These steps are not concrete and may vary from one organization to another according to their suitability to the job, their characteristics and requirements, and the environment.

In the process of conducting a job analysis, the top management team, middle- and lower-level managers, and job analysts must take into consideration the rapidly changing health care environment. Health care organizations are confronting multiple critical environmental factors such as conditions imposed by accrediting entities, laws and regulations, medical services demand, and predicted shortages of health care professional supply. The job analysis team must account for these factors because they can pose a significant threat to the organization. In essence, the systematic approach of job analysis can play a major role in preventing the negative impacts of these threats on and in creating a strategic and sustainable competitive advantage for the organization.

MANAGERIAL GUIDELINES

1. A health care organization and its executives should conduct a job analysis because it helps summarize the human resource needs, provides a guideline for obtaining those needs through a recruitment process, and builds a basic foundation for other activities of human resource management.

2. The methods and processes used to conduct a job analysis are not rigid. Health care executives and the job analysis team must apply the ones that are most appropriate to their needs, circumstances, and the environment.

3. Job analysis can prevent an organization from running into legal problems. An organization is less vulnerable to legal aspects related to human resource functions such as employee selection and recruitment if job analysis is used.

4. As the health care industry is rapidly changing, job analysis should be performed on a regular basis so that an organization is able to effectively respond to the changes as part of the organization's overall strategic plan.

DISCUSSION QUESTIONS

1. What role does a trend in health care professional supply play in the process of job analysis?
2. Define the major types of job analysis methods and their specific approaches.
3. How can you apply job analysis methods to your organization? What kind of human resource programs can benefit from these methods?
4. What kind of environmental information would you need when performing a job analysis? How does this information affect the job analysis and its results?

CASE

You work as an administrator in a small sports medicine practice (five physicians and 30 other staff members). Two physicians, who are the owners, have discussed expanding the practice. They are planning to hire three new physicians. As you walked in through the door this morning, the two physicians asked you to meet with them. They told you their idea and asked you what needs to be done in terms of hiring new physicians. As you walked out of the meeting, you realized that increasing the number of physicians would mean a concurrent increase in the demand for nurses and other administrative staff. The owners have requested to see your recruitment plan in two months. Even though it is very challenging, you know that job analysis can be a useful tool for this project.

CASE DISCUSSION QUESTION

1. Write down the steps you will take and the relevant components you will need to perform the job analyses and describe how this will fit into your recruitment plan.

REFERENCES

Albemarle Paper Co. V. Moody, 422 U.S. 405 (Supreme Court of the United States, 1975).

Brannick, M.T., Levine, E.L., & Morgeson, F.P. (2007). *Job and Work Analysis: Methods, Research, and Applications for Human Resource Management.* Los Angeles: SAGE Publications.

Bratton, J., & Gold, J. (2000). *Human Resource Management: Theory and Practice.* Mahwah, N.J.: Lawrence Erlbaum Associates, Inc.

Bureau of Labor Statistics. (2005). Career guide to industries, 2006-07 edition, health care. Washington, D.C. Retrieved September 15, 2007, from http://www.bls.gov.

Equal Employment Opportunity Commission. (1978). Uniform guidelines on employee selection procedures. 41 CFR 60-3.14 - Technical standards for validity studies. Retrieved October 1, 2007, from http://www.dol.gov.

Gael, S. (1988). *The Job Analysis Handbook for Business, Industry, and Government* (p. xv). New York: Wiley.

Griggs, et al. v. Duke Power Co., 401 U.S. 424 (Supreme Court of the United States, 1971).

He, W., Sengupta, M., Velkoff, V.A., & DeBarros, K.A. (2006). 65+ in the United States: 2005. U.S. Census Bureau – Current Population Reports: Special Reports. Washington, DC. Retrieved October 13, 2007, from http://www.census.gov.

McDonald, J.S., & Dzwonczyk, R. (1988). A time and motion study of the anaesthetist's intraoperative time. *British Journal of Anaesthesia, 61:* 738–742.

National Center for Health Statistics. (2006). *Health, United States, 2006 with Chartbook on Trends in the Health of Americans* (p.61, 76–641496). Washington, DC: U.S. Government Printing Office.

Robert Wood Johnson Foundation. (2007). Engaging nurses in quality improvement. Princeton, N.J. Retrieved August 10, 2007, from http://www.rwjf.org.

Schneider, B., & Konz, A.M. (1989). Strategic job analysis. *Human Resource Management, 28:* 51–63.

Shortell, S.M., & Kaluzny, A.D. (2000). *Health Care Management: Organization, Design, and Behavior* (4th ed.). United States: Delmar Thomson Learning.

U.S. Department of Health and Social Services. (2006). *Physician supply and demand: Projections to 2020.* Washington, D.C.: Lewin Group report prepared for the Bureau of Health Professions, Health Resources and Services Administration. Retrieved September 15, 2007, from http://bhpr.hrsa.gov.

World Health Organization. (1999). *Functional Job Analysis: Guidelines for Task Analysis and Job Design.* San Antonio, Texas: Frank I. Moore. Retrieved September 17, 2007, from http://www.who.int.

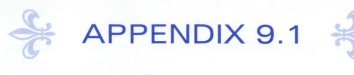

APPENDIX 9.1

RN Description

Department: 6 WEST
Position Number: 14250
FLSA Status: Not Exempt
Access to Protected Health Information: 2

Department: 31312 - 6 WEST
Grade: T15
Type: Job Definition

Job Summary

Description

- Department Job Description: Assess, plan, implement, and evaluate patient care for assigned patients. Collaborate with other members of health care teams efforts to provide patient care in compliance with established standards.

- Age of Patient Served
  - Adolescent: 13–17 Years
  - Adult: 17–65 Years
  - Geriatric: 65+ Years

Department Qualifications

Description

- Education/Experience: Current Alabama License required. Completion of unit specific certification course work within three months required. BCLS certification is required within three months. ACLS certification is required within twelve months. Successful completion of dysrhythmia examination is required within three months unless ACLS certification is current.

- Licensure or Certifications

- Special Skills or Knowledge: Must have knowledge of nursing theory and practice, good oral and written communication skills, effective interpersonal skills, and computer literacy.

- Working Conditions: Work requires exposure to conditions involving skin or lung irritants, cold or heat, poor ventilation, mechanical/electrical equipment, and toxic materials or hazardous waste including blood and bodily secretions.

Physical Demands of the Job

Description

- The following physical activities are routinely required by the position:
  - Stooping: 10%
  - Kneeling: 5%
  - Crouching: 5%
  - Reaching: 50%
  - Standing: 40%
  - Sitting: 15%
  - Walking: 45%
  - Pushing: 50%
  - Repititive motions: 20%
  - Pulling: 50%
  - Lifiting: 25% Up to 75 lbs. An average of 50 lbs.

Department Specific Job Duties

Description

- 25%: Plan patient care utilizing the nursing and medical diagnosis.
- 20%: Implement the Interdisciplinary Plan of Care on Assigned Patients.
- 20%: Provide teaching and guidance to patient, significant others.
- 10%: Assess patient condition on assigned unit.
- 5%: Evaluate patient progress/outcomes.
- 5%: Provide teaching and guidance to staff members.
- 5%: Maintain equipment and supplies and organizes work area.
- 5%: Complete department specific annual competencies.
- 5%: Perform other duties as assigned.

KRA

Rating Scale
Outstanding
Successful
Needs Improvement
Unsatisfactory

1. Plan patient care utilizing the nursing and medical diagnosis. (weight:25)

Description

- a.: Initiate plan of care within 8 hours of admission and develop within 24 hours based on nursing assessment.
- b.: Customize plan of care to include patient specific problems and needs.
- c.: Include patient/family involvement, discharge planning, teaching needs, and measurable outcomes in plan of care.
- d.: Document nursing care, assessment, and resolution of planned goals as per unit guidelines.
- e.: Address changing patient needs, nursing assessment, and the nursing diagnosis in the documentation at least once every 24 hours.

2. **Implement Interdisciplinary Plan of Care on assigned patients. (weight:20)**

Description

- a.: Conduct patient rounds as per unit guidelines.
- b.: Administer medications per hospital guidelines.
- c.: Complete daily plan of care following the medical orders and interdisciplinary plan of care per policy.
- d.: Notify nursing supervisory, medical personnel, and nursing staff immediately of potential crisis situations.

3. **Provide teaching and guidance to patient and significant others. (weight:20)**

Description

- a.: Customize patient/family education to address specific individual needs and level of understanding.
- b.: Evaluate patient/family education for effectiveness and updated as necessary.

4. **Assess patient condition on assigned unit. (weight:10)**

Description

- a.: Complete admission assessment on assigned patients within unit guidelines.
- b.: Complete nursing assessment at beginning of each shift and as patient's condition changes.
- c.: Inform physician immediately of significant deviations from norms.
- d.: Follow departmental guidelines in performing daily patient assessment.
- e.: Record information accurately and legibly.

5. **Evaluate patient progress/outcomes. (weight:5)**

Description

- a.: Revise interdisciplinary plan of care as patient's condition/needs change and as input from other health care providers and family members is received.
- b.: Document crisis situations as they occur to include patient condition preceding, during and after the crisis.
- c.: Provide shift reports to accurately reflect patient status and needs at the beginning and ending of each shift and upon patient transfer.
- d.: Provide pertinent and timely information to all members of the interdisciplinary patient care team.

6. **Provide teaching and guidance to staff members. (weight:5)**

Description

- a.: Assist new employees with orientation and provide feedback.
- b.: Assist pulled staff as needed.
- c.: Assist physicians and other members of the health care team as needed.

7. **Maintain equipment and supplies; organize work area. (weight:5)**

Description

- a.: Ensure safe and appropriate equipment storage.
- b.: Remove defective equipment from patient care area and report to appropriate person for repair.
- c.: Store supplies in safe manner.
- d.: Utilize supplies in a cost effective manner.

8. Complete department specific annual competencies. (weight:5)

Description

- ■ a.: Successfully complete all required competencies within the defined year including femoral sheath removal.
- ■ b.: Any competency not successfully completed is remedied within 60 days and re-testing occurs within the defined year.

9. Perform other duties as assigned. (weight:5)

Description

- ■ a.: Complete all additional duties in an acceptable manner.
- ■ b.: Perform additional duties in a reasonable amount of time.
- ■ c.: Enter all required patient log information legibly.

DEVELOPMENTAL INVENTORY

Rating Scale
Acceptable
Not Acceptable

Description

Determine the applicability of each behavior/skill to the job.

Customer Service Orientation

Description

Meets the external and internal customer needs by providing high quality, courteous and timely service. Listens to, and understands the customer; anticipates customer needs; gives high priority to customer satisfaction.

Job Knowledge

Description

Possesses and maintains adequate knowledge to perform effectively in all areas of the job.

Initiative

Description

Possesses the ability and willingness to think and act indepenently. Originates new ideas.

Communication

Description

Gives and receives information effectively in writing and verbally to enhance productivity and customer satisfaction.

Decision-Making

Description

Exhibits careful analysis, attention to detail, and sound judgement in making decisions necessary for the successful outcome or objectives.

Dependability

Description

Demonstrates reliability in performance or assigned tasks consitently by the use of time management and prioritization of work for optimal efficiency.

Team Dynamics

Description

Relates well with co-workers and customers. Displays a helpful, professional attitude to accomplish team and business objectives. Actively supports departmental and company missions and goals by sharing information and resources with others.

Creativity

Description

Produces innovative ideas that contribute to positive outcomes for quality improvement and cost savings.

Safety

Description

Maintains a safe environment and supports risk reduction activities.

Completion of department specific annual competencies:

Description

Completion of specified Corporate Compliance Training:

Description

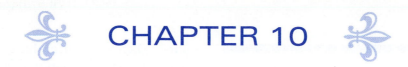

CHAPTER 10

Recruitment and Retention

J. Larry Tyler, FAAHC, FACHE, FHFMA, CMPE and Katrina Graham, MBA

LEARNING OBJECTIVES

Upon completing this chapter, the reader will be able to:

1. Define and discuss the strategic role of human resources (HR) in recruiting and retaining the best qualified applicants for a health care organization.

2. Understand the entire recruitment process from beginning to end and identify internal and external environmental factors that affect the strategic recruitment process.

3. Define recruitment and retention in health care organizations and show how it plays a major role in facilitating organizational success.

4. Enable health care HR executives in strategic decision making; specifically, in developing HR recruitment strategies and retention programs that attract and retain talented employees and allow the organization to meet its short- and long-term business needs.

5. Identify the major challenges in recruitment and retention of health care executives, especially at the CEO level.

KEY TERMS

Off-Limits Policies

Parallel Processing

Severance Package

INTRODUCTION

Begin with the end in mind.
                    Stephen Covey

Ready, fire . . . aim? Sometimes it seems as if the hiring process is so fraught with stops, starts, delays, and mistakes it is a wonder that anyone ever gets hired who is a proper match for the job. This chapter is devoted to helping you find, recruit, and keep good employees and do a much better job in handing a complex situation that seems to defy our organized efforts to be efficient and thorough at the same time.

To put in context the importance of recruiting, one must only refer to the famous *McKinsey Quarterly* article "The War for Talent" (Chambers, et al., 1998). This study by the international management consulting firm McKinsey and Company involved 77 companies and almost 6,000 managers. Released in 1998, the study is still being quoted years later because it had such a profound impact in bringing to the forefront what those in the human capital business already knew. "The search for the best and the brightest will become a constant, costly battle, a fight with no final victory" (Chambers, et al., 1998). One of the co-authors of the report, Ed Michaels, noted that "in the new economy, capital is abundant, ideas are developed quickly and cheaply, and people are willing to change jobs often. In that kind of environment, all that matters is talent. Talent wins" (Chambers, et al., 1998).

Those of us in health care can relate well to Fortune 500 companies trying to fill their pipelines with outstanding people. We are in the same type of boat, but our boat is not always seaworthy. In addition to seeking bright people, we also have to deal with seeking people with the right training and credentials while trying to pay them with scarce dollars. While newly minted MBAs can be had for a dime a dozen, a newly minted nurse is truly a treasure to hold. A newly minted neurosurgeon is even more valuable than a newly minted nurse. Therefore, our problems in recruiting and retention are much more difficult and pervasive than for many other types of industry. This chapter should give you insights that will at least give you a fighting chance at great hires that stay with your organization for years to come.

ESTABLISHING A JOB DESCRIPTION

The first thing one should do when trying to recruit a new employee at any level is to establish a job description that derives from a job analysis. Most of us do not put much time into this, because it is such a boring job that we leave it to the lowest clerk in human resources to put together. This should not be the case. The hiring manager may need resources to help him or her put together a job description because of time constraints or lack of knowledge or experience. Nevertheless, the hiring of a new employee is ultimately the responsibility of the hiring manager and a proper job description is essentially this person's responsibility also.

Generally, job descriptions should include the following information:

1. Job title
2. Reporting relationships—direct and indirect
3. Committee responsibilities and relating responsibilities
4. Educational and professional certification requirements
5. Lists of duties and responsibilities
6. Behavioral characteristics desired of the best candidates
7. Salary range, benefit level, and perks

Job titles should be well thought out. In general, the bigger the title, the more interest will be shown by candidates. For example, an executive vice president (VP) title will be of more interest than a title of director or administrator. Before jumping the title of a position to its highest level, several things must be considered, the biggest of which is the effect of a title on other parts of the organization. A change by one part of the organization can have a ripple effect in others parts that might be damaging to the organization. Therefore, human resources departments usually hold a tight rein on titles and levels of pay within an organization. A second consideration is that if you bring someone into the organization with the highest available title, then there may be no upward mobility for that person, and his or her tenure with the organization may be lessened. A third consideration is that the title must fit the culture and the organization. The title of associate vice-chancellor might have more meaning in an organization than a title of VP because the organization is accustomed to dealing with that title and knows exactly what it means. In Georgia, Dr. Michael Adams, president of the University of Georgia, started referring to himself as the CEO (chief executive officer) of the University. This caused much confusion and ridicule within the tenured faculty. He later dropped the moniker (The Associated Press, 2004).

Reporting relationships are important. Generally, everyone would love to report to the CEO but that is not usually practical, feasible, or wise. Establishing reporting relationships before recruiting begins helps to sort out the working relationships and offers an opportunity to explore other possibilities besides the current situation. As an example, 25% of chief information officers (CIOs) in hospitals report to the CFO (chief financial officer). If your organization utilizes this same relationship, why not consider having the CIO report to the chief medical officer (CMO), or to the COO (chief operating officer), or to the CEO? The development of the job description allows you a new opportunity to explore different reporting structures in order to be more efficient and effective. This statement is also true when it comes to the direct reports to the position. One should always review the list of direct reports and determine if some of the reports should be reporting somewhere else. Or, it should be determined if other departments in the organization should now report to that position.

For example, consider that you are now reviewing and preparing the job description for the new position of VP of quality. The case management department has always reported to the chief nursing officer. As the HR director, you should consider whether or not moving that department over to this new position would be a good idea. You may decide in the end to leave it where it is for good reason. But you should at least ask the right questions and have a discussion beforehand.

Committee responsibilities and relating responsibilities are important also and should not be overlooked. Health care organizations are highly complex matrices, especially in academic medical centers. In order to give both the potential candidates and the hiring organization a realistic and full view of the job, committee and relating responsibilities should be detailed. It also helps to give the candidate a better understanding of the time commitments that may be necessary in order to get the job done. Remember, full disclosure and transparency are important concepts if you wish to keep the candidate you eventually hire.

Educationally and professionally certified employees are perhaps hired more often in health care than in any other field. We are obsessed with education and certifications. Many of these are dictated to us by state licensing laws. Others are thrust upon us by our professional societies or by outsiders trying to assess our quality or our ability to deliver services. When considering the educational qualifications of a potential employee, you must take into consideration the educational levels and certifications of the people who will report to this person. If you are recruiting for a CFO and have a finance department full of CPAs (certified public accountants), you might want your new CFO to not only be a CPA but also have an MBA. The input from the people in the department will be helpful to you as you work on your specifications. It would be embarrassing to put out a job description which missed one of the basic certifications for a position. This might open the floodgates for candidates that you may eventually have to turn down even though according to your job description they are qualified.

The most important section of the job description is the list of duties and responsibilities. This list tells the candidates and the organization what this person is supposed to do and will serve later as the basis for the evaluation of how the candidate is performing. The is perhaps the hardest part of the job description because it requires that one put down on paper as many of the responsibilities that one can think of for the job. It often helps to have a job description for a similar job so that one does not have to reinvent the wheel.

Many organizations have a standard format for job descriptions, so you might also want to follow the prescribed format when developing the responsibilities and duties. In general, it is better to be more specific than general, although there is a trade-off at some point. If a list of responsibilities is too general, then it may allow a new employee to avoid responsibility. Yet if it is too detailed, it may not allow for things that crop up unexpectedly or just evolve into the job. Therefore, the last responsibility should always be "All other duties as deemed necessary." Try to limit the duties to 15–20 so that reading them does not become tedious.

While organizations screen for potential positions based on the technical specifications of the candidate (i.e., education, experience, accomplishments), they hire based on the behavioral competencies. This part of the job description deserves some careful thought and understanding from both the organization and the hiring manager. Many health care institutions have now been able to decipher the behavioral competencies that allow people to be successful in their institutions. If your organization is one of those who has successfully implemented this hiring practice, then congratulations! Much of your job has been done for you. If you are not in that kind of organization, then perhaps we can help you a bit. Many of the professional associations in health care management have conducted behavioral competency studies of their members in order to determine what behaviors result in successful outcomes. They have taken these studies and combined them into one place, the HLA Competency Directory (Healthcare Leadership Alliance, 2008). This would be a good place to look for ideas if you are putting together a job description at the C-level.

In addition, Dr. Andrew Garmin and I conducted a study for the American College of Healthcare Executives on behavior competencies for health care executives (Garman & Tyler, 2002). There are entire books written about behavioral competencies, so our discussion here is very brief. Nevertheless, I would be remiss not to pass on a few tips garnered from 30 years of real-world experience in writing HR briefs. You should know that the number one behavioral competence necessary for survival and success is communication skills. If this is not on your list of job specific competencies, you have made a fatal mistake. This competency should always be listed at or near the top of your list.

Establishing the salary range up front is essential before you begin recruiting. Most HR departments have this information or can get it for you quickly from outside compensation counsel. Remember that when you are recruiting, most individuals will not change jobs for less than a 15% increase in pay, all other things being equal. Therefore, you may find yourself coming in at the top of the range for your new recruits. If things are tight, consider changing the specs so that those with less experience can be considered. Generally, less experienced or credentialed personnel are paid less. Many salary levels are set based upon the job title or the level in the organization. This is another reason why you need to be cognizant of how your recruiting efforts relate to the rest of the organization. Later we will discuss how to deal with a recruiting situation where you want to hire someone outside of the salary range.

THE RECRUITING PLAN

Now that the job description is finalized, a recruiting plan is put together, which is normally composed of both active and passive recruiting components. Usually, one will first start with the passive recruiting components because they can be the most time efficient. Passive recruiting involves posting the employment opportunity on Web sites and job boards, as well as newspaper or journal advertising. Some of the journals and newspapers have a policy that one must advertise the job opening in the publication as well in order to place the job opening on the publication's Web site. Because most positions need to be filled in a hurry, recruiters like to post to a Web site since many publications will have 30- to 60-day lags between the time that you place the advertisement and the time that it runs. Recruiters can utilize their own Web sites for posting of job opportunities too.

A truly effective recruiting program will acknowledge receipt of a resume from an applicant and will provide a mechanism for forwarding more information. Most Web postings will specify that e-mail submission of the resume is best. This is good for several reasons. One, it is quicker than "snail mail," and two, the e-mailed resume can automatically go into the company's database, which will allow for quick sorting and review.

Active recruiting is another matter. This involves figuratively reaching out and tapping someone on the shoulder and saying, "Are you interested in our opportunity?" Active recruiting can be accomplished in the following ways.

Direct Mail

A list can be purchased from a "list house" such as SKA, Billions, and so on. The list is then merged into a letter that is sent by the U.S. Post office or by e-mail to potential job candidates. E-mail is usually the preferred method because it is viral in nature, meaning it can quickly and easily be forwarded on to the interested parties; but e-mail can also end up as spam in the recipient's spam box. The U.S. mail is slower, but paper mail can still have an impact and has a greater chance of actually being seen. However, of course, it is also extraordinarily more expensive than e-mail.

The general tone of a direct mail piece is "We have this opportunity. Do you know someone who might be interested?" Most organizations refrain from asking, "Are you personally looking?" because they are concerned about being criticized by other organizations for poaching. The softer approach is more indirect and less politically charged.

There are direct mail organizations that will provide you with all-inclusive services if you are a larger-volume recruiting organization. You merely have to draft the direct mail piece and they will take it from there. In fact, the direct mail organizations will even draft the letter if you do not have the time or lack the persuasive writing skills to do it yourself.

Networking

This involves telephone solicitation from an internal person charged with the recruitment effort. It is formidably time consuming, so one would normally use it as a last resort. However, a normal recruitment effort should involve at least some telephone work, even if it is limited. For example, if one is recruiting nurses, one should probably make a few calls to nursing schools to get recommendations of potential candidates coming out of school. If one is recruiting a CFO, then the organization should call their external auditors in order to get referrals. Additional calls might be made to the previous auditors and to any auditors in the phone book, whether you know anyone at the firm or not. For many hard-to-find positions, networking may be the only viable way to recruit the candidate. However, an experienced recruiter can only handle three to seven assignments at one time if his or her only source of candidates is through networking.

Networking is enhanced by the availability of information over the Internet. "Googling" for candidate's names and e-mail addresses is very common. Enhanced search engines like Zoom Info can come up with information that allows a recruiter to find hard-to-find and displaced candidates.

Contingency Search Firms

Contingency search firms can be utilized in addition to one's own internal efforts since no fee is usually paid until someone is hired; the fee is "contingent" on placement and so no extraordinary costs are incurred in a search for several candidates. Contingency firms can turn up candidates that may not have been found through your recruiting plan. Usually an organization would use several contingency firms for the recruitment effort, but if a firm has been responsive and successful in the past, you might want to use that firm exclusively for 30 days before you open it up to others. This might also give the firm an incentive to work harder on your behalf. Contingency firms are a good supplement to your own efforts and have the advantage that you can continue your own efforts as well as avoid a fee if they do not produce a successful candidate.

Before you engage or accept resumes from contingency firms, you *must* establish some rules internally for dealing with them, especially since many times you will receive the same resume from multiple firms. If a hire is made, then multiple firms may claim that you owe them a fee. Some of the contingency firms may send you a resume without ever consulting the candidate. There seem to be several ways of determining who gets the fee. Some hiring organizations use a method of posting the date and time that the resume is received and use that information when deciding who gets the fee. Other organizations use another method, the effective procuring-cause method, by designating up front which agency gets the fee based on who actually contacted the candidate and who is scheduling the interviews (Marshall, 2005). It is also smart to have a process in place for arbitrating fees, because many placement situations are not black and white.

Please keep in mind that even though the hiring organization is paying the fee, the contingency firm is in fact working for the candidate. Since the fee is contingent and there is no certainty that a hire is going to be made, the contingency firm tries to send the candidate on as many interviews as possible. To the contingency firm it does not matter where a fee comes from, as long as one is collected.

You should also not expect a lot of background checking from the contingency firm. Do your own reference checks and verifications. In addition, be very specific about the guarantee. Most contingency firms will offer a guarantee of 90 days, which is pro-rated. You should try to negotiate a replacement guarantee (not pro-rated) which encompasses a longer period. You should also make sure that you understand the terms of the contract, such as how the fee is calculated. You should not pay the placement fee until the candidate is actually onboard and working. Enough candidates fail to show up for work such that the industry has a term for it: falloff.

Retained Search

If the position is high enough in the organization (e.g., senior management) then it is possible that the organization may want to use a retained search firm to conduct the search. The retained search process is much like a consulting engagement, so the same types of fees and expenses apply. All retained searches are conducted on an exclusive basis, that is, no other firm is engaged on the search and all candidates are referred to the firm for evaluation, including internal candidates and those who submit their resumes directly to the client. Most retained search firms charge between 30% and 33% of the first year's compensation (salary + estimated bonus + signing bonus). The estimated fee is paid in increments during the search (usually over 90 days) and a settlement is made when the search is completed. The firm also bills for out-of-pocket expenses. Given the financial arrangement, a retained search is a little like a marriage—it should not be entered into lightly.

If you have never done a retained search before or have minimal experience, then you might want to call other health care organizations for recommendations of retained firms that specialize in the health care industry. The American College of Healthcare Executives has an extensive list of health care executive search firms in the career section of its Web site (www.ache.org). Modern Healthcare (www.modernhealthcare.com) has an annual listing of the top health care search firms; however, the listing is of little value since it does not differentiate between retained and contingency firms and little effort is made to verify the reasonableness of the reported numbers. The trade organization for the retained search industry is the Association of Executive Search Consultants (AESC) (www.aesc.org). Not all of the retained search firms are members, but many of the well regarded firms are. The AESC has a client bill of rights on its Web site. This is a great place to start for those who have had no experience with retained searches. When engaging a retained search firm, you might want to ask if they are an AESC member. If they are, you have a place to complain should the firm not live up to its promises.

Once the retained search firm has done a site visit, it will write up a set of specifications for the position and develop a document that reflects the organization, the position, and the criteria for the perfect candidate. You will have to approve this document, because it becomes the document of record for the search. The consultant recruitment plan and evaluation of candidates will be developed from this document.

The search firm will do the recruiting, both active and passive, and present you with a list of several candidates. Depending on the specs, the list may be really long, with over 20 candidates, or really short, with only 2 candidates. After consultation with you, the consultant will interview the selected candidates and process those that seem to be a fit. Most retained search firms will do some sort of preliminary reference checks. Others will do extensive referencing, including degree verification and credit/criminal/driving checks before the candidates are presented to you. Make sure you understand up front which checks the search firm is responsible for and which ones you are responsible for. Regardless of who does the preliminary checks, you should be prepared to do some referencing yourself and also to make the offer contingent on a satisfactory reference from the candidate's current employer.

There are two issues that are important to organizations hiring retained search consultants. These are **off-limits policies** and **parallel processing**. The standard of ethics for search consultants is that a client will remain off-limits for recruiting purposes for a certain period of time. That is, the search firm will not solicit candidates from the organization without the permission of the organization. In large organizations, there may be also a definition as to what parts of the organization are off-limits. For example, an individual hospital in a

multihospital system may be off-limits, while other hospitals in the system, as well as the corporate offices, are not. UPMC in Pittsburgh makes all of their organization off-limits for one year from the completion of the last search. The off-limits policy should be discussed up front with your search firm and made a part of the engagement letter. No organization wants a recruiter walking its halls, recruiting away its best people, and then soliciting it to replace them.

A retained search firm should give you an exclusive on the candidates. Once the candidate has entered your process, that candidate should be exclusively yours and not be introduced into another search until your search is concluded. Introducing a candidate to multiple clients is called parallel processing and is a problem (Executive Search Review, 2002). Parallel processing was prohibited by the AESC, but in the 1990s the prohibition was somewhat watered-down, such that it is not prohibited as long as the clients understand and agree to allow parallel processing (Executive Search Review, 2002). As a hiring organization, parallel processing is not generally in your best interests as it places the search firm in the position of representing the candidate and not you. Who does the search firm represent when two retained clients want the same candidate? The conflict of interests is substantial (Executive Search Review, 2002). Nevertheless, there are circumstances when parallel processing is appropriate and your interests are not harmed. For example, is it really fair to penalize a candidate when you put your search on hold for six months and may not fill it? Is it fair to put all the candidates in limbo with a search firm when other opportunities could be pursued by them?

THE INITIAL SCREEN

Once a resume gets to the organization, an initial screening call is important. Depending on how the resume was obtained, the interest levels of the candidate vary widely. Perhaps the person submitting the resume saw your posting. Maybe they did not see it and just submitted the resume blindly. However the applicant chose your organization, someone who knows something about the job and has been charged with the screening should call the applicant to get more information.

Most contacts with potential employees are made during business hours. Because of this, the screening needs to be done with some degree of decorum and confidentiality. If the work phone number is not on the resume, you can assume that the candidate does not want to be contacted at work. Call the home number and leave a message or e-mail the candidate and ask the candidate to call you.

It has been my experience that candidates are looking for three broad things when they are changing jobs. These are Money, Opportunity, and Location. It is important to remember these three things when you are doing your screening call. If you can offer at least two of these as positive to the candidate then you might have a possible match. This is especially true if location is one of the matches. As you begin your call, you should keep this information in mind because it will be important to you to remember it when the time comes to make the offer. A good screening call will elicit the following information:

1. Why is the person interested in your opportunity? What is the motivation to change jobs?

2. What is it about the person's current situation that is a dissatisfier? Is the person currently employed or in the process of exiting his or her organization?

3. What makes the person qualified for the position?

4. What is the person's current compensation?

5. Why is the location of the employer attractive?

6. Is the candidate looking at other employment opportunities? At what stage are these opportunities?

7. What are the potential dates that this person could come for a face-to-face interview?

A good screening call will establish the interest level of the candidate and how well the candidate meets the position specifications. After screening a group of candidates you will then have to decide which ones to bring in for interviews at the organization. It is important that you contact those candidates that you screen initially and let them know of their status. Some organizations fail to follow up with candidates and leave them uninformed. It has been my experience that frankness with candidates is most appreciated by them. If your search falls apart, you may want to reconnect with a candidate. The candidate is likely to return your call if you have been a responsive communicator previously. Remember, good candidates always have other options.

THE ON-SITE INTERVIEW

The interview onsite is extremely important and needs to be coordinated carefully. In addition, one might have a gift basket placed in the candidate's hotel room with a welcoming note from either the hiring manager or the human resources contact. Effective coordination can dramatically increase candidate interest. Conversely, ineffective coordination can be a candidate turn-off. Candidates make value judgments about how they are treated during the interview process. It behooves an organization to put its best foot forward.

As a prelude to putting the best foot forward, the internal coordinator should make sure that all of the people who are interviewing the candidate understand what position the candidate is interviewing for. Each interviewer should receive the resume of the candidate, the full itinerary of interviews, the job description, and an evaluation form with instructions. Some organizations also provide a set of questions to be asked or have a pre-interview meeting to decide which person is going to ask which question. Sometimes these questions are structured around the values of the organization or around the behavioral competencies identified as necessary and important to the organization. The higher the position in the organization, the more elaborate and deliberate is the interview preparation. Relevant information can be distributed to your least accomplished interviewers so as to facilitate the interview process.

Most organizations have moved toward asking behavior-based questions. These questions are usually phrased something like this: "Describe a situation where you encountered an angry physician. What were the circumstances and how did you deal with the situation?" These types of questions can elicit how a candidate thinks and are much more revealing than the standard questions that one might put forward, such as "Tell me about yourself" or " Tell me about your strengths and weaknesses." In addition, some interviewers like to ask the "left field" question, such as "I have a curio in my office. I have cleared the top shelf and have given you the opportunity to put something important to you on the shelf. It will be there for all to see. What are you going to put on the shelf and why is it important to you?" Left-field questions are often very revealing because the candidate has not prepared for them. In addition, we can find out how the candidate thinks on his or her feet and, occasionally, what the candidate values in his or her personal life.

Clear instructions and directions are essential for the candidate, as well as an itinerary listing the names and position titles of the people that the candidate will meet. At the executive level, it can be useful to include biographical sketches of the management team so that the candidate knows a little more about the team and each introduction is not an uninformed one. Generally, a candidate will meet with the hiring manger first. An initial interview usually lasts an hour or two. Other interviews follow with various people within the organization. Usually, human resources are involved at some point in order to explain benefits and the compensation parameters. There may also be some kind of testing that human resources might administer. At the end, there is usually a reconnect with the hiring manager to answer any questions that might have come up and to say goodbye.

Feedback is very important to the hiring manager. Most organizations have some type of interview evaluation form which they use as the feedback mechanism. This is usually a stock form that focuses on values or behavioral competencies that are generic to the organization. A better way of getting feedback would be to customize each evaluation instrument according to the job. Unfortunately, the customization process is time consuming and therefore should only used sparingly, such as in the case of evaluating a CEO candidate or a C-suite executive. It is helpful to also include a final recommendation on the evaluation form forcing the interviewer to make a choice between options such as (1) Move forward to the next phase, (2) Move forward to the next phase with reservations noted, and (3) Do not move forward. Such direct questions will indicate the level of enthusiasm of the interviewer for the candidate.

When coordinating site visits, provisions must be made for the unexpected. We have had candidates end up in the emergency room of the hospital with appendicitis or get involved in a car wreck and be hospitalized. The person within the organization who is coordinating the interview should obtain the candidate's cell and home phone numbers in case the organization needs to contact him or her for any reason, for example, in the case of emergency.

Candidate feedback should be garnered by someone before moving to the second interview. If working with a search firm, the search firm will handle that for you and let you know of the candidate's continuing interest or lack thereof. Some organizations have a recruiting contact in the organization get the feedback; others use feedback from the hiring manager. When gathering feedback, one should ask the candidate about the interview process. Were there any glitches? How was the candidate treated? The feedback gathering should also cover any concerns the candidate has about the job, especially with regard to the money, opportunity, and location aspects of the candidate's thinking. Finally, as a gauge of the candidate's interest level, ask the candidate: "At this point, can you give me an idea of your interest level on a scale of

1 to 10?" A seven or better is usually pretty good. Obviously a ten is a wonderful response, and a response of "six" should cause concern. Given a low response, the next question might be, "What would it take to make this opportunity a 10?" This should draw out the concerns the candidate has. Some of the concerns may be remedied by adding or subtracting another department or changing the reporting structure for the final position. Others, such as location, may not be easily changed. Normally, one would bring back for secondary interviews those who have a high interest in the job. At other times, you may want to encourage those with less interest to come in for a second interview because they offer outstanding experience and you want a second chance to sell them on your position. Maybe the candidate did not get to see someone who you would have liked for them to see. Or maybe something got misinterpreted that caused the candidate to have a less than favorable opinion of the organization. At any rate, you need to know the candidate's interest level so as to allow you to make your judgment about returning the candidate for the second interview.

THE SECOND INTERVIEW

Second interviews tend to be somewhat different from first interviews. The candidate has met the hiring manager and the peers. In most organizations, the candidate now gets to meet the subordinates and other parties that might have an interest in the candidate, such as board members or physicians. Whereas the first interview might have had several one-on-one meetings, the second interview has more group meetings.

There can also be another person on this interview—the candidate's spouse. The arrival of the spouse throws another dimension into interview process. One cannot forget that the spouse is also a participant in the candidate's life and may have veto power over what job the candidate takes. An organization must consider the needs of the spouse on the second interview and structure the interview process with those needs in mind (Mayo & Mathews, 2006). It is hard to know what those needs are unless someone has contacted the spouse and asked about those needs. Whoever is assigned to the coordination of the second interview needs to do this. Most often those needs reside around real estate issues, then schools, then job potential for the spouse. Occasionally, there are needs that you would have never guessed, such as the presence of a symphony orchestra or a competitive swim team for an athletic child. Again, you will not know until you ask, and we recommend asking the spouse directly without going through the candidate (Mayo & Mathews, 2006). In this way, you can establish communication with the spouse and also gauge the enthusiasm or reluctance of the spouse for the move.

Real estate issues can be difficult. Your organization should have a few real estate agents that you can recommend and connect to the candidate and spouse. The agent should contact the couple ahead of time, develop a rapport, and provide opportunities to look at housing in their price range. The agent should also give you a heads-up on issues that come up from conversations with the couple. This will give you additional insight into the thinking of the candidate. Special real estate considerations might also be made for single parents, whose children may be heavily involved in the relocation of a good candidate.

Periodically, the real estate market goes south and candidates start to have trouble selling their houses. This presents a particular bind for the candidate and a similar bind for the organization. It is extraordinarily important for the candidate and the candidate's family to relocate as soon as possible. To make the transition easier for the candidate, most companies offer some type of relocation assistance. A typical relocation assistance program would include:

a. Six months' temporary living for the candidate. This is usually a furnished apartment or a hotel suite that allows the ability to cook meals in the suite.

b. Two or three house-hunting trips with the spouse. These would include the cost of transportation and food.

c. Two or three trips home for the candidate before the spouse moves.

d. Movement of household goods. Usually the candidate is the one who contacts the moving companies. The candidate is usually required to get three bids and accept the lowest one.

"Bonuses to sign" have become a common technique in health care in order to land the preferred candidate. As is often the case in other industries, the preferred candidate is usually the most expensive. Hiring the candidate at the salary the preferred candidate needs might upset the internal equity of the salaries in the organization. A way around this issue is to give a one-time bonus to sign, which will allow the candidate to receive the total income needed without unsetting the internal pay equity.

A bonus to sign can also be used to offset the loss of bonus a candidate might be leaving behind at the previous employer. This is known as "making the candidate whole." Making the candidate whole can become an expensive proposition. Candidates often leave behind at the former employer long-term and short-term bonuses, accumulated paid time off, unvested retirement plans, and stock options. An organization needs to think seriously about the wisdom of making a candidate entirely whole because the costs mount up quickly and may in the end make the candidate less cost effective. This is especially onerous if the candidate for which the organization "moved heaven and earth" turns out to be an ineffective employee and gets fired. Note the controversy surrounding the firing of Bob Nardarelli from The Home Depot. The disclosure of his **severance package,** which included a number of items that were agreed to ahead of time in order to entice him from General Electric, even drew attention in Washington when House Financial Services Committee Chairman Barney Frank, D-Mass., cited it as more evidence that lawmakers should deal with CEO pay. The pattern of CEO pay "appears to be out of control," Frank said in a statement. Frank has tapped CEO pay and wage inequality as priorities during his term as chairman of the financial panel (Waters & Moore, 2007).

SEVERANCE PACKAGES

Severance packages have become common place in health care. Once only the provenance of the CEO, severance agreements now are prominent in the C-suite and are moving downward through the organization. As they move lower in the organization, the severance agreements become less lucrative. Most organizations will have some type of severance policy for the rank and file that will call for a modest continuation of salary and benefits.

Severance packages are in place for several reasons. First, a severance package provides a degree of protection for employees who, through no fault of their own, are released from the organization. Their release may be caused by internal reorganization, a merger with another organization, or some other cause for the redundancy. Second, a severance package also serves as a form of protection for those in the organization taking on risks that may have negative consequences. An example might be that of a CEO taking on an on-call issue with the medical staff. A CEO without a severance agreement may be unwilling to take any risk. Third, a severance agreement says to the organization, those leaving, and those who are being recruited, that the organization is fair to its employees regardless of their employment status. Fourth, the severance agreement provides some protection for the organization in that most health care organizations require the recipient of the severance package to sign a waiver agreeing to not disparage the organization and to not discuss the circumstances surrounding his or her departure or even the agreement itself. Failure to follow the waiver guidelines will call for the severance to cease and prior payments to be refunded.

A great deal of thought should go into the severance agreement. A policy or an individual agreement should never be concluded without legal input. For example, many agreements call for dismissal with cause, such as a conviction for a felony, to void the severance package agreement. The organization should ask itself, "What if the employee is convicted of a misdemeanor. What is our policy?" Should the C-suite be held to a higher level of accountability than the rank and file? These are all important considerations when developing a severance package.

At the CEO level, the model contract for health care executives as proposed by the American College of Healthcare Executives calls for 24 months of salary and benefit continuation (www.ache.org). Other perks such as continued use of the company car, access to secretarial services, and outplacement assistance are usually included.

A caveat on severance agreements: While it is a good thing to grant a severance package to an employee, too long of a severance payment period may be a detriment to an executive. For example, a CEO with 24 months of severance may think that he has 24 months to find a job and therefore the executive may make only a token effort to find a job in the first 6 to 12 months, or take a 6-month sabbatical.

WELCOME ABOARD

Relatively new to the recruiting and retention process has been the development of onboarding programs in order to help a candidate get off to a good start (Morel, 2007). Unfortunately, a bad start can set a new employee up for future failure because early impressions tend to be lasting impressions, so the costs of not having an onboarding program can be high (Gierden, 2007). Early intervention when things are falling apart can save the employee and keep the organization from having to start the recruiting and hiring process all over again (Morel, 2007). Onboarding processes tend to focus on the first 90 days of employment.

Oftentimes, an outside coach is hired to make sure that onboarding proceeds appropriately.

Coaching addresses issues that orientation and training alone may not be able to address (Gierden, 2007). Internally, the human resources department will take control to make sure that the employee is given a proper orientation to the organization, has been introduced to the appropriate internal resources and customers, and has a plan for getting things done so as to establish a good reputation early in the game. Periodic feedback is important to a new employee, so many organizations do a multirater evaluation during this early time period so the new employee can have feedback regarding how he or she is viewed by subordinates, peers, and the supervisor.

Loss of productivity or loss of interest in a company on the part of the employee can have a significant impact on an organization. This is especially true if an organization does not support a comprehensive introduction phase for new employees (Snell, 2006). This initial phase is critical, because 64% of new executives hired externally will fail in the job, and the average CEO is in the job for less than four years (Snell, 2006). A progressive organization will not only recruit well but also make sure that a new hire has all of the opportunities for success that the company can provide.

There are some benefits from efficient onboarding processes and technologies that can affect the organization's bottom line (Snell, 2006), for example:

- Reduced time and effort by HR and others involved in onboarding
- Improved data collection and transfer of information between payroll and HRIS systems
- Compliance and consistency with legal and policy mechanisms inside and outside the organization
- Improved tracking of metrics for greater process efficiency
- Improved manager and employee communications

A well designed and controlled onboarding process reduces costs and improves retention of employees, who are more quickly involved in the organization and more immediately productive

(Snell, 2006). Ultimately, such employees remain over the long run because of their satisfaction with the onboarding process.

RETENTION

After onboarding has taken place, the next issue that arises is the long-term employment of the candidate. Hiring a candidate is one thing, but keeping that person long term involves a multifaceted approach. Obviously, if an organization can keep an employee for the long term, the cost of its recruiting efforts drops dramatically.

The multifaceted approach to retention will involve resolving the following issues.

Pay

Almost every survey of why people leave jobs finds that pay is not necessarily a "satisfier." That is, a 50% increase in pay doesn't necessarily make people stay in a job, but a 50% decrease in pay makes them leave in a hurry. Recruitment and retention should not be based solely on compensation, because a person lured into an organization by a big pay offer will almost certainly leave for an even bigger one (Bartlett & Ghoshal, 2002). Employees have to pay their bills, but will accept less pay if there is something else in the organization that emotionally rewards them. An organization must maintain an adequate compensation program that keeps its pay competitive with the field; otherwise, turnover will result.

Benefits

Benefits are sometimes more important than pay to an employee. Many benefits, like health care costs, are not taxable to the employee. Some benefits are beneficial to one set of employees, but not to others (Numerof, Abrams, & Ott, 2004). As an example, an educational reimbursement program might be very attractive to a young person set on moving up in the world, but not attractive to another person who has already attained the necessary educational credentials for the field. Surveys of the different classes of employees often uncover the benefits that are important to them (e.g., reasonable day care for the children of nurses). Some organizations have taken the step of lumping benefits into a "cafeteria" plan such that the employee is given an amount of money to spend on benefits and can pick and choose which benefits are personally important to the employee.

Education and Career Advancement

Most of the best employees of an organization want to get ahead. This may mean that they want and need additional education in their field in order to prepare them for the next level. Or they may want education to prepare them for another aspect of the health care field. Benefits like tuition support, scholarships, and initiation of loan repayment are increasingly a part of the best retention programs in the country (Rick, 2001). A well-thought-out training program gives employees the opportunity to learn new things and be able to compete for the top jobs when they come up. All employees at all levels need to have the opportunity to learn. Organizations that scrimp on their training budget often find that their turnover increases.

Work Environment

A good work environment and empowerment in the workplace play a larger role than benefits and wages in retention of staff (Spetz & Adams, 2006). For employees, just having a say in what is going on for them can have a beneficial impact on the individuals as well as the organization. Retention programs should also included employee satisfaction surveys as a part of the overall program. Truly enlightened organizations post the survey results for everyone to see. This is very difficult to do when things are not going well in a department or in the whole organization. The tendency is to deal with such issues quietly. Unfortunately, this can also create the attitude that management is not going to do anything about the results, so why bother completing the survey? In addition to employee surveys, the human resources department should also be conducting exit interviews in order to determine the reasons that individuals are leaving the organization. Oftentimes, these interviews can reveal weaknesses in management or other issues that need to be addressed.

Sense of Mission and Accomplishment

People will stay with an organization even if the benefits are bad and the pay is poor if they feel that they are accomplishing something, especially something good for mankind. People like to be surrounded by people of like mind. Hiring those that fit in the organization and understand its mission will go a long way toward motivating employees to excel and reducing turnover.

SUMMARY

The workplace is evolving, and it is necessary for human resource professionals to remain up to speed. The best practices of the past may no longer be relevant to the recruitment, onboarding, and retention needs of organizations today. Nowhere is this need more prevalent than in the health care industry. From nurses to CEOs, organizations are being faced with new issues in recruiting and retaining the best and most talented professionals for their organizations. Human resource professionals should be ready to hire the best, and this begins by having a recruitment and retention strategy specifically designed for the organization.

New mechanisms for gaining a competitive advantage through hiring the best and the brightest are available. From direct mail advertising to the Internet, employers now have the most technologically advanced methods for advertising open job positions and are no longer constrained by geographical limitations. Contingency search firms and retained search firms offer hiring managers additional weapons for their use in recruiting for all levels of the organization without placing a strain on already overburdened HR departments. Finally, from initial employee benefits to severance packages, there is an increasing number of perquisites being offered to employees before they start on day one. Having knowledgeable HR professionals to manage all of these competing demands can help organizations to best leverage their options in gaining the most talented personnel available to help grow their organization.

MANAGERIAL GUIDELINES

1. *Establish a job description.* Job descriptions should include job titles, reporting relationships, committee responsibilities, required educational background, professional certifications, and duties and responsibilities. Developing the job description provides an opportunity to explore different structures in order to become more efficient and effective. Committee responsibilities offer candidates a realistic job preview and time commitments necessary to get the job done. Educational and professional certifications provide baseline qualifications for the job. Duties and responsibilities indicate what the person is supposed to do in the job and later serve as the basis for performance evaluation.

2. *Develop a recruitment plan.* Recruitment plans are composed of both passive and active components. Passive recruiting involves posting a position on Web sites and job boards, as well as newspaper and journal advertising. Active recruiting involves reaching out to prospective employees and includes such activities as direct mail, networking, and contingency/retained search firms.

3. *Conduct an initial screen of candidates.* The initial screen will indicate the interest level of the candidates and how well they meet the position specifications.

4. *Conduct an onsite interview.* All people interviewing the candidate should understand what position the candidate is interviewing for. They should receive the candidate's resume, interview itinerary, job description, and an evaluation form, and they should know ahead of time the specific questions they are going to ask.

5. *Apply a multifaceted approach to retention.* Long-term employment issues typically revolve around aspects of the job such as pay, benefits, education and career advancement, work environment, and sense of mission/purpose. A comprehensive program should be in place to address these issues.

DISCUSSION QUESTIONS

1. List and describe the characteristics of a good job description.

2. How are retained search firms and contingency firms different? What issues are important when using their services to recruit talent to an organization?

3. What is onboarding and how could an onboarding program be incorporated into an organization's best practices?

4. Why is "making the candidate whole" such an expensive proposition, and how would an organization manage candidate expectations in such a situation?

5. What issues are involved in the retention of health care executives? How can these issues be best resolved?

6. Discuss the major differences between first and second interviews.

REFERENCES

Bartlett, C.A., & Ghoshal, S. (2002). Building competitive advantage through people. *MIT Sloan Management Review, 43*(2): 34–41.

Chambers, E., Foulon, M., Handfield-Jones, H., Hankin, S.M., & Michael, E. (1998). The war for talent. *The McKinsey Quarterly, 3*: 44–57.

Executive Search Review. (2002). *Revised AESC Guidelines Designed To Clarify Best Practices For Industry.* Riverside, CT: Hunt Scanlon Corporation.

Garman, A., & Tyler, L. (2002). *360 Feedback for Leadership Development in Health Administration.* Chicago: American College of Healthcare Executives.

Gierden, C. (2007). Get on the right track with executive onboarding. *Canadian HR Reporter, 20*(13): 14.

Healthcare Leadership Alliance. (2008). HLA Competency Directory: 2005–2007 American College of Healthcare Executives; American Organization of Nurse Executives; Healthcare Financial Management Association; Healthcare Information and Management Systems Society; and Medical Group Management Association and its certifying body, the American College of Medical Practice Executives.

Marshall, B. (2005). Pre-prep is the key, *The Fordyce Letter.* New York City: ERE Media.

Mayo, E., & Mathews, M. (2006). Spousal perspectives on factors influencing recruitment and retention of rural family physicians. *Can J Rural Med, 11*(4): 271–276.

Morel, S. (2007). Onboarding secures talent for the long run. *Workforce Management, 86*(12): S9.

Numerof, R.E., Abrams, M., & Ott, B. (2004). What works . . . and what doesn't. *Nursing Management, 35*(3): 18.

Rick, C. (2001). Warp-speed innovation. *Nursing Management, 32*(7): 14.

Snell, A. (2006). Researching onboarding best practice. *Strategic HR Review, (5)*6: 32.

Spetz, J., & Adams, S. (2006). How can employment-based benefits help the nurse shortage? *Health Affairs, 25*(1): 212–218.

The Associated Press. (2004). After no-confidence vote on Adams, UGA faculty trying to improve communication. Accessed Thursday, March 25th, 2004, at 3:30 a.m., from *AccessNorthGA.com.*

Waters, J., & Moore, A. (2007). Home Depot chairman, CEO Nardelli resigns, *MarketWatch.* Chicago: The Wall Street Journal.

CHAPTER 11

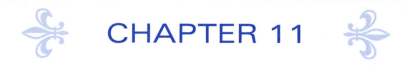

Personnel Selection and Onboarding

Andrew N. Garman, PsyD, MS and Daniel P. Russell, MS

LEARNING OBJECTIVES

Upon completing this chapter, the reader will be able to:

1. Describe personnel selection within the context of the broader hiring cycle, which includes position design, position marketing, prescreening, interviewing, reference checking, hiring, onboarding, and retention.

2. Identify legal issues associated with hiring decisions, with particular focus on the United States.

3. Describe how the concepts of reliability and validity are related to selection tools.

4. Analyze the return on investment associated with making more accurate hiring decisions.

5. Identify appropriate approaches to hiring based upon the unique needs of different positions, including frontline positions, nurses, physicians, and other health professionals, as well as leadership positions.

6. Recognize the pros and cons of various approaches to selection and identify the right approach for the situation.

7. Assess the quality of a new hire's onboarding experience to plan improvements in that process.

KEY TERMS

Adverse Impact

Content Validity

Construct Validity

Criterion-Related Validity

Disability

Essential Job Function

Fair Discrimination

Inter-Rater Reliability

Job Applicant

Onboarding

Reliability

Reasonable Accommodation

Selection Process

Talent Acquisition Process

Title VII of the Civil Rights Act of 1964

Undue Hardship

Unfair Discrimination

Uniform Guidelines on Employee Selection Procedures 1978 (UGESP)

Validity

Jill and Fred

Jill and Fred were old friends from their college days. After several years at separate institutions, they were now working for the same medical center; Fred worked in the radiation oncology practice and Jill in the geriatric care facility. They both made a point of getting together for lunch at least once a month. Sometimes they found time to be social; often they used the opportunity to discuss the many management challenges they each faced. A recent conversation focused on hiring decisions.

"So, Jill, did I hear that the new administrative assistant you hired is gone already?" Fred asked.

"That's right," Jill answered. "That position's back on the market. Know any good candidates?"

"Not off-hand," Fred replied. "What went wrong with your last person?"

"She just wasn't working out, on a variety of fronts. Basically, she looked a lot better on paper than she ended up being in person. But you know, Fred, the worst part of it was that I had my doubts about her from the beginning."

"Wow, that *is* too bad. You still decided to hire her?"

"Yes—you know how it is—we were getting pretty desperate. The position had been vacant for months, and we just weren't seeing any decent candidates. She was far from perfect, but she at least looked like she *might* work."

Fred tried to give Jill a sympathetic smile, but it just annoyed her.

"I don't suppose I can expect you to understand, Fred—everyone you hire has a license of some kind, and the professions are pretty tightly knit—word gets around about who's good and who's not. There's no degree or licensure for administrative assistants, and unless you have an employee vouch for them personally, you just never know what you're getting until they're on the job."

Fred laughed, "Okay, Jill, we *do* get a lot of candidates—but come on now, hiring clinicians is

no picnic either. Just because someone makes it through school is no guarantee they'll be good with patients—or that they'll work well in a team! And when they *do* work out," Fred continued, "within six months the suburban hospitals try to poach them, and suddenly they're gunning for a higher salary!"

Jill looked surprised—she had assumed her hires were more difficult than Fred's. Now she wasn't so sure. She decided to change subjects.

"So, Fred, are you ready for my big news?"

"Lay it on me, Jill."

"I got selected for LDP!"

"Oh… congratulations," Fred said, half-heartedly.

"LDP" was the medical center's internal Leadership Development Program. It was designed to help the center develop and retain its "up and comers"—managers thought to have executive potential. Participation was highly coveted, and the selection process was mysterious at best.

"When did you find out?" asked Fred.

"Last Friday. Gee Fred, your congratulations really weren't all that convincing. What's the matter?"

"Well, it's just… I thought they were going to announce the nominations next week."

"They're going to, but they reached out to the nominees already, because they needed to know… oh, oh my goodness," Jill's face fell, "I'm sorry Fred. I'm really sorry—god I can be so insensitive. You were probably in the running too?"

"Guilty as charged," Fred replied. "My third year in the running, in fact."

"It's probably just a political thing—gender balance, or something like that."

"Yeah, something like that. Anyway, I am more happy for you than down for me. Congratulations, Jill—you really deserved it."

"Thanks, Fred. Look, I'll see what I can find out about how the whole process worked. Whatever I can learn, I'll let you know next time we have lunch."

INTRODUCTION

The example that started this chapter illustrates several major dynamics associated with hiring decisions in health care. Health services positions tend to have high demands for specific skill sets; many professional positions go through periods of marked staffing shortages; and frontline positions, whose pay may not be competitive with other service industries, can suffer from high turnover as well as substantial numbers of poor-fit individuals in the applicant pool.

Modern personnel selection techniques provide a viable strategy for improving the quality and stability of the health care workforce within an organization, and while they do not provide a panacea for all staffing challenges (workforce-level shortages, in particular), they can often yield substantial benefits for the health care organizations that adopt them.

What defines effective personnel selection? A good working definition for our purposes is *the evidence-based process of systematically using information about positions and position candidates to make informed decisions about who is most likely to be successful in which roles.* Note that this definition includes all decisions related to considering people for positions, including internal transfers and promotions. It can also include traineeships and internal development programs, such as the LDP described in the opening vignette. Essentially, any process that has at its end a judgment about a person's fit for a future position can be considered a selection decision, one in which effective practices can help—and ineffective practices can hinder or even put the organization at risk.

Why Managers Use Formal Selection Approaches

There are few areas of HR research for which the evidence is as clear as this one: unstructured, informal approaches to making hiring decisions are *significantly* less effective than structured, formal approaches (Schmidt & Hunter, 1998; Weisner & Cronshaw, 1988). The case has been so strongly made in the research that one has to wonder why every manager has not adopted formal selection approaches, opting instead to continue with a less systematic approach. It may be because unstructured approaches tend to feel more natural—more like getting to know a new person, sizing them up to judge whether you would enjoy spending more time with them. The problem that arises is that almost anyone with the slightest degree of professional training will have mastered the basic etiquette of the interview process—they will have the basic social skills down—so what's left in an informal interview is an assessment of advanced social skills and little else. So in the end there is a trade-off in using more systematic approaches—especially at first, when the process can feel less natural, less intuitive. But for the managers willing to use them, and the organizations who adopt these approaches system-wide, the yield in terms of higher performance and improved retention can be substantial.

To best understand selection, however, it needs to be described in the context of the full staffing cycle, also known as the Talent Acquisition process.

THE TALENT ACQUISITION PROCESS

The overarching goal of the **Talent Acquisition Process** (sometimes also called Staffing) is to fill each open position with the best person possible. Often, the mission is distorted into just filling positions with *any* person, or, at least, a minimally qualified person. At the other extreme, positions can remain unfilled for too long because the hiring standards are too high. Recruiting and selection must be balanced

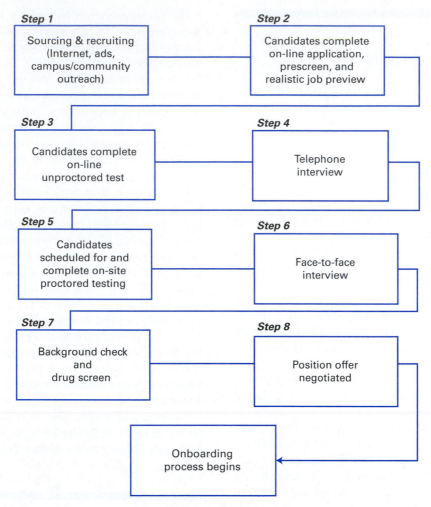

Figure 11.1. **Sample Best-In-Class Hiring Process**

SOURCE: Adapted from Russell (2007).

within an organization to have an effective talent acquisition process.

Consider the broad talent acquisition process shown in Figure 11.1. Each step feeds the one following and none can be considered in isolation from the others. All the various parts of the process are closely interrelated. There are aspects of recruiting and selection within each step of the process. Recognizing this will help executives design and better manage the overall talent acquisition processes.

Talent acquisition begins with sourcing and recruiting. While these topics were covered in detail in the previous chapter, it is sufficient to say here that strong sourcing and recruiting enables an organization to be more selective in the talent it hires. If both recruiting and selection are strong, the organization will have high-quality talent. If either is weak, it will face talent challenges such as unfilled positions and/or unqualified employees.

Alignment around the Position Description

Job analysis methods and outcomes were covered in Chapter 9 in detail. Thorough and accurate documentation of position activities and requirements is vital to the success of the talent acquisition process. The position description (also known as success profile or competency model) is the primary guide for designing each step in the talent acquisition process. Working backwards from **onboarding** will show not only how vital the position description is to process design, but also how interdependent the various steps are within the process. The process includes the following steps:

1. The onboarding process should include information about how new hires will be evaluated on the job—based on the position description. Training provided during the onboarding process will be tied to the specific knowledge needed for the job as well as how competencies that are required upon entry are demonstrated through everyday job activities.

2. Hiring decisions are made by determining which job candidate has the highest probability of successfully executing the activities described in the position description.

3. Various assessments (e.g., tests, interviews, reference and background checks) are designed or selected to measure candidates' profiles based on the competencies required upon entry to the job (i.e., will not be trained after hire). These competencies should be explicitly listed in the position description along with how they are demonstrated in the course of performing daily job activities. The best assessments will measure the relevant competencies while taking into account the context of how they are demonstrated on the job.

4. Recruiting and sourcing strategies are designed to contact individuals who have a high likelihood of possessing the competencies required for the job (thus increasing the likelihood that they will pass the selection steps

of the process). The best recruiters target their efforts based on the position description rather than simply getting the word out to everyone (many of whom will not be interested or qualified for the position).

It should be clear based on this explanation that the position description is the "glue" that ensures that the entire talent acquisition process works together cohesively. If all the phases of the process focus back on this description, everything will be aligned and successful. Conversely, misalignment around the position description will cause the talent acquisition process to fail, as well as promoting disagreement among the various stakeholders of the process.

Selection and Retention

Retention of talented staff is an ongoing challenge for many health care organizations—particularly for organizations in competitive markets and for positions that may be experiencing regional or national shortages. A substantial body of research has been conducted on the drivers of employee retention. While some factors affecting retention are outside the influence of the individual (e.g., pay, benefits, supervisor competence), many factors involve characteristics of individual employees and can be predicted using high-quality selection tools (Arthur, Jr., et al., 2006). Often, a selection system designed to predict on-the-job success will also have an indirect positive impact on both voluntary and involuntary turnover. Most "job fit" assessments fall into this category; they assess job-relevant competencies such as work orientation and teamwork and learning agility. Employees who are successful on the job will have more positive experiences on the job and, therefore, will stay with the company.

Often the most effective predictors of retention are these types of direct assessments that are specifically designed to predict tenure regardless of job. For example, Barrick and Zimmerman (2005) found several factors that can be measured during the selection step and are predictive of employee retention:

- Tenure at previous employers
- Having friends or family at the current employer
- Clear intention to quit after a short period of time
- Desire for the job
- Self-confidence
- Decisiveness

However, retention-focused **selection processes** do typically involve additional time, as well as cost. Assessment costs and candidate time should be weighed against the value of more highly qualified talent who stay with the company longer, which can be quite substantial. By one conservative estimate, turnover costs may represent 5% or more of a hospital's total operating budget (Waldman, et al., 2004).

LEGAL CONSIDERATIONS IN PERSONNEL SELECTION

Because selection decisions directly impact a candidate's ability to work and to earn a living, there is an ethical as well as a legal imperative to ensure that these decisions are fair and unbiased. Although biases in hiring are typically unintended (few hiring managers would say they consciously set out to make discriminatory hiring decisions), in the eyes of the courts it is the consequences rather than the intent that get organizations into trouble. In other words, ignorance of the law or of hiring practices will not shield an organization from legal trouble. Some of the laws and guidelines regulating hiring processes include:

- Title VII of the Civil Rights Act (CRA) of 1964, as amended in 1972; Tower Amendment to Title VII
- Age Discrimination in Employment Act of 1967 (ADEA)

- **Uniform Guidelines on Employee Selection Procedures**—1978
- Title I of the Civil Rights Act (CRA) of 1991
- Americans with Disabilities Act (ADA)—1990
- State and local employment laws
- Landmark cases setting legal precedents

We will touch on some of these briefly in this section, but it is advisable to have legal counsel participate in, or at least review, any personnel selection system to ensure it is legally defensible.

In general, all these laws and regulations are in place to prohibit **unfair discrimination** against **job applicants** in any protected group. Employers need to understand the difference between unfair and **fair discrimination.** Making personnel decisions based on job-relevant knowledge, skills, abilities, or other competencies is fair discrimination. The law has provided for companies to fairly discriminate between qualified and unqualified applicants in personnel decisions, based on the organization's business necessity to employ individuals who can successfully perform the job. Making personnel decisions based on gender, race, ethnicity, age, or **disability** is unfair discrimination, and opens an organization up to potential lawsuits.

Title VII of the Civil Rights Act of 1964 is landmark legislation that prohibits unfair discrimination in all terms and conditions of employment based on race, color, religion, sex, or national origin. The employment practices covered by this law include:

- Recruitment
- Transfer
- Performance appraisal
- Disciplinary action
- Hiring
- Training
- Compensation
- Termination
- Job classification
- Promotion
- Union or other membership
- Fringe benefits

The law applies to all employers having 15 or more employees, as well as employment agencies and labor unions. The Tower Amendment to Title VII specifically allows that workplace assessments can be used to make employment decisions. However, it stipulates that only assessments that do not discriminate against any protected group can be used.

The Age Discrimination in Employment Act of 1967 (ADEA) prohibits discrimination against employees or applicants who are age 40 and older. ADEA applies to companies with over 20 employees, but certain public safety positions are exempt, such as police, fire, and uniformed military personnel.

Uniform Guidelines on Employee Selection Procedures 1978 (UGESP) is a set of specific requirements governing the development, implementation, and use of assessments for employee selection. UGESP was developed jointly by the U.S. Equal Employment Opportunity Commission, the Civil Service Commission (now known as the Office of Personnel Management), the U.S. Department of Labor, and the U.S. Department of Justice to ensure consistency among the various federal agencies regulating employment practices. Adherence to the detailed guidance in the UGESP is absolutely critical when planning and administering the talent acquisition processes.

One of the most common principles outlined in the UGESP is **adverse impact.** It is unlawful to use any selection procedure that demonstrates adverse impact against a protected group, unless its use has been justified by a validation study. The simplest and most common way to determine if a selection procedure has adverse impact is the *80% rule* (also known as the *4/5ths rule*). Specifically, a selection process is said to violate the 80% rule if the pass rate for a specific protected group is less than 80% of the pass rate for the majority group. For example, say the pass rate for women is 75% and the pass rate for men is 85%. When you divide 75% by 85%, the result is a pass rate ratio of 0.88 (88%)—no adverse impact. If, on the other hand, the pass rate for women was 60%, the ratio would be 0.71, which is below the 80% threshold and indicative of adverse impact.

Many employment attorneys and statisticians have developed more sophisticated ways of identifying adverse impact (e.g., two standard deviation analysis) that have been upheld by the courts. Detailed explanation of these methods is beyond the scope of this text. However, it is important to know that an organization may be asked by federal enforcement agencies (e.g., EEOC, OFCCP) to conduct multiple types of analyses to review its selection procedures for adverse impact.

If an assessment tool demonstrates adverse impact, the organization does not necessarily have to stop using it. UGESP only states that where a total selection procedure shows adverse impact, the company must be able to produce documentation supporting the criterion-related, content, or construct validity, of each step in the selection process. The guidelines also detail which types of validity are most appropriate for different assessments as well as the standards for each type of validity evidence.

Specific recordkeeping requirements are described in the UGESP and were updated in 2004 and 2005 by the federal Government (U.S. Department of Labor, 2005). Specifically, employers with more than 100 employees must maintain information showing whether or not the overall talent acquisition process has adverse impact on any job in the organization. Adverse impact must be calculated for each group listed on the Federal EEO-1 report. These rules require organizations to gather and maintain records on all "applicants" (as defined by the federal government). The recordkeeping requirements were revised to reflect the popularity of using the Internet for hiring purposes. Given the relative fluidity of how applicants search for jobs and how recruiters search for resumes on job boards, the definition of an applicant was revised to include four specific criteria:

1. A job seeker makes an expression of interest in the job, following the company's standard procedures (e.g., posts resume for a specific job opening)

2. The organization considers the individual for a particular position (i.e., a specific opening)

3. Information provided in the expression of interest indicates that the individual possesses the basic qualifications for the position

4. The individual does not remove himself or herself from consideration

In addition, companies are required to keep records on the disposition (hired or not hired) of all applicants meeting these four criteria.

Americans with Disabilities Act (ADA) of 1990 prohibits discrimination in employment decisions based on an individual's disability status. ADA introduced four new concepts that must be considered when making any sort of employment decision: disability, **reasonable accommodation, essential job function,** and **undue hardship.**

A *disability* is defined broadly to include any physical or mental impairment that substantially limits one or more of an individual's major life activities, such as caring for himself or herself, walking, talking, hearing, or seeing (U.S. Department of Labor, 2000). Examples of disabilities include visual or hearing impairments, mobility impairments, alcoholism, cancer, AIDS/HIV, and mental illness.

Individuals with disabilities may request a reasonable accommodation to be able to perform the essential functions of the job. An essential job function is a primary work activity that is necessary to perform the job. To be defined as an essential job function the activity usually must be (1) performed by every employee holding that specific job title; (2) performed frequently, relative to other job activities; and (3) critical to accomplishing the goal of the job. A reasonable accommodation can be any type of modification to enable the individual to perform the job. Examples of reasonable accommodations include schedule modifications, improving work location accessibility, or providing specialized equipment. Finally, companies can elect not to accommodate a disability if the requested accommodation imposes an undue hardship on the organization. Claims of undue hardship may be based on unrealistic financial investment, number of employees insufficient to share job activities, safety of overall workforce, or significant impact on production or quality.

Applicants must make a request of the company to make reasonable accommodations during the talent acquisition process. It is a good practice to ask applicants if they need accommodation to be able to complete the hiring process only (asking for notice of accommodations to be able to complete job activities at this stage would be a violation of ADA). The company can make determinations on a case-by-case basis about these accommodation requests. A good rule of thumb when considering requests for reasonable accommodation in the selection process is to accommodate in the selection process the same ways the company provides accommodation for the job in question.

Another important impact of ADA is that medical examinations or inquiries prior to making a job offer are expressly prohibited. The company may require a medical examination of employees only when the information gathered is job relevant and a business necessity. It is important to note here, also, that some psychological assessments were designed to be used in the mental health setting rather than for employee selection. Using one of these assessments (e.g., a Minnesota Multiphasic Personality Inventory (MMPI) or a clinically-focused interview with a psychologist or psychiatrist) puts the organization at risk for claims under ADA, as well as invasion of privacy laws.

ASSESSMENT OF RELIABILITY AND VALIDITY

Reliability and validity are the two primary properties used to determine the quality and usefulness of selection tests. Both dimensions are measured using common statistical tests; professional test developers will typically have analyses of reliability and validity available upon request. Reliability and validity are the most important factors to consider when evaluating the appropriateness of an assessment for a specific application.

Reliability

If a person takes the assessment again or is interviewed by a different interviewer using the same guide, will he or she get a similar score or a much different score? Reliability is a measure of the extent to which a test can be expected to yield dependable and repeatable results for candidates. For organizations with multiple locations, reliability is particularly important for ensuring consistent standards across the enterprise.

The statistical property of a test that is used to determine reliability is called a *reliability coefficient.* This statistic ranges between 0.0 and 1.0, with higher numbers indicating a more reliable test. Most tests demonstrate reliability between 0.60 and 0.97 (a perfect reliability of 1.00 is extremely rare). Reliabilities over 0.80 are typically considered to be good; reliabilities between 0.70 and 0.80 are considered acceptable (U.S. Department of Labor, 2000). Assessments with a reliability coefficient below 0.70 may have limited applicability. Test developers, publishers, and consultants should be able to report the reliability of their assessment test.

Interviews, assessment centers, and other assessments involving ratings have a statistical property called **inter-rater reliability** (sometimes called *inter-rater agreement*). This statistic measures the amount of agreement among the various raters involved in the assessment. Because inter-rater agreement is affected not only by the quality of the assessment tools but also by the effectiveness of the raters, it can only be calculated after an assessment has been implemented and data are available from the raters' judgments. One important way to improve rater quality is through training.

Validity

Validity is the most important characteristic of any assessment. Validity measures how effectively an assessment measures the competency it is intended to measure. Although the terms validity and validation are used commonly within human resources,

they have very specific technical and legal meanings when applied to assessments.

An assessment is valid if it measures a characteristic that is job relevant (i.e., necessary for successful job performance). Assessment results are meaningful and useful only if they are valid. If an assessment is valid, its results will be predictive of success on the job. There are three ways test developers demonstrate validity:

- **Criterion-related validity** is the statistical relationship between assessment results and actual on-the-job performance. In other words, individuals who score higher on the assessment generally perform better on the job. Typically, criterion-related validity is demonstrated using a statistical correlation between the assessment score and some measure of job performance.

- **Content validity** means that the content of the assessment is relevant to the content of the job. For example, if data entry is required for the job, a data entry assessment would be content valid. Content validity is usually demonstrated by documenting the judgments of subject matter experts who have been asked to determine if the content of the assessment is an effective measurement of a job-relevant competency.

- **Construct validity** encompasses both criterion-related validity and content validity and is generally the demonstration that the assessment measures the characteristic that it purports to measure and that that characteristic is relevant to job performance.

There is another validity construct that is also worth mentioning here: *face validity.* Face validity is simply the extent to which a test appears—on the face of it—to be job relevant. Face validity is not a technical basis of validity or a basis for legal defensibility; however, it may actually be one of the most important types of validity in applied settings. Tests that are face valid are more widely accepted by internal stakeholders (e.g., hiring managers, recruiters); their use is also far less likely to be challenged on legal grounds in the first place.

APPROACHES TO SELECTION

In the last section, we described how selection tests are evaluated. We now turn to a consideration of some of the major types of selection assessments in use today.

Prescreens

Prescreening questions (also called "knock out" questions) can be another effective step in the talent acquisition process. Questions typically used as prescreens include:

- Legally required certifications
- Willingness to complete required background and drug screens
- Willingness to perform essential job functions
- Willingness to work required shifts
- Minimum education requirement
- Minimum experience requirement

Companies must be careful to include only validated, job-relevant content in prescreens. Educational requirements, job experience, and skill requirements must be validated to ensure both usefulness and legal defensibility. In addition, willingness and ability to perform essential job function questions must meet all the requirements described above for essential job functions. Prescreening questions are typically validated using a content validation approach.

Incorporating job-relevant and objective prescreens will select out individuals who do not possess the minimum qualifications and will greatly increase the efficiency of the hiring process. For example, a short questionnaire incorporating only objective job requirements and willingness to perform essential job functions will often eliminate 10 to 25% of those expressing interest in the position who do not meet minimum qualifications for the job.

Realistic Job Previews

Realistic job previews (RJPs) are an important part of an organization's talent acquisition process and are included in this chapter because they can be an effective selection tool. RJPs are oriented toward giving the candidate the full picture of the job in both work activities and job context. They focus on helping candidates really understand the kind of position they would be taking on, the work environment in which they would spend their days or nights, and the essence of the company's culture. Essentially, RJPs tell candidates "what it's like to work here and do this job." Marketing and recruitment pieces focus much more on just the positive aspects of the job and organization. They are intended to help with the critical need to generate quality applicant flow. But once that step has been accomplished, the immediate need is to engage candidates in the screening process by explaining to them both the perceived positives and the negatives of the job. This is where RJPs contribute to self-screening and to improvements in selection process efficiency and effectiveness (McEvoy & Cascio, 1985; Phillips, 1998).

Realistic job previews can be as sophisticated as Web-based, interactive programs that incorporate multimedia clips or as low-tech as written highlights or "talking points" for recruiters or hiring managers. Some companies even provide tours or job "tryouts." The best RJPs incorporate information from job incumbents in their own words as well as information from HR and business leaders.

RJPs are most often used to reduce organizational turnover by helping job candidates gain a better understanding of the job. However, RJPs also have added benefits in making the talent acquisition process more efficient and enhancing the organization's employment brand. When RJPs are implemented at the beginning of the talent acquisition process (e.g., during recruiting), candidates can self-select out of the process earlier—saving the trouble of processing uninterested applicants.

Interviews

Interviews are the most commonly used assessment in talent acquisition processes. At a high level, most job interviews last between 30 and 120 minutes. The number of questions included in the interview can vary widely depending on the type of question. Interviews can be conducted face to face or over the phone and typically include:

- *Opening*—building rapport and explaining the interviewing process
- *Questions and Answers*—eliciting job-relevant information from the candidate
- *Closing*—selling the candidate on the position and answering the candidate's questions about the job, the organization, and the talent acquisition process
- *Evaluation*—after the candidate leaves, making judgments about the candidate's responses

There are two general types of interviews in use today to evaluate job applicants. Unstructured interviews are typically not consistent across candidates applying for the same job or across interviewers and include questions that may not be job relevant, not predictive of job performance, and carry a high degree of legal risk. Structured interviews are consistent, reliable across interviewers and job candidates, predictive of job performance, and utilize legally defensible methods to assess candidates' competencies. In addition, structured interviewing makes it easier for interviewers to conduct interviews and evaluate candidates.

A structured interview approach:

- evaluates the candidate on criteria that are important to success on the job
- eliminates redundancy, overlap, and potentially illegal questions
- treats all candidates fairly by being systematic, consistent, and uniform

Further, good structured-interview questions include lead questions, probing questions, and rating scales with specific behavioral examples. Lead questions are open-ended, do not signal a correct answer, and elicit a detailed response. Probing questions request additional detail, are also open ended, and usually begin with who, what, where, when, how, why, or explain. Specific behavioral examples are used to help the interviewer evaluate the skill level of the candidate's response. Figures 11.1 and 11.2 are examples of structured interview questions.

Within structured interviews, there are behavioral and situational interviews. Behavioral interviews, also called *experience-based* interviews (Garman & Lesowitz, 2006), ask the candidate to describe what he or she has done (or failed to do) in a given past situation. Behavioral interviews focus on using past behavior as a predictor of future behavior. Focusing on past behavior can make the interview more valid, reliable, and legally defensible. Example behavioral interview questions are provided in Figure 11.2. When conducting a behavioral interview, the interviewer should be looking for a complete behavioral example of how the candidate addressed a situation relevant to the question. A good way to remember this is "Take CARE," as illustrated below (Aon Consulting, 2007):

- *Circumstance*—the event, activity, or situation
- *Action*—specifically how the candidate responded
- *Results*—impact (effective or ineffective) of the candidate's action
- *Evaluation*—compared to the examples provided, how well the candidate's response demonstrates the target competency

In addition to the principles of CARE, keep in mind that behavioral evidence is usually provided when the candidate:

- speaks in the first person and uses past tense
- speaks confidently
- shows behavior that is clearly consistent with other known facts
- provides enough detail to fully explain answers

Focusing on job-relevant information and clarifying facts reduces misunderstanding of information.

CUSTOMER FOCUS	
LEAD QUESTION Describe a time when it was particularly important for you to build a strong relationship with an internal or external customer. **NOTES**	**SUGGESTED PROBES** • How did you build this relationship? • Has this developed into a long-term relationship? • Why was it important to build a strong relationship with this customer? • What was the result?

Specific Examples	Rating (Circle One)
Creates and maintains strong relationships with customers Sees all customers as individuals with unique/specialized needs Appears highly committed to customer satisfaction even when it is convenient or difficult Anticipates and successfully fulfills customer needs; persists until customer is fully satisfied	Outstanding
Creates some strong relationships with customers Generally sees some customers as individuals with unique/specialized needs Appears committed to customer satisfaction Responds quickly to customer requests	Acceptable
Does not create strong relationships with customers Does not see customers as individuals with unique/specialized needs Does not appear to be committed to customer satisfaction Does not appear value to the customer; fulfills only the most basic and urgent customer demands	Less Than Acceptable

Copyright 2007 Aon Consulting—Used with permission.

Figure 11.2. Example Behavioral Interview Question

In addition, probing for behavior discourages candidate "faking." Behavioral evidence provides a clearer picture of the candidate's skills and abilities, and looking for "factual" behavior minimizes the impact of interviewer bias.

In contrast to behavioral interviews, *situational interviews* ask the candidate to state what he or she would do if put in a given situation. While not quite as effective as behavioral interviews

(Taylor & Small, 2002), well-designed situational interviews have been found to be valid and legally defensible, particularly for positions of lower complexity (Huffcutt, et al., 2004). Situational interviews are the most useful when the applicant pool includes a majority of candidates with little or no previous job experience. Examples of situational interview questions are provided in Figure 11.3. The structure of the candidate's

COMMUNICATION	
LEAD QUESTION You have been given the assignment of presenting a new technical procedure to two audiences—one technically-oriented and the other one non-technical. How would you prepare for these two presentations? **NOTES**	**SUGGESTED PROBES** • Which audience will be more difficult to communication your ideas to? • What would you do differently in each? • Which would be more difficult for you? • What presentation format would you use for each group? • What media would you use for each group?

Specific Examples	Rating (Circle One)
Relays information at a high level of proficiency across contexts Presents complicated or technical information in an organized and articulate manner Organizes information into the most simple intuitive format to facilitate understanding Uses the most concise style/terminology possible given the subject matter to be communicated	Outstanding
Presents information clearly and concisely Typically uses the simplest terminology possible Creates and follows a general outline or structure for formal communications Acknowledges audience characteristics and adjusts style accordingly	Acceptable
Fails to successfully get points across Presents information in a confusing way Relies excessively on complex terms and/or lengthy sentence structure Ignores audience needs/characteristics in determining presentation style	Less Than Acceptable

Copyright 2007 Aon Consulting—Used with permission.

Figure 11.3. Example Situational Interview Question

response is similar to that elicited with a behavioral question; the main difference is that the candidate is asked what they "would do" in a given situation, rather than what they "have done" in the past. As with other types of interview questions, it is important to probe for additional details to ensure that the candidate thinks through the possible actions and realistic outcomes to the hypothetical situation.

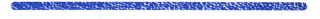

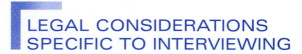

LEGAL CONSIDERATIONS SPECIFIC TO INTERVIEWING

Like all assessments used for employee selection, interview questions must be tied back to the competencies required for successful job performance.

When writing or choosing interview questions, it is important to ensure that only job-relevant questions are included in the guide. In practice, professionally developed interview guides are typically validated using a content validation approach by having subject-matter experts review the interview content and make ratings endorsing its relevance to the job.

The legal risks of interviews increase when organizations do not use professionally developed structured interviews or when interviewers stray from the approved interview content. Interviewers can stray into risky areas just by making small talk. In addition, interviewers often ask illegal questions when making assumptions about the candidate's ability to meet job requirements based on his or her age, sex, ethnicity, religion, or other status. Examples of such questions include:

- Are you and your husband (or wife) planning on having children?
- Do you have reliable childcare?
- Do you have a car?
- Would working on Saturdays interfere with your religion?
- What is your native language?
- Do you have any friends or family members who work here now?
- What are your hobbies?

The goal of the interview is to understand if the candidate will be able to meet the requirements of the job. Asking job-relevant questions is good—as long as they do not include presumptions. For example, an interviewer should ask if the candidate can get to work on time rather than asking if he or she has a car. The best rule of thumb is: If you aren't sure that the question is job related, don't ask it!

Selection Tests

Selection tests come in a myriad of formats. There is a wide variety of selection tests available for purchase from specialized test developers, and organizations also have the option of creating customized assessments for unique applications. However, proper test selection and implementation can be tricky, requiring a great deal of specialized knowledge and judgment, as well as knowledge of the legal considerations. Administration and interpretation of some kinds of tests also requires specialized training, education, or experience.

In general, tests can be broken down into categories by what they measure and how they measure it:

- *Cognitive ability* or *mental ability tests* are among the most effective (i.e., reliable and valid) tests available (Schmidt & Hunter, 1998). They are also sometimes called intelligence tests. These tests may measure general mental ability or specific facets of mental ability such as math, reading, or spatial ability. Although these tests are among the most useful, they also tend to demonstrate adverse impact when used alone.

- *Personality tests* are also commonly used for selection today, but are more typically called "behavioral," "fit," "profile," or "potential" tests due to the social stigma associated with personality testing. Most personality tests designed for use in selection settings focus on facets such as achievement orientation, conscientiousness, dependability, teamwork/agreeableness, persuasiveness, and stress tolerance. Personality assessments can be moderately to highly predictive of job performance and are often particularly effective when used in conjunction with cognitive ability assessments, since the two measure such different constructs. However, executives need to be careful to only use personality tests designed for employment settings; use of clinical personality tests is likely to run afoul of ADA and privacy laws.

- *Biodata inventories* or *biographical data questionnaires* ask candidates about job-relevant experiences in a multiple-choice, rather than interview, format. Example questions might include number of extracurricular activities pursued in high school or average time spent studying per week. Like behavioral interviews, biodata inventories are based on the principle that past performance is the best predictor of future performance. Well-constructed biodata inventories have been shown to be very effective predictors of job performance (Bliesener, 1996), particularly when they emphasize independently verifiable information (Harold, McFarland, & Weekley, 2006) and focus specifically on those competencies relevant to job performance (e.g., Schmidt, Ones, & Hunter, 1992). Depending on the construction of the biodata inventory, the test may actually measure constructs very similar to what is measured on a personality assessment except the items "look" very different to the test taker.

- *Honesty* or *integrity tests* are a specific type of personality test, but are generally called out separately by test users and vendors. When polygraph testing was banned in 1988, employers sought a legal option to assess candidate honesty. These tests are particularly widely used in retail or other settings where employees handle cash or financial and other highly sensitive information. *Overt* or *objective* integrity tests include transparent questions concerning the candidate's attitudes toward and involvement in illegal activities. *Personality-based* integrity tests are more subtle in nature and are used to predict a broader range of counterproductive behaviors (e.g., absenteeism, turnover, breaking rules). Honesty tests have not been as successful in predicting overall job performance as some of the other types of tests discussed in this chapter. It is particularly difficult to demonstrate criterion-related validity or return on investment for these tests due to the relatively low occurrence rate of employee theft in the health care industry. Caution should be used when considering honesty testing given the tests' mediocre utility and narrow applicability.

- *Situational judgment tests* include questions that ask the candidate to choose the most appropriate response to a given situation from among a number of alternatives. Some tests ask the candidate to rate the effectiveness of or prioritize the responses to the given situation or to select the "best" and "worst" choices concerning how to handle a given situation. If the situations posed to the candidate are realistic and job relevant, a situational judgment test can also act as a type of realistic job preview. Well-constructed situational judgment tests are typically moderately to highly predictive of job performance, but tend to have lower reliabilities than other types of tests discussed in this chapter.

- *Knowledge tests* are usually customized for a particular job within the organization or industry and measure how much the candidate knows about a particular content domain. Knowledge tests usually have a very narrow application and are often very good predictors of job performance in the specific domains they assess. A nurse licensing test is a good example of a knowledge test.

Most commercially available tests will have reliability statistics and criterion-related validity evidence documented and available. Many tests also have return-on-investment results available from criterion-related validity studies conducted with objective measures. Remember also to consider the face validity of the test. When weighing these various pieces of information about a test, criterion-related validity against objective metrics should be given the highest importance followed by other criterion-related validity evidence, reliability, and face validity. All these factors are important, but tangible outcomes are paramount.

Reference Checks

Reference checking involves someone in the hiring organization, usually either a recruiter or the hiring manager, contacting individuals that a candidate has worked with previously for information about how effectively they have performed in the past.

Although reference checks are widely used, particularly for candidates of leadership positions, the usefulness of reference checks is under a great deal of debate today by experts in talent acquisition (Mullich, 2007). Some say that references are the best source of information about the candidate, while others say that the little information gathered is not worth the effort. Many are concerned that those contacted for a reference will not provide any detailed information out of fear of being sued by the candidate. Others believe that references only provide positive information because they may have been previously coached by the candidate. Since in most cases candidates are the ones who identify their own references, there is also an inevitable self-selection bias, in which candidates will tend to "nominate" those most likely to have had favorable experiences with them in the past.

Regardless of the ultimate usefulness of reference checks, we do know that the threat of verifying education, employment, and past behaviors will typically cause applicants to be more honest during earlier phases of the process (Mabe & West, 1982). In addition, checking references can reduce the risk of lawsuits based on negligent hiring (U.S. Department of Labor, 2000).

Simulations

Simulations include any assessment techniques in which candidates are placed in a situation analogous to what they might face on the job, and their responses are recorded for evaluation. (In fact, "situational judgment tests," discussed earlier, are considered a form of "low-fidelity" simulation (Motowidlo, Dunnette, & Carter, 1990).

Simulations are becoming more popular today as companies are finding ways to deliver simulations more efficiently. Simulations provide, perhaps, the best combination of realism and prediction among all potential selection assessments. Specifically, well-designed, job-relevant simulations offer:

- Realistic job preview
- Excellent face validity
- Strong prediction of future job success
- Broad competency coverage in a single assessment

Simulation assessments come in a variety of formats, including Web-based job simulations, work samples or job tryouts, role plays, group activities, and in-baskets (paper-based exercises simulating job-relevant paperwork). Assessment centers are a specific type of simulation that combine several different assessments (often an in-basket, role plays, and group activity) together in a face-to-face session.

Of the various types of assessments discussed in this chapter, simulations tend to be the most resource intensive, and as such tend to be used primarily with particularly high-stakes hiring decisions. One challenge with simulations is having enough properly trained assessors available to administer an in-person process. Often companies elect to outsource administration and assessment of simulations. Simulations requiring in-person human assessors (as opposed to telephonic or computerized simulations) may cost the organizations thousands of dollars per candidate. Therefore, remote simulations using the Internet or telephone simulations have become very popular.

EVALUATING ASSESSMENT TOOLS

Daniel (2005) estimated that there are over 2,500 commercially available selection tests on the market. Unfortunately, in practice many organizations make buying decisions with no more research than performing an Internet search on "employment testing." Misuse of tests is frequent, and the ability to administer tests over the Internet has seemed to add an unwelcome air of legitimacy to tests published by irreputable vendors. Despite all the warnings, policies, and legal guidelines, unqualified hiring managers and human resource (HR) staff continue to be able to purchase, administer, and attempt to interpret psychological assessments of varying quality.

Several large organizations have recently seen their inappropriate use of tests successfully challenged in court (Heller, 2005). For example, multiple organizations have lost lawsuits based on their use of clinical assessments (e.g., MMPI) in employment settings. Other organizations have lost lawsuits by implementing cognitive assessments (without validation evidence) that resulted in adverse impact. Ultimately, the use of any assessment without evidence of job relevance is risky. Although actual lawsuits are rare, federal regulatory agencies (e.g., OFCCP, EEOC) are becoming more aggressive in their enforcement of guidelines and regulations around employment testing.

The inappropriate use of assessments and the use of low-quality assessments seem like obvious problems to avoid. However, salesperson claims of large returns on investment and other testimonials and compelling case studies can seem like reliable evidence to unsophisticated buyers. Executives need to know how to evaluate which assessments are best for their organization.

Confirming Validity and Reliability

In considering the use of selection tools, *demonstrated validity* is the most important factor to keep in mind. Test vendors should be able to report how their test has predicted job-relevant criteria in the past, such as supervisory ratings of performance, absenteeism, turnover, or objective performance data unique to the organization or industry. Reputable vendors will supply this information to you readily; if they cannot, consider it a red flag.

Criterion-related validity is usually reported as the validity coefficient (r) and ranges between 0 and 1.00. Validity coefficients typically range between 0.20 and 0.35 and are rarely higher than 0.40 for a single test. Tests with validity coefficients below 0.11 are unlikely to be useful, coefficients between 0.11 and 0.20 are questionable, and coefficients above 0.20 are likely to be valuable. (Coefficients that are quite a bit higher than 0.40 may also be suspect.)

Criterion-related validity using objective ratings is often reported as "return on investment" outcomes showing how the test can yield financial returns through increased production and quality or decreased cost of turnover. This information may

also be reported as validity coefficients, or it may be translated into dollar savings. Both should be reviewed to determine the potential impact of the test (from the validity coefficient) as well as the practical value of that impact (from the financial analysis).

Reliability analyses of tests should also be reviewed prior to purchase. While reliability is an important piece of data to consider, most practically minded test experts will suggest weighing validity evidence over reliability. As cited earlier, a reliability coefficient above 0.70 is typically acceptable, and above 0.80 is good. Unlike validity, where "higher is always better," the 0.80 threshold can be considered a ceiling on yield; in other words, an unusually high reliability (e.g., 0.96) will not necessarily mean it is a more valuable test.

Ongoing Monitoring

After implementation, it is important to monitor the performance of the assessment periodically. Most organizations will monitor pass rates and adverse impact ratios on a quarterly to annual basis. However, most never assess the validity or utility of the assessment after it is launched. Best-in-class organizations track assessment return on investment by correlating assessment scores with key business metrics. Typically, companies conduct these studies annually by pulling performance indicators for employees hired since the assessment was implemented. Turnover is one popular metric to monitor and is applicable to nearly every organization. Other metrics specific to health care settings include training outcomes, patient satisfaction scores, reduced waste, and employee satisfaction (that is, satisfaction of the employees within a manager's work unit correlated with the manager's assessment scores). If your organization includes a call center, these systems can offer an abundance of metrics. For example, average handle time, first-call resolution, and call-monitoring ratings are common measures used to validate assessments on a continuous basis. Most of these metrics can be translated into bottom-line results showing real business impact of the assessment.

Managing a Successful Assessment Implementation Project

For hospitals and health care organizations, like most other types of organizations, it is more efficient to "buy" rather than "make" selection systems. Designing and implementing talent acquisition processes involve large-scale technology projects that usually require significant changes in management efforts. Current users may be reluctant to change the way they are doing their jobs, and various stakeholders may have conflicting opinions about the optimal solution. Even more basic than this is simply the need to understand organizational capabilities from a human, IT, and financial perspective. The successful project leader will have a good understanding of these constraints and will strike a careful balance among them in designing the new process.

For example, a large multinational company initiated a project to develop and implement a new web-based recruiting and staffing system. While there was a clearly defined need to develop improved assessments (e.g., prescreens, tests, and interviews), the technology aspects of the project began to take precedence over assessment development and had not been communicated to other project stakeholders. As the project entered the pilot phase, the project team discovered that there was no Internet access at any of the locations slated for participation! Ultimately, the vast majority of the company's locations did not have reliable Internet access and the system's users were not at all comfortable with computers or the Internet. The company's recruiting team was also not involved during the process and system design phases of the project. Recruiters were first exposed to the system during a vendor-led training workshop. Within six months of launch of the pilot, the technology solution was discontinued due to recruiter dissatisfaction.

Careful planning and talent acquisition process design are critical for ensuring a successful implementation of a project. Before issuing a request for proposals/information or engaging internal resources to begin developing a solution, it is important for the organization to clearly and completely define the scope of the project, as well as the corporate and selection-specific goals it is intended to support. Often an outside consultant is contracted for assistance at this stage, to help define the problem or simply to cut through internal politics to get an objective viewpoint of the problem and project goals. Project team members should plan to spend considerable effort gathering information and system requirements from key stakeholders. The project leaders should begin by (1) describing the organization's current hiring processes in detail; (2) seeking to understand what is and is not working, along with what portions of the process are and are not regularly adhered to; (3) gathering data about the current and future environment of the user population; and (4) defining success for the project.

By considering issues such as technology changes that may be required and future business challenges, leadership will be in the best position to design a process that will meet its current needs while keeping in mind potential growth and other organizational changes. Internal and external change agents will be forced to challenge assumptions about how things have been done in the past and if things can change in the future. Armed with this information about the current state of affairs and potential near-term changes, the organization can construct revised process maps including the new assessment solutions. It is important to circulate these new processes in order to get feedback and buy-in from all key stakeholders. Often, input from end users will uncover a flaw in the initial design that can be corrected before it becomes a costly mistake.

SPECIAL CASES IN SELECTION

Although most of the content of this chapter has applicability across positions of all types in the health care industry, two position types—physicians and executives—typically involve a substantial number of additional steps and considerations.

Physician Selection

Although all of the above considerations typically apply also to physicians, in private-sector settings the selection process is both advantaged and complicated by the opportunity to analyze the net contribution of a physician's practice to the fiscal health of the organization. Physician recruits also typically involve a significant investment on the part of the organization in establishing the practice itself, and as such can involve a significant financial risk. Hiring of physicians thus overlaps the business planning function in a very direct way. The following illustration, "Hiring Physicians at Rush University Medical Center," provides an example of physician-recruiting practices in a large academic medical center.

 Hiring physicians at Rush University Medical Center

Much of the focus of selection involves identifying the right person for a role that has already been created. In some circumstances, however, the position specification and the selection process are tightly intertwined. This is often the case when academic medical centers hire new physician faculty. While every hiring decision an organization makes is an investment decision, physician recruits in particular can involve very substantial investments in order to support the institutional goals the hire is intended to fulfill. Given the high-stakes nature of these hiring decisions, some academic medical centers have moved toward maintaining more formal decision-support processes to aid in their effective execution.

Rush University Medical Center, in Chicago, recently went to such a model. Historically, department chairs, in collaboration with the dean, bore ultimate responsibility for all aspects of physician recruiting, hiring, and onboarding. Through process-improvement discussions, the senior leadership of the medical group (Brian Smith and Armen Gallucci) determined that by developing a more systematic review process, one with a greater breadth of accountability to the stakeholders and greater depth of financial pro forma analysis, they could provide the dean as well as the department chairs with more useful support prior to hiring

decisions being made. Such a business review process could not only assist the medical center in making more informed selection decisions, it could also provide more accurate projections concerning patient volume and associated revenues.

The approach they developed starts with a department chair, who makes or concurs with an initial decision that a new physician faculty member is needed. The chairperson and/or his or her staff then communicates this need to the Recruitment Work Group (RWG), utilizing the "Intent to Recruit & Hire Form" the group developed. The RWG reviews the form, along with initial pro formas, hospital financials, and the like. Although the request could be accepted based on the strength of the initial application, like most external review processes the RWG often identifies complexities not initially seen by the originator of the request. Additional data (e.g., market data, hospital financials) may need to be identified, and original assumptions may need revision. With additional data and review, if the hire makes sense to the RWG committee, the application will be reviewed by the full Executive Recruitment Committee (ERC), who will make the final determination regarding whether the position will be approved. Membership of the ERC includes the Provost, the Senior VP of the Medical Center, as well as three additional physician leaders and

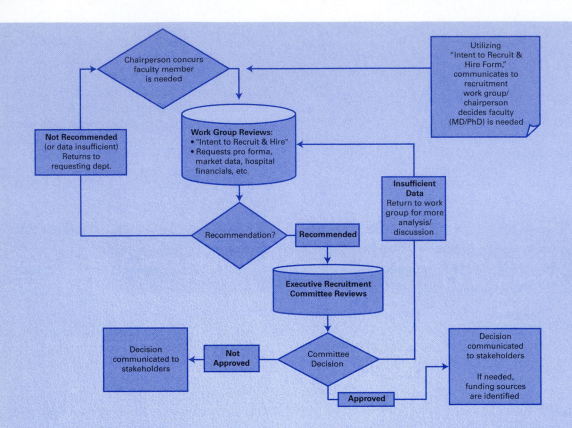

seven administrative leaders; as a group they are in the ideal position to review proposed hires in terms of how they will support the organization's mission, vision, and corporate goals. If the ERC approves, the selection function of the committee changes to a recruiting and onboarding function; the goals, similarly, change from vetting to supporting efficient execution of the recruitment and a smooth start-up process.

Evaluation

For the new approach to be successful, Smith and Galluci recognized that it would need to provide useful decision support but also be sensitive to the complicated timing associated with many recruitment decisions. They have been able to serve both goals by pursuing a clear understanding of the time parameters associated with recruitment proposals, by continually streamlining the process (for example, by moving toward electronic proposal systems), and by adding additional resources as needed. They also recently created and filled a Director of Physician Recruiting role to provide a higher level of ongoing support to the process as more volume began coming through it.

In shifting away from a model in which department chairs needed to autonomously make their own hiring decisions, the approach has so far been well received, as evidenced by the ongoing support of the medical school dean.

Executive Selection

In general, as managers reach higher organizational levels, technical competencies provide less power in predicting high performance (Freedman, 1998). In health care settings in particular, success at higher levels begins to depend much more on behavioral and other leadership competencies, such as building trust and communicating a compelling vision (Garman, Tyler, & Darnall, 2004). As such, selections for executive levels tend to favor candidates with a combination of successful experience in similar roles in the past, as well as an assessment of the candidate's leadership style and/or interpersonal skills (Garman & Tyler, 2007).

Candidate source (within the organization vs. outside vs. a combination) is also an important dynamic in executive-selection decisions. Internal candidates may have a substantial advantage in the extent to which they have already forged important relationships with key people within the organization; conversely, they may have a more difficult time taking the organization in a different direction if that is what is called for. However, although external candidates may come in to a position without the burden of this history, they still carry the burden of "proving themselves," needing to establish relationships of trust with others who will be essential to their success in their new roles.

Executive-selection decisions also tend to be highly politicized processes, which can make an objective determination of what is best for the organization very difficult at best. For this reason, many organizations will involve multiple decision-makers in the selection decision, including at least one individual who will not be working directly with or for the person being hired. Also, there is some evidence to suggest that having more decision makers involved improves the perceived effectiveness of the selection process (Garman & Tyler, 2007).

External consultants are often used to provide a more objective assessment of a candidate's qualifications and competencies. Executive search consultants, who are often also involved in the sourcing of candidates, often provide a preliminary assessment of strengths and limitations of the candidates they refer; consulting psychologists may also be used to develop a more comprehensive assessment of individual candidates.

Reference checks can be a particularly important part of the leadership-selection processes (e.g., Prien, Schippman, & Prien, 2003); unfortunately, in practice this step is often either neglected or poorly executed. It can be difficult to get good-quality reference information about candidates; some employees are counseled to limit evaluative comments about prior employees for fear of lawsuit. However, there are methods which can ameliorate these concerns and yield higher-quality responses (e.g., Smart, 1999; Taylor, et al., 2004), which are worth the trouble to pursue.

Larger health care organizations and health care systems may have internal leadership development programs that, in addition to providing developmental opportunities for their leadership personnel, can also serve as a valuable source of performance data to inform selection decisions. A recent survey of U.S. hospital systems found that performance in internal leadership development/talent management programs was the most frequently used formal method for selecting senior executives (Garman & Tyler, 2006), followed by interviews, assessment centers, and peer nomination, in that order.

ONBOARDING

So far in this chapter we have been discussing effective approaches to selection; however, there are also important steps for managers to take after they have selected a candidate and the candidate has accepted an offer. The process of helping new hires to reach their optimal productivity, often called "onboarding," can make a big difference in how quickly a person acclimates—or even to their ultimate success in the role.

One of the most common forms of onboarding is to provide an initial structured training program, often of short duration, which is typically referred to as an "orientation." In hospitals and other health care settings, a standard orientation is provided to all or almost all new employees. Such an orientation may cover mandatory training modules (e.g., OHSA, HIPAA) as well as rudimentary overviews of topics such as parking and employee benefits.

It is easy to underestimate the amount of new learning associated with taking a new position in a new organization, and, unfortunately, in some organizations the onboarding process does not extend far beyond these initial steps. Since it is sometimes easiest to see the value of effective onboarding by considering what *poor* onboarding looks like, an example is provided in the following illustration, "Diary of a troubled onboarding process."

⚜ Diary of a troubled onboarding process

Imagine, for a minute, that you were offered a practice management position in a prestigious academic medical center. You excitedly accept, and within two weeks you receive a letter indicating your orientation date.

The day of your orientation comes. You spend most of the day in perfunctory training sessions. You realize that the sessions are a necessary part of working in a hospital, but you question the value of using this valuable face-to-face time in sessions of this type (your last employer, a small community hospital, had offered similar sessions in an at-your-own-pace e-learning format). You then receive a voucher for lunch in the hospital cafeteria. Some people you were sitting with in the morning invite you to sit with them during lunch; you instead elect to see if you can reach your new manager to touch base. You call him on your cellphone, but you get his voicemail. You wait a few minutes to see if he will call back; when he doesn't, you return to the cafeteria, which now has a line going out the door.

After lunch, you return to the orientation room for several sessions about benefits. The sessions contain several unpleasant surprises. For one, you learn that there are no employee parking spaces left on the campus. You can rent one that is a "relatively short walk" away, but you will need to be put on a waiting list for the on-campus spots. For another, you learn that your health insurance will not

start until 30 days after you begin work. Last but not least, you will receive fewer vacation days than you were originally led to believe.

It is now the day after orientation, and despite all of these unfortunate experiences, you are still glad to have this new position and are eager to get started. However, when you show up to your new office, you find the desk and file drawers filled with the files of the last person who had occupied it. From the dates on the files, it appears that she left this office two years ago; you think she was in a position that had some relevance to the one you were hired for, but the value of her files to you is unclear.

At this point, you start a "to do" list, and begin it with "clean out office." You're not sure which of these files your department may need to retain for legal purposes, and you're not sure who to call to ask, so you decide to call your manager. You look around the office for a few moments and then realize there isn't a phone. Luckily, there at least is a computer in the office, so you decide to e-mail your manager. You switch the computer on, and after waiting for it to power up, you are asked for login information. Having none, you check your instructions from the orientation about how to contact information services. You locate a phone number... but then you remember that you have no phone.

Running out of options, you come out of your office to find another phone you might use. Your search leads you eventually to the receptionist, who tells you that the other staff are away at the monthly all-staff meeting, and asks, "Shouldn't you be attending as well?" Since the first hour of the 90-minute meeting is already over, and you are unclear on how to get to the meeting room, you decide to skip it and instead inquire about using the receptionist's phone to make some calls. She invites you to return at noon when she'll be on break, but you remember that you are supposed to have lunch with your manager at noon, so you instead arrange to come by at the end of the day.

Over the course of the morning, it begins to dawn on you that you will need to be much more proactive in getting yourself set up in this new role than you had originally assumed. Thus begins your quest to arrange for your own telephone, computer access, software installations, e-mail account, business cards, and office supplies, as well as learning how to access the online directory, financial reporting system, and time-and-attendance system. You eventually line up every last thing you need, and within six weeks, with all of the basics set aside, you are now ready to start making the internal contacts you need to be fully productive in your new role (Smith, et al., 2007).

If you were the new hire in this case example, you would probably feel that in many ways you had been left to "fend for yourself"—practically the antithesis of a message that the organization appreciates you as a new employee and values your contributions.

Managers and organizations that get onboarding right recognize the importance of taking a more involved, "high touch" approach to the process. There are needs common to all employees that can be addressed through a structured process, but there will also be relationship needs, unique to each employee, which are often best addressed by making sure that new employees get opportunities early on to meet with their new manager, to hear from leadership that their contributions are important and valued, and to understand how their role fits in to the bigger picture. Taken together, an effective onboarding process should include the following elements.

Pre-Start Preparation

Most organizational roles require a set of job-related tools and resources to be available in order to achieve full productivity. Hiring managers can help new employees by making sure all of these resources are available from the beginning. Specific needs will differ substantially depending on the nature of the role, so managers may find it most efficient to develop a position or departmental checklist of new employee needs. Common examples include:

- *Workstation* (e.g., dedicated physical location, office furniture and supplies)
- *Telecommunications* (e.g., telephone and/or PDA, access account, voicemail, directory listing, and access instructions/training)
- *Computers* (hardware, software licenses, login, and entry in appropriate e-mail group listings)

In addition to these tangible items, it can be helpful to think about the interpersonal aspects of the role—who will new employees need to know to get their work done? Depending on the nature of the position, a list of key contacts or even a series of planned introductions may be very helpful.

Early-Days Acclimation

The first days of a new role can feel very chaotic for a new employee; managers and coworkers can help employees acclimate faster by developing methodical approaches to "teaching" new employees about how things are done. Examples of useful information include:

- *Organization structure*—organization charts, discussions of who reports to whom, and how the department relates to broader operating departments
- *Historical context*—how long the department has been in place; changes that have taken place over time—particularly as they relate to current employees
- *Current climate*—departmental goals and initiatives, and how they are going; departmental policies
- *Operating guidelines*—walk-through of how decisions of various types are made; schedules of standing meetings; other ongoing scheduling considerations

Beyond having this information available, giving a new employee dedicated time to review and learn it can be very helpful. Many departments will formalize this process by setting aside a "departmental orientation" day or days, where these activities can be plugged in to a set schedule so they do not compete with other task demands.

SUMMARY

There are two very good reasons for organizations to follow sound personnel selection practices: (1) they are more likely to keep the organization out of legal trouble, and (2) they will yield better hires and better retention. Given the very high costs associated with turnover in health care organizations, particularly among clinicians and executives, investments in effective personnel selection and onboarding practices typically pay for themselves very quickly.

MANAGERIAL GUIDELINES

Selecting assessment tools

1. *Request technical reports.* When considering the adoption of selection tools, always ask vendors for validity studies and/or technical reports associated with the tools. If the vendor cannot provide this information, seek a different vendor or at least a different test.

2. *Assess reliability and validity.* In considering tests, consider validity to be the most important factor. The ideal for tests is to find criterion-related validity coefficients above 0.20. For valid tests, favor those with reliabilities (Cronbach's alphas) of at least 0.70, and preferably at or above 0.80.

3. *Consider the adverse impact risks.* Review any information provided about adverse impact. Be very cautious about adopting any assessments that might have substantial adverse impact.

Conducting job interviews

1. *Structure your approach.* Prepare a core set of interview questions ahead of time, to assess specific competencies related to the position. Use experience-based questions where possible and structured situational questions when experience-based questions cannot be used (e.g., for candidates with little or no relevant work experience).

2. *Check your questions.* Review legal guidelines before conducting interviews, to ensure questions are legally defensible.

3. *Document applicant responses.* During the interview, take notes on the candidate's responses for evaluation later. Evaluate the candidate's responses after the interview is over.

Onboarding

1. *Keep track of what new hires need to know.* Review needs and experiences of new hires on an ongoing basis. Use this feedback to keep an updated list of new-hire knowledge needed.

2. *Plan for onboarding.* Before a new hire starts, determine the knowledge, skills, and relationships they will need to develop, and make a plan for how the new hire can develop them. Where possible, provide goal-focused "protected time" to deliver these learning opportunities.

DISCUSSION QUESTIONS

1. Think about one or two memorable interviews you have had— either positive or negative. What aspects of the interviews made them more positive (or less positive)?

2. Based on the information you learned in this section, what suggestions might you make to a friend who is applying for a job with a strong selection process?

3. A university orientation is an important form of "onboarding" experience; its success can make a big difference in how effectively new students get started in their studies. List the things a new student to your university (or academic department) needs to know or be able to do to be most effective. Now identify whether each should ideally be a "preboarding," and "orientation," or an "early days" (or "on your own") learning opportunity.

4. The decision to use selection assessments should be based on business impact. However, the most useful and valid selection processes sometimes will demonstrate adverse impact once they are implemented. What are some things to consider when faced with making this kind of decision?

5. Imagine that you have been asked to evaluate the effectiveness of a selection process that is already in place at your organization. What are some outcomes (e.g., metrics produced by the employees hired using the selection process) that you might use to evaluate the process?

CASE

Imagine you have been asked by a director of support services for help in selecting an assessment tool, or tools, to help the organization improve its hiring of handymen. The director gives you the names, contact information, and Web sites of three vendors of selection tools (Alpha Selection, Best Bet Assessments, and Cartagena Consulting Services), who at least on the surface look like they may be useful for this application.

CASE DISCUSSION QUESTION

1. Design a set of criteria to help yourself and the director select the most appropriate tool. Format the criteria as a decision grid, one that you could fill out after reviewing appropriate background information from each of the three companies, and describe how you would use the responses you collected to inform your final decision.

REFERENCES

Aon Consulting. (2007). *Structured Interviewer Training.* Chicago, IL: Author.

Arthur, W. Jr., Bell, S.T., Villado, A.J., & Doverspike, D. (2006). The use of person-organization fit in employment decision-making: An assessment of its criterion-related validity. *Journal of Applied Psychology, 9*: 786–801.

Barrick, M.R., & Zimmerman, R.D. (2005). Reducing voluntary, avoidable turnover through selection. *Journal of Applied Psychology, 90*: 159–66.

Bliesener, T. (1996). Methodological moderators in validating biographical data in personnel selection. *Journal of Occupational and Organizational Psychology, 69*: 107–120.

Daniel, L. (2005). Use personality tests legally and effectively. *Staffing Management, 1.* Retrieved March 13, 2009, from http://www.shrm.org.

Freedman, A.M. (1998). Pathways and crossroads to institutional leadership. *Consulting Psychology Journal: Practice & Research, 50*: 131–151.

Garman, A.N. (2002). Assessing candidates for leadership positions. In R. Lowman (Ed.), *Handbook of Consulting Psychology.* New York: Wiley/Jossey-Bass.

Garman, A.N., & Johnson, M.P. (2006). Leadership competencies: An introduction. *Journal of Health Care Management, 51*: 13–17.

Garman, A.N., & Lesowitz, T. (2005). Research update: Interviewing candidates for leadership positions. *Consulting Psychology Journal: Practice & Research, 57*: 266–273.

Garman, A.N., & Tyler, J.L. (2004). *Succession Planning Practices and Outcomes in Freestanding U.S. Hospital Systems: Final Report.* American College of Healthcare Executives. Retrieved October 1, 2006, from Garman, A.N., & Tyler, J.L. (2007). Succession planning practices and outcomes in U.S. hospital systems: Final report. *American College of Healthcare Executives.* Retrieved October 1, 2006, from http://www.ache.org.

Garman, A.N., & Tyler, J.L. (2007). *Succession Planning Practices and Outcomes in U.S. Hospital Systems: Final Report.* American College of Healthcare Executives. Retrieved October 1, 2006, from http://www.ache.org.

Garman, A.N., Tyler, J.L., & Darnall, J.S. (2004). Development and validation of a 360-degree feedback instrument for health care administrators. *Journal of Health Care Management, 49*: 307–322.

Harold, C.M., McFarland, L.A., & Weekley, J.A. (2006). The validity of verifiable and non-verifiable biodata items: An examination across applicants and incumbents. *International Journal of Selection and Assessment, 14*: 336–346.

Heller, M. (2005). Court Ruling That Employer's Integrity Test Violated ADA Could Open Door to Litigation. *Workforce Management.* Retreived October 22, 2007, from http://www.workforce.com.

Huffcutt, A.I., Conway, J.M., Roth, P.L., & Klehe, U-C. (2004). The impact of job complexity and study design on situational and behavior description interview validity. *International Journal of Selection and Assessment, 12*: 262–273.

McEvoy, G.M., & Cascio, W.F. (1985). Strategies for reducing employee turnover: A meta-analysis. *Journal of Applied Psychology, 70*: 342–353.

Mabe III, P.A., & West, S.A. (1982). Validity of self-evaluation of ability: A review and meta-analysis. *Journal of Applied Psychology, 67*: 280–296.

Motowidlo, S.J., Dunnette, M.D., & Carter, G.W. (1990). An alternative selection procedure: The low-fidelity simulation. *Journal of Applied Psychology, 75*: 640–647.

Mullich, J. (2003, September). Cracking the Ex-Files. *Workforce Management.* Retrieved October 22, 2007, from http://www.workforce.com.

Phillips, J.M. (1998). Effects of realistic job previews on multiple organizational outcomes: A meta-analysis. *Academy of Management Journal, 41*: 673–690.

Prien, E.P., Schippman, J. S., & Prien, K.O. (2003). *Individual Assessment: As Practiced in Industry and Consulting.* Mahwah, NJ: Erlbaum.

Russell, D.R. (2007). Recruiting and staffing in the electronic age: A research-based perspective. *Consulting Psychology Journal: Practice & Research, 59*: 91–101.

Schmidt, F.L., & Hunter, J.E. (1998). The validity and utility of selection methods in personnel psychology: Practical and theoretical implications of 85 years of research findings. *Psychological Bulletin, 124*: 262–274.

Schmidt, F.L., Ones, D.S., & Hunter, J.E. (1992). Personnel selection. *Annual Review of Psychology, 43*: 627–670.

Smart, B.D. (1999). *Topgrading: How Leading Companies Win by Hiring, Coaching, and Keeping the Best People.* New York: Prentice-Hall.

Smith, B.T., Higgins, C., Klumpp, J., Rubin, A., & Sibert, T. (2007, February). *Successful Faculty Recruitment and Retention Strategies.* Presentation at the UHC Ambulatory Care and Group Practice Joint Council Meeting, Oak Brook, IL.

Taylor, P.J., Pajo, K., Cheung, G.W., & Stringfield, P. (2004). Dimensionality and validity of a structured telephone reference check procedure. *Personnel Psychology, 57*: 745–772.

Taylor, P.J., & Small, B. (2002). Asking applicants what they *would* do versus what they *did* do: A meta-analytic comparison of situational and past behavior employment interview questions. *Journal of Occupational and Organizational Psychology, 75*: 277–294.

U.S. Department of Labor (2000). *Testing and Assessment: An Employer's Guide to Good Practices.* Washington, DC.

U.S. Department of Labor (2005). Obligation To Solicit Race and Gender Data for Agency Enforcement Purposes. *Federal Register 41 CFR Part 60–1, Vol. 70* (No. 194), pp. 58946–58963.

Waldman, J. D., Kelly, F., Arora, S., & Smith, H. L. (2004). The shocking cost of turnover in health care. *Health Care Management Review, 29*(1): 2–7.

Weisner, W.H., & Cronshaw, S.F. (1988). A meta-analytic investigation of the impact of interview format and degree of structure on the validity of the employment interview. *Journal of Occupational Psychology, 61*: 275–290.

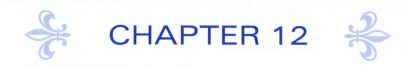

CHAPTER 12

Training and Development

Connie Schott, MBA, SPHR and Christy Harris Lemak, PhD

LEARNING OBJECTIVES

Upon completing this chapter, the reader will be able to:

1. Understand employee training and development and how they differ.

2. Identify how health care organizations can use training and development to improve employee performance.

3. Recognize how training and development can assist health care organizations in the change process.

4. List the basic elements of training needs assessment, design, implementation, and evaluation.

5. Describe the unique challenges of training and development in the health care sector and identify ways to overcome those challenges.

6. Recognize the importance of leadership support for employee training and development.

KEY TERMS

Ability

Failure Mode Effects Analysis (FMEA)

Instructional System Design (ISD) Model

Knowledge

Needs Assessment

New Employee Orientation

Performance Consulting

Skill

Training

Training Motivation

INTRODUCTION

One of the biggest challenges facing health care leaders is how to put together a team of employees that is composed of the best people doing their best work. Various human resources functions contribute to the creation of the team, as described in other chapters of this book. Now, with the team in place, what actions can health care leaders take to ensure that all employees have the opportunity to do their best work? **Training** and development are important ways of ensuring that employees have the **skills** they need, the understanding of how to employ those skills, and the opportunity to learn and use new skills that will allow them and the organization to achieve higher levels of success. This is especially true for health care organizations, where new **knowledge,** new technologies, new clinical care processes, and new customer expectations mean constant demands for human resources to learn, grow, and develop. The core activities of any health care organization are performed by people. These key human resources must be ready and able to do the job well. Excellent health care organizations know that this goes beyond technical expertise and skill to include caring, compassion, and listening to patients and families. To achieve the Institute of Medicine's Committee on Quality of Health Care in America's goals for safe, effective, patient-centered, timely, efficient, and equitable care (Institute of Medicine, 2001), health care organizations will need to put more emphasis on training and development. In general, studies show that employee training translates to improved organizational performance (Mathieu & Leonard, 1987). Truly, training and development become powerful tools to meet current and future challenges in the health care system.

So why training *and* development? How are they different? In a nutshell, *training* addresses the skills that an employee needs in his or her current position. For example, ongoing training can help a nursing assistant or billing clerk to be the very best

nursing assistant or billing clerk possible. In any industry, employees must update their knowledge, skills, and work habits (Ilgen & Pulakos, 1999). This is particularly true in health care, where direct care providers and other staff must be made aware of new clinical guidelines, changing legal and regulatory requirements, and other new organizational initiatives, including customer service, quality of care, and patient safety programs.

Development is geared toward adding new skills or experiences, usually to prepare an employee for a promotional opportunity or a different career path. For example, the nursing assistant may be provided with the opportunity to learn how to read telemetry—not a normal part of the nursing assistant role. With this new skill, she can advance to a higher level in her career. The billing clerk may be provided with the opportunity to lead a work team and to develop and demonstrate leadership skills. This gives him new opportunities as team leader or supervisor. Organizations must consider human resources as valuable assets and invest in the development of their human capital (Ilgen & Pulakos, 1999).

The best leaders in health care constantly seek to identify talented people in the organization. Providing opportunities for training and development ensures that employees are engaged in their organizations and resilient when faced with organizational changes. As a result, patients and visitors enjoy excellent customer service, caring interactions, and outstanding patient care. When leaders create an environment where employees can do their best work and have opportunities to learn and grow, they take a big step toward overcoming the effects of shortages in critical health care professions. Employers who create great work environments—such as Griffin Hospital in Derby, CT—have waiting lists for jobs, with people willing to drive miles out of their way for the opportunity to work there (Frampton, Gilpin, & Charmel, 2003).

Each health care organization must identify the training and development needs of its workforce. A large integrated health system offers more training programs than a small physician group practice or nursing home. Most health care organizations, however, must consider training and development in the following five major categories: (1) orientation and new employee training; (2) training for job-specific skills, concepts, or attitudes; (3) in-service training programs on organization-identified topics; (4) continuing education provided outside of the organization; and (5) employee career development to add new skills or enable employees to perform new jobs and take on additional responsibilities. In today's environment, successful health care organizations view training and development as essential to organizational learning and achievement of the mission, vision, and values.

This chapter explores how health care leaders can use training and development to improve employee performance, create ongoing opportunities for employees, and successfully implement changes to maintain or improve the organization's competitive position. Models for training program development and evaluation are presented, as well as key issues for implementing training programs in the health care environment.

USING TRAINING AND DEVELOPMENT TO IMPROVE EMPLOYEE PERFORMANCE

Training and development strategies can address a broad spectrum of organizational needs and challenges. Hospital leaders who understand the full spectrum of training and development increase their personal success and the success of their organizations by using training and development to build the skills of both teams and individuals and by understanding both the strengths and limitations of training-based solutions. A review of training and development literature found that "health care organizations that develop strong retention cultures often adopt unique human resource workplace practices that stress employee participation, empowerment, and accountability. . . . In addition to high commitment practices and a decision-making culture to enable them to work, employees

require additional training and development if they are to be effective in their work" (Rondeau & Wagar, 2006, p. 247).

Traditionally, training and development have been thought of as the best answers when a health care organization needs to build or change an employee's knowledge, skill, or **ability** to perform effectively on the job. Knowledge, skill, and ability are similar in that they each involve learning; however, each requires a specific approach in the learning process. *Knowledge* is familiarity, awareness, or understanding. *Skill* is the capacity, facility, or dexterity acquired through experience or training. *Ability* is the mental or physical power to get something done, in other words, the quality of being able to do something (The American Heritage Dictionary, 2007). Because of the differences in knowledge, skill, and ability and how they are acquired, training approaches will differ based on the desired outcome. And in some cases, training will not be the most effective way to address a performance need.

Training is an ideal solution for the employee who has demonstrated a lack of task-related skill. For example, an environmental services worker who is turning over an inpatient hospital room between patients follows a prescribed plan for completing each cleaning task. Training can address issues where tasks are missed, such as the wastebasket not emptied or brochures not placed on the bedside table. Training can also improve skills when a task is completed incorrectly, such as the proper way to make the bed. Many health care organizations now include standard training on a very specific skill—how to consistently and effectively wash hands and use disinfecting gels before and after entering a patient room.

New employee orientation is a classic example of task-related skill building that typically combines classroom instruction with on-the-job teaching. Employees learn important information about the organization and its expectations in an initial orientation that occurs in a classroom setting. Then, a more experienced employee is assigned to the new person to "show him or her the ropes" and to guide learning. The introduction of new procedures often follows a similar pattern, with some employees trained to be the trainers of other employees on the team.

Moving beyond basic skills and embracing the idea of development allows health care leaders to drive the organization to higher levels of performance. Training and development are an important part of the continuum of employment, providing the opportunity for the employee to learn new skills and achieve higher level positions with the company. Developing employees in this way not only enhances organizational performance, it also increases the employee's level of engagement and connection to the employer. Studies show that engaged employees lead to decreased turnover, increased customer satisfaction, and increased quality of care (Rondeau & Wagar, 2005).

Is training *always* the best approach? Can training be used to improve performance? In answering these questions, health care managers must work with human resources professionals and consider at least two important issues. First, each situation must be evaluated to determine whether training and development can work and what might be the most effective training and development strategy. Second, managers must realize that some skills and behaviors cannot be taught effectively.

More specifically, managers must consider the first issue: training strategies. Some topics are ideally suited to traditional classroom training. The transfer of knowledge, such as regulatory requirements related to patient safety, diversity awareness, sexual harassment, and benefits program changes are all well-suited to training and can be conducted effectively in a classroom setting. The addition of skills-practice opportunities, such as Resusci-Annie or computer work station exercises expands the ways in which classroom training can be effectively used to transfer knowledge to employees.

Training encompasses much more than sitting in the classroom and other purely didactic methodologies, however, and other approaches can be used for employee training. Mentoring and **performance consulting** provide the opportunity to target individual needs and specific competencies. Mentoring typically provides a one-on-one experience in which an employee is able to observe an expert and ask questions in real time about real situations. Here, the teaching and learning are geared to development of skills in a safe and personalized environment.

Performance consulting is geared to teams and team dynamics. Conducted with intact work teams, performance consulting occurs in the real world environment, providing a way to observe and respond to how a team functions. By using empirical data, performance consulting effectively changes team behaviors and reinforces changes in skills and process in the work environment. Other team training programs such as Crew Resource Management and Team Strategies and Tools to Enhance Performance and Patient Safety (TeamSTEPPS) have been implemented to address patient safety and reduce medical errors (Alonso, et al., 2006). Team development initiatives are critical ways to encourage and facilitate "local learning" in health care settings (Edmondson, 2004).

Finally, it is essential to recognize that some skills and behaviors cannot be taught. Training is not an effective response when a person has been hired into a job that does not match his or her current ability. While many people can and do continue formal education while working, health care organizations cannot hire staff members "on spec," that is, without some evidence of a minimal level of skill to perform in the position. Thus, the rehab aide who plans to go to nursing school is not hired as a nurse with the expectation that he or she will learn the requisite skills on the job. So, training is not the correct response when the employee's skill level does not meet the minimum qualifications for a position.

It is far better to recruit and select potential employees to the jobs which best match their personal style. Further, certain behaviors, such as responding consistently with a smile and a helpful demeanor to customers, are difficult (though not impossible) to train. Having a "curmudgeon" at the front desk is bad for business, even if he or she does have excellent clerical and administrative skills. When specific behaviors and attitudes are critical job components, training dollars are best spent on equipping those who will be doing employee interviewing and hiring to recognize job-relevant skills in potential employees.

TRAINING TO SUPPORT ORGANIZATIONAL CHANGE

Organizational change is often described as one constant in the health care system. Successful organizations must respond quickly and effectively to changes in the business environment. A well-designed strategy for implementing change typically includes training. Employee training is an effective way to move the organization through the change process. The following example describes one community hospital's experience of implementing the "Planetree" approach.

Bringing Planetree to a community hospital

Many community hospitals provide highly regarded patient care with caring staff who work in a physical environment designed years ago. Some hospitals' physical plant and décor may be old and sterile. Equally important, processes were developed for the convenience of the caregivers, with little understanding of the impact that they have on patients and families. A classic symbol of the hospital experience, and the basis of many jokes, is the hospital gown. Designed to provide easy access for caregivers, the typical patient gown provides little dignity for the patient. Driven by customer input, and the emerging trend throughout hospitals toward patient-centered care, one community hospital CEO became enamored of the "Planetree" model for the provision of patient care.

Planetree has 10 components that address every aspect of the patient experience. This is a radical shift in that it requires that the hospital redefine its expectations and processes from the point of the view of the patient (Frampton, et al., 2003). Planetree can easily be seen as creating additional work or inconvenience for health care providers. It also encourages patients to actively participate in their own care—a significant challenge for practitioners who are accustomed to being the unquestioned experts.

One may wonder why a hospital would undertake the culture shift required to adopt Planetree philosophies and components. Taking the Planetree approach to patient care has resulted in increased patient satisfaction, technical quality, and the satisfaction and engagement of employees.

For organizations that can successfully negotiate the change process, the rewards of Planetree can far outweigh the risks of maintaining the status quo. Effective leaders know that the status quo is not a viable long-term strategy.

The implementation of a culture change of this magnitude involves several employee training challenges. To transition into a Planetree model, 100% of current employees must be trained on the Planetree approach. At one Community Hospital, this was accomplished with a series of 25 offsite, full-day programs devoted to creating understanding and acceptance of Planetree and patient-centered care. Second, maintaining the culture change required ongoing training for current staff to reinforce the components of the Planetree model and the hospital's new performance expectations. Periodic refreshers and new training programs to support the culture change were implemented. Recognition programs were designed around the Planetree components rather than old standbys like perfect attendance and length of service. As hospital programs and procedures were changed, they were supported by various training and development activities. And, finally, new-employee orientation was revised to reflect the Planetree commitment to patient-centered care. This constant infusion of new employees with the expectation of a Planetree-style work environment further reinforced the culture change, and ensured that employees did not revert to old work habits. In summary, the organization used employee training methods to support and maintain this large-scale organizational transformation.

Ensuring quality in patient care settings involves special challenges. Manufacturers have the ability to set the specifications and tolerances on a process and then allow robots and computers to routinely (and mindlessly) complete the same task thousands of times without errors. In health care, both the person performing the task and the person on whom the task is being performed represent opportunities for inconsistent applications and errors.

Building a culture of quality requires both proactive and reactive reliance on training and development. Continuous quality improvement programs seek to transfer the process methodologies of manufacturing assembly operations to the health care arena. The programs rely on employees who have been trained to approach the patient care interactions as processes, so that when errors or unexpected outcomes occur, the point of failure can be identified and studied. While many versions of the quality improvement process exist, all share similarities with the process popularized by Dr. Edwards Deming and depicted in the Shewhart cycle of plan, do, check, act (Schultz, 1994).

Focusing on process, rather than on individual performance, as the source of errors helps organizations use training to create lasting process improvements and increase employee commitment. This type of quality-based training is also a key part of the health care organization's regulatory compliance strategy (Motwani, Frahm, & Kathawale, 1994).

From time to time, even with a fully developed quality program, errors occur in health care. In the case of serious errors or when a patient's course of treatment results in an unanticipated outcome, regulatory oversight and sound management practice will require a reactive response. Thorough review of the actions taken and the processes involved will uncover opportunities for training to address the mistakes in knowledge, skills, and ability. For example, **Failure Mode Effects Analysis (FMEA)** may be used to identify the potential for errors and to provide appropriate corrective actions before they occur. FMEA is a very powerful

needs assessment tool because it can highlight areas where focused training may be used to proactively prevent an error (for more on FMEA, please see the Institute for Healthcare Improvement Web site, www.IHI.org).

Effective training supported by health care leadership benefits the organization and its employees. Ensuring that employees have the knowledge, skills, and ability to perform their jobs effectively and safely is one important part of effective health care leadership. For hospitals and health systems, the Joint Commission (JC) requires that "Hospitals must also provide the right number of competent staff to meet the patient's needs. . . . The hospital provides ongoing in-service and other education and training to increase staff knowledge of specific work-related issues" (JCAHO, 2006, CAMH HR-1, overview). Thus, quality training is an essential element in achieving most health care organizations' strategic and operational objectives.

TRAINING DESIGN AND IMPLEMENTATION

The **instructional system design (ISD) model** provides a framework for designing and implementing effective training programs (Goldstein, 1986, 1991). In essence, ISD suggests that training programs begin with a comprehensive training needs assessment. Next, training objectives and strategies are developed to address identified training needs. After implementation, an explicit training evaluation is conducted. Studies have found important linkages among personal training needs, various instructional methods, and learning effectiveness (Chen & Klimosk, 2007).

Kirkpatrick (1998) offers a useful framework for planning and implementing effective training programs that includes 10 critical steps (see Table 12.1). In this chapter, we focus on training needs assessment (Step 1), training design and delivery (Steps 2–9), and training evaluation (Step 10).

Table 12.1. Critical Steps in Training Planning and Implementation.

1	Determining needs
2	Setting objectives
3	Determining subject content
4	Selecting participants
5	Determining the best schedule
6	Selecting appropriate facilities
7	Selecting appropriate instructors
8	Selecting and preparing audiovisual aids
9	Coordinating the program
10	Evaluating the program

SOURCE: Kirkpatrick, D.L. (1998). (2nd ed.) *Evaluating Training Programs (electronic resource): The Four Levels.* Berrett-Koehler Publishers.

TRAINING NEEDS ASSESSMENT

Organizations must continually and systematically assess training and development needs. Needs assessment is a diagnostic process in which the organization identifies performance gaps and determines whether and how training can be used to improve performance.

Training and development needs assessment occurs at the organization, department, and individual levels.

At the *organization* level, key human resources issues, including training and development needs, may be discussed during the strategic planning process. Training and development needs may be identified from inside the organization, for example through routine surveys of managers and employees or from new organization-wide initiatives such as adapting the Planetree model or implementing the Studer Group BEST Approach (www.studergroup.com). Similarly, when new equipment or technology is purchased, training is a key part of the implementation process. The

organization's chief human resources officer annually summarizes key employee indicators, such as job satisfaction, turnover, grievances, and the like. Analysis of these data may reveal training and development needs for the organization.

The impetus for new training programs may come from outside the organization, as regulatory or compliance requirements change or as national organizations issue recommendations or requirements. For example, *Keeping Patients Safe: Transforming the Work Environment of Nurses*, issued by the Institute of Medicine's Committee on the Work Environment of Nurses and Patient Safety Institute, specifically recommends that health care organizations dedicate financial resources to support nurses' "ongoing acquisition and maintenance of knowledge and skills." The report includes not only nurse education and training programs but also recommends that each licensed nurse and nurse assistant have an individualized plan and resources for educational development (2004, Recommendation 5-5). As health care executives establish strategic organizational priorities, training and development opportunities must also be included.

At the *department and work-unit* level, training and development needs can also be systematically identified through the annual employee evaluation process from patient and stakeholder surveys, grievances, reports of patient safety problems or near misses and as leaders and staff members continually identify ways to improve care delivery or business functions. Each department and work unit identifies the skills, knowledge, abilities, and attitudes that are essential for achieving department and unit goals and objectives. Department head analysis of job descriptions, vacancies, and other employee data will help identify training opportunities. As performance gaps are identified, the next step to consider is how training can be used to build, maintain, or enhance performance.

Finally, as recommended by the Institute of Medicine for nurses, each *individual* employee should have a written, individualized employee training and development plan that is evaluated annually. Employees must be rewarded for keeping training up-to-date and for attending customer service and other available training programs. Annual training and development goals are ideally linked to overall job performance and monitored during the annual performance appraisal process. Employees, human resource professionals, and direct supervisors can work together to establish training goals, develop and schedule training sessions, and track employee progress. Further, as employees become trainees, human resources professionals should consider key personality and situational attributes that may affect **training motivation** and training outcomes. For example, anxiety has been found to be negatively associated with training motivation and training outcomes (Colquitt, LePine, & Noe, 2000). Thus, employees who are under a great deal of pressure or experiencing other sources of stress are not good candidates for training or may need a chance to reduce or eliminate stressful situations in order to succeed in training.

After training and development needs are identified at the organization, department and work unit, and individual employee levels, these needs are synthesized and prioritized. A key question is, how would addressing each identified training need contribute to achieving the organization's mission, vision, and strategic objectives? In this way, limited training resources are dedicated to the most strategically relevant training and development activities.

TRAINING METHODS AND APPROACHES

As suggested by Kirkpatrick's 10 steps, the next phase of training planning and implementation involves setting objectives, determining subject content, selecting participants, schedules, facilities, instructors, and needed audiovisual and other learning tools. At this point, it is critical for managers and human resource professionals to carefully match training needs, objectives, methods, and materials.

Each type of training offered by health services organizations—(1) orientation; (2) in-service training for job-specific skills, concepts, or abilities (typically a technical focus); (3) in-service training programs on organization-identified topics (often more interpersonal in nature); (4) training and education provided outside of the organization; and (5) employee career development—will have unique training goals and require specific objectives. Table 12.2 outlines common objectives of four of these major types of training and the potential types of methods and attendance policies that can be used to achieve them. Managers and human resources professionals work together to design and deliver training to achieve organizational and training objectives.

TRAINING EVALUATION

Comprehensive, rigorous evaluations of employee training programs are essential, but are often not done or not done well. This is typically due to limited resources and lack of leadership support for evaluation (Lilly, 2001). Today's health care environment emphasizes evidence-based clinical and managerial decision making. Health care organization leaders and human resources professionals must demand comprehensive evaluation of employee training programs in order to develop a body of evidence in this arena.

Kirkpatrick (1998) recommends four levels of training program evaluation: reaction, learning, behavior, and results (Table 12.3). The levels follow a sequence, so that results (Level 4) depend on changed behaviors (Level 3) and learning (Level 2), and similarly, learning and behavior change are more likely to occur when trainees react favorably to the training program (Level 1).

Table 12.2. **Training Programs in Health Care: Typical Objectives, Potential Methods, and Attendance Policies.**

Type	Typical Objective(s)	Potential Delivery Method(s)	Attendance
Orientation	Introduce organization's mission, vision, and values Provide organization and job information Begin employee socialization and integration Describe organizational ethics Increase knowledge of hazardous waste disposal, fire safety, other issues related to physical safety Inform staff about patient safety, patient rights, confidentiality, HIPAA, other patient issues Present human resources information (benefits)	Web-based, combined with group sessions Videos Presentations by leaders General organization portion and specific department or work unit portion	Required for all new employees May be required for all employees at a specific tenure mark (e.g., every 5 years)
In-service *technical* training	Comply with federal and state regulations, such as Occupational Safety and Health Administration (OSHA), Environmental Protection Agency (EPA), and others Learn to use key technologies, information systems, and other tools Improve knowledge and skills related to quality of care, patient safety, medical errors Enhance existing knowledge, skills	Web-based Other electronic formats (CD, DVD) Classroom, group settings On-the-job, interactive Team based	Required for specific jobs and job categories May be required for all employees to achieve strategic objectives, such as BEST, Planetree, etc.
In-service *interpersonal* training	Address particular problems or situations Improve working relationships Develop problem-solving skills Develop new skills for employee advancement Develop skills for dealing with patients and families Modify employee attitudes Enhance supervisory skills Develop learning culture	Simulations Role plays Group activities On-the-job, interactive Team based Multiple methods	Optional, as part of employee training and development plans
Offsite training	Wide range of objectives Often best choice for smaller organizations without large training staff May offer training tools and techniques that are too expensive to develop in-house	Multiple methods offered Use when highly specialized techniques or specific credentials of trainers are needed	May be required or optional, depending on area of training and as part of employee training and development plans

Table 12.3. **Levels of Training Program Evaluation.**

Level	Description	Examples
1. Reaction	Participants' reaction to and satisfaction with the training program	▪ trainees enjoyed the program ▪ participants would recommend it to others ▪ training materials were helpful
2. Learning	The extent to which participants change attitudes, improve knowledge, and/or increase skills as a result of attending the program	▪ increased awareness of hazardous waste disposal methods ▪ identify steps in patient room turnover process ▪ ability to describe patient confidentiality rules
3. Behavior	The extent to which change in behavior has occurred because participants attended the training program	▪ improved team functioning ▪ zero mistakes in patient admission process ▪ asks visitors or patients if they need help finding a location in the hospital
4. Results	The final results that occurred because participants attended the program; the impact of training on business activities and processes	▪ increased productivity ▪ reduced patient errors or near misses ▪ reduced staff turnover ▪ improved employee satisfaction ▪ improved patient satisfaction

SOURCE: Based on Kirkpatrick, D.L. (1998). (2nd ed.) *Evaluating Training Programs (electronic resource): The Four Levels.* Berrett-Koehler Publishers.

As training programs are developed, managers and human resources staff must identify objectives and standards for each of the four levels. For example, what *reactions* to the training are most important? Examples include trainee reaction to the facilities used for the training, the schedule of training sessions (e.g., time of day, day of week, length), the exercises conducted in training, training materials, and the participant's perceived value of the training. It is important that reaction forms be distributed to 100% of those in the training program, that the forms be turned in immediately, and that trainees be encouraged to go beyond the formal questions to add written comments and suggestions. A key part of all evaluation is to use the information provided to improve the training in future sessions.

When evaluating *learning,* it is important to have specific, written objectives identified before training begins. Ideally, learning (that is, knowledge gained,

skills developed or improved, attitudes changed) should be measured before and after the training using a pre-test/post-test approach. When feasible, a control group of employees who did not receive the training is used to isolate the effects of training on knowledge, skills, or attitude change. In many organizations and settings, a control group may not be possible. In some cases, a staggered training schedule can be used, so that control group members for early sessions are trainees in later sessions (Kirkpatrick, 1998).

The third level of training evaluation involves measuring *behaviors,* that is, what employees take back to the job after training ends. This training outcome is very difficult and complex to measure. In fast-paced, complex patient-care environments, it is often very difficult to carefully and accurately assess behaviors before and after training occurs. In the best case, multiple perspectives are used to assess behavior change: supervisors, subordinates, coworkers and others can be asked to evaluate trainees' behaviors following a training program (Kirkpatrick, 1998) As discussed in a later section, many factors combine to determine whether and how trainees can transfer what is learned in training to actual performance on the job.

The final level of training evaluation is assessing *results*, that is, the impact that training has on the overall work unit, department, or organization's business processes and outcomes. As with evaluation of learning and behavior, a pre-post test design is ideal. There are many challenges to identifying, isolating, and quantifying the effects of training on organizational performance. Excellent health care organizations know that there are various potential effects of training, including improved quality of care, enhanced productivity, reduced staff turnover, improved employee satisfaction, greater patient satisfaction, improved financial performance, and other strategic organizational indicators. For some, however, the relationships are difficult to precisely and accurately identify. It is important to remember that the effects of training programs on organizational results may take time to manifest or become evident (Kirkpatrick, 1998). Strategic human resources managers know that the key is to measure often, track trends, and identify how employee training and development are linked to achieving the organization's mission, vision, and strategic objectives.

THE RETURN ON INVESTMENT FROM TRAINING

Precisely calculating the *return on investment* (ROI) for training programs is something that is rarely done. It is estimated that training ROI is conducted for about 10–20% of all training programs. The following four-step approach is a recommended way to compute training ROI (Lilly, 2001). First, the effects of training must be isolated. To truly identify

and accurately quantify training effects, it is important to have data gathered before training begins, with pre- and post-test and control group designs. For many health care organizations, this data may not be readily available or tracked, but "hard data" are preferred, including quantitative measures of training effects on productivity, quality, labor hours, absenteeism, turnover, worker's compensation claims, time required to fill vacancies, market share, patient satisfaction, and so on. In some cases, however, manager and employee perceptions and other "soft data" are also used in calculating the training ROI. Next, training effects must be converted into monetary values. Managers can assist in the process of attaching costs and revenue figures to training effects on turnover, satisfaction, compliance, and other outcomes.

The third step of calculating training ROI involves estimating the cost of conducting the training program. This includes the costs to develop the program; wages and salaries of trainers, support staff, and trainees (sometimes called the cost of "seat time"); fees paid to outside trainers or consulting; the costs of instructional materials, equipment, facilities, marketing, documents, and logistics (e.g., food, lodging, shipping); and travel time to and from the training location. Finally, the training ROI is calculated by comparing the effects, or benefits, of training to the incurred costs.

While it is difficult to measure ROI, human resources professionals should begin to think about training in this manner. Considering the short-term, mid-range, and long-term effects of training is critical to a strategic human resources process. Moving in the direction of determining ROI will begin to get the organization thinking about the value of training. As recommended by Lilly, "sometimes you may need to focus on the big picture, the changes that are occurring, rather than a line-by-line item of cost benefit analysis or ROI" (2001, p. 3). In this way, human resources professionals can shift their emphasis "from being the 'keeper and distributor of people information' to the more critical role of 'developer of people and productivity'" (Lilly, 2001, p. 5).

TRAINING MOTIVATION AND TRAINING TRANSFER

So far, this chapter has focused on the strategic and structural aspects of training and development in health care organizations. In addition to considering the appropriate objectives, methods, materials, and evaluation of training, it is also critical for managers and human resources staff to keep in mind that individual employees—people—are being trained, and their level of motivation will play a key role in obtaining desired training outcomes and organizational results.

Training motivation is defined as the "direction, intensity, and persistence of learning-directed behavior in training contexts (Colquitt, et al., 2000; Kanfer, 1991). A recent review of the training literature found that attributes of individuals (including self-confidence), attributes of the job, and attributes of the situation were important predictors of training motivation and outcomes. Trainers should consider and measure aspects of individual trainees as they design, deliver, and evaluate training programs. For example, trainees with a more internal locus of control were consistently found to be more motivated and achieved better outcomes in training. Those who were more conscientious reacted more favorably to training and achieved better training outcomes. In addition, employees who were more involved in their jobs, those with greater organizational commitment, and those with defined career plans experienced higher levels of training motivation and showed greater training outcomes. Several studies demonstrated that employees who believe they can achieve the behaviors and skills targeted in training are more motivated and learn more (Colquitt, et al., 2000). Managers and trainers should emphasize that trainees are capable of the desired behaviors. Finally, research has shown that attributes of the trainees' work environments are key predictors of whether and how much trainees can bring the knowledge, skills, attitudes, and behaviors they acquired in training back to their everyday work settings. Support for training by immediate supervisors and peers is critical, as is a climate that supports learning and personal growth. This suggests that even the very best training programs will not succeed if the organization's work settings do not embrace and reward training and development at all levels.

UNIQUE TRAINING AND DEVELOPMENT CHALLENGES IN HEALTH CARE

Health care work environments can pose unique challenges for the delivery of training and the successful implementation of new skills, knowledge, and abilities. These challenges include scheduling, ensuring full participation by trainees, support in the workplace, and overcoming resistance from several sources.

Scheduling training is the first challenge. How does the health care manager find a time that is convenient for all? The solution for this problem starts long before the selection of training dates and times. Rather, at the point that a needs assessment or change initiative points toward a training solution, it is critical to also obtain the support of the senior leaders for the training. Then, it is a matter of selecting the least disruptive dates and times by avoiding critical patient care times. In the same way that executives manage their personal calendars by protecting specific "golden" times, scheduling for training should take account of "golden" times in the organization's operations. For example, training should not be provided to bedside caregivers during the change of shift or on days of high admitting and discharge activities (typically Mondays and Fridays).

Getting the physical presence of the trainees to the training location at the scheduled time is only the first step. Equally important and challenging is ensuring that the participants have the opportunity to bring their full attention to training. Rules about silencing cell phones and pagers should be made and enforced. Ideally, participants should be relieved of all job-related responsibilities for the duration of the training. Managers and participants should imagine that the training is taking place in a distant location, even when it is just in the training room in the adjacent building. This can help leaders and participants plan for full commitment to the training process.

For many reasons, some organizations find training to be more disruptive than helpful. Leaders, in such cases, talk about the disruptive impact of the newly trained workers returning to the workplace. Again, leadership support and preparation are key to creating the necessary conditions in the work environment for the new learning to be carried back and applied.

When introducing a new work process or a change in the culture or work expectations into a group, the performance consulting approach of *intact team training* is recommended. In this case, all employees are trained at the same time and change occurs simultaneously rather than incrementally. And, as research shows, teamwork plays a major role in the delivery of care. Teams need to know and use effective communication and coordination behaviors. Team training, especially when focused on effective communication, is an important part of error prevention. Research supports the claim that "scenario-based training is important in improving the performance of teams in high-risk settings where technology is at a premium" (Alonso, et al., 2006, p. 402).

It is the responsibility of the health care leader to understand the value of training and to create a supportive environment for it. Training can and may disrupt the flow of work. However, such disruptions are temporary, and their impact can be minimized with effective planning. The longer-term impacts from a well-designed and implemented training effort include increased customer satisfaction, increased quality outcomes, and increased employee engagement and retention.

LEADERSHIP IS THE KEY TO EFFECTIVE TRAINING AND DEVELOPMENT

There is no doubt that effective training and development depends on leadership support. Recent literature reviews and meta-analyses conclude that leadership support contributes to enhanced learning and improved training transfer (Chen & Klomisk, 2007).

In health care settings, organizational leaders must establish training and development as critical to achieving the organization's mission, vision, and values. By establishing a compelling organizational vision that includes organizational learning and an emphasis on people and continuous improvement, leaders will make training and development an organizational priority. They must also provide resources for training and reward those managers who successfully develop the skills and abilities of their staff. Organizational executives should specifically identify future leaders and formalize employee development plans. Leaders must also model learning and development by participating in training programs themselves, by continuing their own career and professional development, and by supporting managers who wish to do so.

In addition to that of senior leaders in the health care organization, there is also an important role for "local leaders" to encourage and support training and development. Managers at all levels of the organization should share best practices for training and development, identify and inform employees who are chosen for development and training initiatives, and support employee training by removing barriers to participation and training transfer. It is crucial that managers reward those who learn and grow and not punish those who attend training by giving them more work to do when they return from training programs. Managers at all levels must also model learning and growth by taking time to attend training and advance in their own career development. Perhaps most importantly, managers and direct supervisors can work to get employees involved directly in training and development planning. There is strong evidence that trainees react more positively to training when they themselves decide to participate, instead of their boss making that decision for them (Mathieu, Tannenbaum, & Salas, 1992). Successful health care leaders will encourage and support organizational efforts to grow and develop human resources.

SUMMARY

Employee training and development are powerful tools to meet the current and future challenges in the health care system. Training and development are important ways of ensuring that employees have the skills they need, the understanding of how to employ those skills, and the opportunity to learn and use new skills that will allow them and the organization to achieve higher levels of success.

Training addresses the skills that an employee needs in his or her current position; *development* is geared toward adding new skills or experiences, usually to prepare an employee for a promotional opportunity or a different career path. Training and development strategies can address a broad spectrum of organizational needs and challenges. Hospital leaders who understand the full spectrum of training and development increase their personal success and the success of their organizations by using training and development to build the skills of both teams and individuals and by understanding both the strengths and limitations of training-based solutions.

Effective training design and implementation includes comprehensive training-needs assessment, thoughtful training design and delivery, and rigorous training evaluation. Training-needs assessment is a diagnostic process in which the organization identifies performance gaps and determines whether and how training can be used to improve performance. Ideally, training programs are evaluated on the four levels of reaction, learning, behavior, and results. Health care work environments can pose unique challenges for the delivery of training and the successful implementation of new skills, knowledge, and abilities. A key element of successful training and organization is support from leaders and managers at all levels of the organization.

MANAGERIAL GUIDELINES

1. Providing opportunities for training and development ensures that employees are engaged in their organizations and resilient when faced with organizational changes.

2. Health care organizations typically consider training and development in the following major categories: (1) orientation and new employee training; (2) training for job-specific skills, concepts, or attitudes; (3) in-service training programs on organization-identified topics; (4) continuing education provided outside of the organization; and (5) employee career development to add new skills or enable employees to perform new jobs and take on additional responsibilities.

3. After training and development needs are identified at the organization, department and work unit, and individual employee levels, these needs are synthesized and prioritized. A key question in this process is, how would addressing each identified training need contribute to achieving the organization's mission, vision, and objectives? In this way, limited training resources are dedicated to the most strategically relevant training and development activities.

4. Managers must remember that the effects of training programs on organizational results may take time to manifest and become evident. Strategic human resources managers know that the key is to measure often, track trends, and identify how employee training and development are linked to achieving the organization's mission, vision, and strategic objectives.

5. Health care leaders and human resources professionals should begin to think about calculating the return on investment (ROI) of training. Moving in the direction of determining ROI will begin to get the organization thinking about the value of training.

6. Attributes of the trainees' work environments are key predictors of whether and how much trainees can bring back the knowledge, skills, attitudes, and behaviors to the everyday work setting. Support for training by immediate supervisors and peers is critical, as is a climate that supports learning and personal growth. Even the very best training programs will not succeed if the organization's work settings do not embrace and reward training and development at all levels.

7. By establishing a compelling organizational vision that includes organizational learning and an emphasis on people and continuous improvement, leaders will make training and development an organizational priority.

8. Health care leaders must provide resources for training and reward those managers who successfully develop the skills and abilities of their staff.

9. There is an important role for "local leaders" to encourage and support training and development. Managers at all levels of the organization should share best practices for training and development, identify and inform employees who are chosen for development and training initiatives, and support employee training by removing barriers to participation and training transfer.

10. Managers and leaders must also model learning and growth by taking time to attend training themselves and advance in their own careers.

DISCUSSION QUESTIONS

1. How are training and development related to a health care organization's mission, vision, and values?

2. What are key steps in planning and developing effective training programs?

3. How can leaders support training and development?

4. Some health care organizations are very small; how can such organizations effectively provide training and development for their employees?

5. What are the main types of training offered by health care organizations? How are they the same? How are they different?

6. How can managers improve training transfer?

7. What factors of the person, situation, supervisor, and organization are related to training motivation and training outcomes?

8. Write a short (500 words or fewer) memo to the board of trustees that describes why you believe the organization should triple its investment in training and development this year.

9. How can you analyze the ROI for a patient safety training program targeting pharmacy and nursing staff?

10. Convince the CFO that the training budget will "pay off" over time.

CASE: NEW OPERATIONS DIRECTOR AT HYBRID MEDICAL CENTER

Marianne Bundt has just landed the job as director of operations at Hybrid Medical Center, a full-service community hospital. She is excited about the opportunity to prove herself and believes that if things go well, she will be on her way to the CEO job she has dreamed about since graduate school.

Marianne has read Hybrid's web page:

"You're not a number or "just another patient" at Hybrid Medical Center. You are a special individual and your needs will be cared for by our compassionate health care professionals who are dedicated to their community hospital.

Our 112-bed, acute care medical center is in downtown Smallville, a historic community of strategic importance during the American colonial period. Our area's historical significance and easy access to popular tourist attractions make us a popular vacation stop.

Providing convenient and compassionate care to those living in and visiting our area is our #1 goal. Everyday we offer a healing touch to those who choose Hybrid Medical Center for their health care needs."

After a few weeks of work, Marianne is beginning to feel that Hybrid's reality doesn't consistently match the hype. As with many community hospitals, the Emergency Room (ER) is the primary portal for entry into the continuum of care. In fact, more than 50% of admissions start in the ER. Hybrid enjoys the well-deserved reputation of having the best ER among all of the regional hospitals—shortest wait times, nicest and most caring staff members, and skilled physicians. Now that ER visits have soared to more than 35,000 per year, the workload is stressing the whole hospital.

Hybrid currently employs 800 employees and vacancy rates are low. However, the management team has been in flux for the past year, with reorganization and the elimination and/or replacement of about 60% of Hybrid's key leaders.

Marianne's challenges are to (1) maintain the volume in the ER; (2) keep patient satisfaction high; (3) demonstrate high quality care; and (4) hit all budget targets (revenues and costs).

CASE DISCUSSION QUESTIONS

1. How can Marianne create an effective team or teams to address the ER issues? What type of support from human resources will ensure that the many departments and disciplines needed to address ER growth are able to spend their time problem solving and not finger pointing?

2. Some members of the medical staff are using direct admits to bypass the increasing delays in the hospital admissions process. Heavy workload is also causing increased errors in admissions paperwork. How can training be used to address these issues?

3. How can training and development help make Hybrid's "walk" match its "talk" as described on the hospital web page? What are key steps that must be taken, and how can Marianne overcome potential barriers?

REFERENCES

Alonso, A., Baker, David P., Holtzman, A., Day, R., King, H., Toomey, L., & Salas, E. (2006). Reducing medical error in the military health system: How can team training help? *Human Resource Management Review, 16:* 396–415.

Chen, G., & Klimosk, R.J. (2007). Training and development of human resources at work: Is the state of our science strong? *Human Resource Management Review, 17*(2): 180–190.

Colquitt, J.A., LePine, J.A., & Noe, R.A. (2000). Toward an integrative theory of training motivation: A meta-analytic path analysis of 20 years of research. *Journal of Applied Psychology, 85:* 678–707.

Edmonson, A.C. (2004). Learning from failure in health care: Frequent opportunities, pervasive barriers. *Quality and Safety in Health Care, 13*(6, supp. 2): ii3–ii6.

Frampton, S.B., Gilpin, L., & Charmel, P.A. (2003). *Putting Patients First: Designing and Practicing Patient-Centered Care.* San Francisco, CA: Jossey-Bass.

Goldstein, I.L. (1986). (2nd ed.). *Training in Organizations: Needs Assessment, Development and Evaluation.* Monterey, CA: Brooks/Cole.

Goldstein, I.L. (1991). Training in Work Organizations. In M.D. Dunnette & L.M. Hough (eds.) *Handbook of Industrial and Organizational Psychology, Vol. 2* (pp. 507–620). Palo Alto, CA: Consulting Psychologists Press.

Ilgen, D.R., & Pulakos, E.D. (1999). Introduction: Employee Performance in Today's Organization. In D. R. Ilgen & E. D. Pulakos (eds.) *The Changing Nature of Performance: Implications for Staffing, Motivation, and Development* (pp. 1–18). San Francisco, CA: Jossey-Bass.

Institute for Healthcare Improvement. *Failure Modes and Effects Analysis Tool.* Retrieved November 14, 2007, from http://www.ihi.org.

Institute of Medicine Committee on Quality of Health Care in America. (2001). *Crossing the Quality Chasm: A New Health System for the 21st Century.* Washington, DC: National Academies Press.

Joint Commission on Accreditation of Healthcare Organizations (JCAHO). (2006). *Comprehensive Accreditation Manual for Hospitals (CAMH).* Chicago, IL: Joint Commission Resources.

Kanfer, R. (1991). *Motivation Theory and Industrial and Organizational Psychology.* In M.D. Dunnette & L.M. Hough (eds.) *Handbook of Industrial and Organizational Psychology* (Vol. 1, pp. 75–170). Palo Alto, CA: Consulting Psychologists Press.

Kirkpatrick, D.L. (1998). *Evaluating Training Programs: The Four Levels.* San Francisco, CA: Berrett-Koehler Publishers.

Lilly, F. (2001). *Four Steps to Computing Training ROI.* (whitepaper). Alexandria, VA: Society for Human Resource Management.

Mathieu, J.E., & Leonard, R.L. (1987). Applying utility concepts to a training program in supervisory skills: A time-based approach. *Academy of Management Journal, 30*: 316–335.

Mathieu, J.E., Tannenbaum, S.I., & Salas, E. (1992). Influences of individual and situational characteristics on measures of training effectiveness. *Academy of Management Journal, 35*: 828–847.

Motwani, J.G., Frahm, M.L., & Kathawala, Y. (1994). Quality training: The key to quality improvement. *Training for Quality, 2*(2): 7–12.

Rondeau, K.V., & Wagar, T.H. (2006). Nurse and resident satisfaction in magnet long-term care organizations: Do high involvement approaches matter? *Journal of Nursing Management, 14*: 244–250.

Schultz, L. (1994). *Profiles in Quality.* New York: Quality Resources.

The American Heritage® Dictionary of the English Language. (2007). (4th ed.) Retrieved November 13, 2007, from http://dictionary.reference.com.

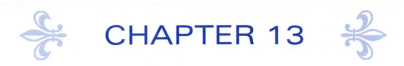

CHAPTER 13

Performance Appraisal

Grant T. Savage, PhD and Naresh Khatri, PhD

LEARNING OBJECTIVES

Upon completing this chapter, the reader will be able to:

1. Appreciate the important role that performance appraisal plays in managing human resources (HR) in health care organizations.

2. See the connection of performance management function with other key HR functions of recruitment/selection, training/development, and compensation and rewards.

3. Have an appreciation of the legal implications of performance appraisal.

4. Describe the problems inherent in the performance appraisal process.

5. Place performance appraisal in the context of continuous quality improvement (CQI) and the mandated standards of the Joint Commission (JC).

6. Describe the key features of 360-degree feedback and team appraisals.

KEY TERMS

Absolute Standards

Alternation Ranking

Comparative Methods

Forced-Choice Method

Forced Distribution

Graphic Rating

Management By Objectives (MBO)

Paired Comparison

Performance Appraisal

Performance Management System

Personality-Based Appraisal Systems

Straight Ranking

Supervisor-Only Based Appraisal Systems

Total Quality Management (TQM)

Weighted Checklists Method

INTRODUCTION

Today's health managers are under extreme pressure to contain costs and improve the efficiency of operations. They may be the most constrained of all corporate executives. To be competitive in the health care industry, these managers must use methods and techniques to improve the performance of their organizations. Much has occurred in recent years to push the management of for-profit and not-for-profit health care organizations into positions of strength regarding the transfer of management knowledge and technology to health care organizations.

One area of health care management not yet developed to its potential is **performance appraisal.** Interestingly, this topic holds great opportunity for improving the management of health care organizations and yielding sizable dividends at both the individual and organizational level. Through proper design, implementation, and maintenance of a dynamic performance appraisal system, individual and organizational performance may be monitored and enhanced, resulting in a more efficient and effective organization.

The need to develop a superior and effective performance appraisal system in a health care organization can be described in clear and simple terms. Indeed, health care organizations are so "employee intense" that salaries and wages that comprise as much as 60 to 70% of their operating costs are not unusual. Such data reveal the clear linkage between the successful operation of the organization and the effective and efficient performance of its employees. A good performance appraisal system can help the organization to attract and retain highly qualified employees. Health managers should understand the reasons for implementing a performance appraisal system that is effective in promoting organizational goals as well as in developing human resources.

Performance appraisal and management, along with recruitment and onboarding, training and development, and compensation and reward systems, constitute the four core functions of human resource management in organizations. Like any other human resource management activity, it appears simple and straightforward, but research and practice in the past 20–25 years has shown that performance appraisal and management is very complex and elusive. Nonetheless, organizations have to get it right not only to retain their high-performing employees but also to keep them motivated and performing at their full capacity.

There is a distinction between performance appraisal and performance management. Performance management is a broader term and encompasses performance appraisal. Performance management is the integration of performance appraisal systems with broader human resource systems as a means of aligning employees' work behaviors with the organizational goals. It should be an ongoing, interactive process designed to enhance employee capability and facilitate productivity. Most systems of performance management have several parts: (1) performance definition, (2) appraisal process, (3) performance measurement, and (4) feedback and coaching (Fisher, Schoenfeldt, & Shaw, 2006). Performance appraisal is that part of the process in which an employee's contribution to the organization during a specified period of time is assessed. Performance feedback lets employees know how well they have performed in comparison with the standards of an organization. In practice, however, when health care managers talk about performance appraisal, they usually mean both the appraisal and feedback process.

Delivering and receiving performance feedback during performance appraisal is usually an emotionally charged process that affects employees' attitudes toward both the organization and themselves (Fisher, et al., 2006). If used effectively, performance assessment and management can increase employee motivation and performance. If used inappropriately, it can be disruptive, de-motivating, and frustrating to employees, and can potentially lead to low satisfaction and high turnover in the workforce.

Performance appraisal is a complex activity that confronts even the most well-meaning appraiser with a maze of interactions that frustrate the assignment of clean, accurate, and merit-based ratings. Moreover, appraisals become progressively more complicated with the introduction of additional variables and quality demands.

As a result, performance appraisal is not an inexpensive activity. The average cost of appraisal per employee ranges between $1,500 and $2,000 (Dutton, 2001).

Performance appraisals in health care organizations can be described as a "necessary evil" that can create barriers between the appraiser and the appraisee (Chandra & Frank, 2004). Conducting performance appraisals is often considered one of the most difficult aspects of a manager's job and is often an area of much confusion and discomfort for both the manager and the employees being appraised. Despite their importance, performance appraisals are often met with negative feelings. Moreover, some researchers have found current performance appraisals to be ineffective (Longnecker, Sims, & Gioia, 1987; Nelson, 2000).

The remainder of the chapter is organized as follows: In the next section, we discuss the purpose of performance appraisal, followed by a discussion of the strategic importance of performance appraisals in managing human resources. We then discuss common performance-appraisal methods, newer and more health care-specific performance-appraisal methods and issues, and common problems encountered in the performance-appraisal process. We end the chapter with a summary.

PURPOSE OF PERFORMANCE APPRAISAL

Organizations evaluate performance of their employees for many purposes, including compensation, counseling, training and development, promotions, staff planning, retention/discharge, and validation of selection techniques (Cicek, Koksal, & Ozdemirel, 2005). Other purposes include communicating company objectives, providing feedback to employees, identifying talent, and documentation for legal protection.

More broadly, performance assessment has two purposes. In the first purpose, as an employee development tool, performance appraisal is used to set goals, reinforce performance, improve performance by correcting wrong employee behaviors, determine career paths of employees, and to identify training needs in the workforce (Fisher, et al., 2006). In the second purpose, as an administrative tool, performance appraisal is useful in linking rewards to performance and evaluating human resource management (HRM) policies and programs.

STRATEGIC IMPORTANCE OF PERFORMANCE APPRAISAL

Organizations strive to (1) design jobs and work systems to accomplish organizational goals, (2) hire individuals with the abilities and desire to perform effectively, and (3) train, motivate, and reward employees for achieving high performance and productivity (Fisher, et al., 2006). Each of these activities is dependent to a significant extent upon performance management as a control mechanism.

Numerous examples exist of reward systems that commit the folly of rewarding for a particular activity while actually hoping for another outcome (Kerr, 1995). These unintended consequences often can be traced to poorly aligned human resource management practices, and occur because of the misfit between organizational strategy and employee behaviors and/or the misfit between organizational values and employee job behaviors (Fisher, et al., 2006).

Unfortunately, fragmented HR functions often occur in health care organizations. Such fragmentation results from the lack of an overarching framework in the form of an HR strategy. For example, payroll and compensation may be performed by the finance/accounting department, some crucial HR functions may be carried out in the units where people are working (e.g., assigning work and projects, setting up teams, performance appraisal and promotion), and even within an HR department or division, each activity, function, or program may run autonomously, with no unity of purpose.

Organizational and Human Resource Strategy and Performance Appraisal

HR strategy is necessary to guide HR policies and practices. Tyson defines HR strategy as "the intentions of the corporation, explicit and covert, towards the management of its employees, expressed through philosophies, policies, and practices" (1995, p. 169). In the absence of an HR strategy clearly linked with organizational strategy and culture, HR programs and practices are likely to lack the direction, coherence, and support for required employee behaviors.

Human resource management practices are more effective as a bundle and less effective when individual practices are instituted (Ichniowski & Shaw, 2003; MacDuffie, 1995). It is vital that the core HR functions of recruitment and onboarding, compensation and rewards, training and development, and performance appraisal

and management are aligned properly with each other. Performance appraisal and management has critical interdependencies with three other core HR functions (see Figure 13.1). For example, performance appraisal and management should inform the recruitment and selection processes about which selection criteria to use and which selection methods are the most effective. On the basis of the actual performance of hired employees, HR managers can then determine which selection criteria have a stronger relationship with performance. Similarly, the performance appraisal process can identify the training and development needs of employees. The immediate supervisor, in consultation with the employee, can figure out what factors are causing subpar performance of an employee and accordingly recommend an appropriate training program.

In fact, we have come across many organizations that use performance appraisal to determine training and development needs. In the appraisal interview, supervisors discuss with their subordinates what is causing the shortfall in the subordinate's performance and what measures can be taken to rectify it. Also, the success of pay-for-performance compensation strategies hinges critically on measuring performance accurately. If the performance of individuals cannot be measured correctly, the basic premise of the pay-for-performance—that performance can be measured accurately and rewarded accordingly—does not hold true. Consequently, the

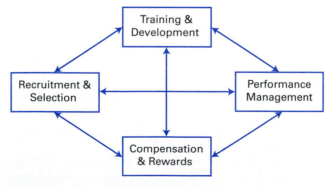

Figure 13.1. **Inter Relationships among Major HR Functions**

pay-for-performance strategy is likely to fail, leading to a demoralized, frustrated workforce instead of a motivated and high-performing workforce, which is the intent of the strategy.

Joint Commission requirements, as well as malpractice and employee lawsuits, have made legal and regulatory issues in performance appraisal of strategic importance. Thus, the legal aspects in performance appraisal require special mention.

Legal and Regulatory Issues in Performance Appraisal

Performance appraisal has become a regulatory necessity in health care. For example, the Joint Commission, a voluntary accrediting body for over 15,000 health care organizations, mandates that all personnel receive performance appraisals on a consistent periodic basis. At the same time, performance appraisals frequently figure in malpractice and wrongful discharge litigations.

While physicians as independent contractors may be the initial focus of a malpractice lawsuit, the organizational workplace in which physicians carry out their practice is also liable. Thus, health care organizations, such as hospitals and long-term care facilities, bear the risk of litigation for malpractice. The competencies of nurses, nurse aids, technicians, and other direct employees of the health care organizations often are scrutinized in such lawsuits. Significantly, performance appraisals and timely managerial actions, such as appropriately disciplining and terminating low-performing employees, can avert or minimize the malpractice liability of the health care organization.

Understandably, layoff and firing decisions will often trigger lawsuits. When an employee is terminated for reasons related to job performance or is preferentially chosen for layoff and the action is contested, performance appraisal documents in the personnel file become a central concern. Appraisals should support the manager's decisions. Thus, many wrongful discharge lawsuits are a consequence of inadequate performance appraisal procedures. To avoid litigation and associated legal costs, subjective assessments in performance appraisal that are hard to defend legally are best kept to a minimum (Fallon & McConnell, 2007).

Hence, many managers and human resource professionals in health care organizations are concerned about legal issues, which may partly result from an inflated perception of the organization's litigation risk. A fundamental danger associated with legal-centric decision making is that its focus on salient litigation threats and what is legally defensible occurs at the expense of other legitimate criteria for organizational performance (Roehling & Wright, 2006). Ironically, legal-centric decision making may lead to an increased risk of employee litigation because of its sole focus on salient legal threats, and generating favorable evidence in order to avoid litigation may, inadvertently or purposefully, divert attention from underlying, systematic problems that contribute to either employee or malpractice litigation. By following an "organizationally sensible approach," human resource professionals may create a more motivated and higher-performing organization, as well as minimize litigation costs.

COMMON PERFORMANCE APPRAISAL METHODS

Numerous methods exist for evaluating performance; these generally are classified as **comparative methods, absolute standards,** or **management by objectives.** An organization should choose a method based on at least two criteria: (1) the key competencies or behaviors the organization desires from its employees, and (2) the method that best suits the organization's purpose for assessing performance.

Comparative Methods

As their name suggests, *comparative methods* compare one employee to another in order to determine performance ranking. **Straight ranking** merely asks the rater to list employees, beginning with the strongest employee and ending with the weakest. This method utilizes overall job proficiency on predetermined job dimensions or characteristics (Timmreck, 1989). In **alternation ranking,** the most common ranking method, the rater repeatedly chooses the strongest then the weakest employees, each time choosing from the names remaining in the list until all employees have been placed on the ranking list, with the last two ranked in the middle (Ivancevich & Glueck, 1986; Timmreck, 1989).

In **paired comparison,** one employee at a time is compared to all other employees. Each time an employee is ranked higher than another employee, a tally is placed by the higher-ranking person's name. The employee with the most tallies is considered to be the most valuable, and the others are placed in order according to the number of tallies by their name. **Forced distribution** asks the rater to assign a certain proportion of the employees to one category on each criterion. For example, 10% of employees might be in the "superior" category, 20% in the "good," 20% in the "average," continuing on to "poor" as the lowest category (Ivancevich & Glueck, 1986). While these methods of performance comparison are often used to determine merit raises, promotion opportunities, or layoffs, they are open to extensive criticisms, many of which are discussed later in this chapter.

Absolute Standards

Through the use of standards, each individual is evaluated against written standards, and several factors of performance are measured. In one such method, the **weighted checklists method,** the rater identifies and assigns a weight to each of the tasks to be evaluated. The employee is then scored on each task to determine overall performance.

In the **forced-choice method,** the rater selects statements that best fit the performance characteristics of the individual employee. The rater does not know the value assigned to each characteristic, and consequently forced choice can reduce bias. However, this advantage can become a disadvantage if the rater is offended by the confidential weights assigned to the statements.

Graphic rating is the most commonly used method for performance appraisal. The scale requires the rater to choose a value or statement along a continuum that best fits the employee for each criterion being reviewed. The advantage of a graphic scale is that it shows the degree to which an employee performs a job or task (Douglas, Klien, & Hunt, 1985).

The *critical incidents technique* was developed in response to the faults of essay and behavioral trait methods. In the essay method, a supervisor periodically describes employee performance at whatever length is considered necessary. It is time consuming and highly subjective. The employees that are sycophants may be evaluated more favorably. In the behavioral trait method, a list of personality/disposition traits are numerically rated. Traits may include items such as cooperation, flexibility, and attitude. The trait approach is found to be quite unreliable and invalid. In the critical incident method, the rater records critical behaviors of employees that are related to both good and poor performance. This method, however, does not indicate the frequency with which a particular behavior is performed, nor the degree to which it is performed (Douglas, et al., 1985). It is a nonquantitative technique.

As a result of the shortcomings of the critical incidents method, the *behaviorally anchored rating scale* (BARS) was developed. BARS uses characteristics judged to be critical to job performance and rates the degree to which each characteristic is attained by the employee. The employee's performance is determined by summing the values assigned to each of the critical indicators and/or characteristics.

A system developed from the BARS model, the *behavioral observations scale* (BOS), attempts to eliminate some of the disadvantages of BARS. The development of BOS also begins with the identification of critical incidents, which are then categorized according to behavioral dimensions. Each behavioral dimension usually contains five to eight items, and these items are then used to rate employee performance. A frequency format is developed in which the highest number corresponds to "almost never." Unlike the BARS method, BOS does not require the appraiser to record the occurrence of critical incidents regularly. Instead, BOS asks the rater to evaluate the employee on a variety of behaviors that have been determined to be critical to good or poor performance (Douglas, et al., 1985). Thus, BOS is a more structured and quantitative approach in which critical incidents serve as anchor statements on a scale.

Management by Objectives (MBO)

Management by Objectives (MBO) is a result-based evaluative program in which goals are mutually determined by supervisors and subordinates, and employees are rated on the degree to which these goals are accomplished. MBO stresses the value and importance of employee involvement and encourages discussion of employees' strengths and weaknesses. However, in a clinical health care setting, patient-oriented treatment goals represent performance standards that may be extremely difficult to determine in advance. Given the variable nature of patient care, performance goals must be flexible enough to allow the caregiver latitude in resources consumption while stressing cost containment measures. This obviously presents a potential dilemma in the health care environment.

MBO became popular for several reasons. First, it promotes communication and interaction between the superior and subordinate. Additionally, the process of MBO development forces the organization and individual units to recognize and coordinate goals. Second, employees gain an understanding of work objectives and learn what is expected of them. This goal-setting emphasis provides the opportunity to integrate MBO with the performance appraisal by connecting standards and objectives to subsequent performance levels (Beck, 1990). Because of its focus on goal-setting and goal attainment that are aligned with organizational strategy, MBO is, perhaps, most suitable for assessing the performance of managers and supervisors.

RECENT HEALTH CARE-SPECIFIC PERFORMANCE APPRAISAL METHODS AND ISSUES

A major issue for performance improvement is the movement by health care organizations toward some form of continuous quality improvement (CQI). As a result, there is an emerging trend away from organizational structures with many hierarchical levels of command-and-report toward flatter organizational structures. Two forms of performance appraisal methods have emerged that are compatible with continuous quality improvement: 360-degree feedback and team appraisals. These two methods have also gained prominence because of heightened emphasis on the quality of patient care and these methods' capabilities to improve communication and information sharing in health care organizations.

Continuous Quality Improvement (CQI) and Performance Appraisal

A CQI or **total quality management (TQM)** philosophy entails improvement of organizational processes; use of structured problem-solving processes that incorporate statistical methods; use of interdisciplinary teams as the major focus for improvement processes; employee empowerment; and a focus on customers, both internal and external. Within the past decade, there has been a movement within large health care organizations toward improving health care quality and ensuring patient safety that is premised on CQI.

As a result, for many hospitals and health care systems, CQI has become central to their organizational culture. Nonetheless, CQI requires adjustments to be made in all the management systems within the health care organization, especially human resources management (Haddock, et al., 1995). The importance of HR philosophy and practice for quality improvement is reflected in the Malcolm Baldrige National Quality Award's inclusion of "Workforce Focus" as one of the seven categories in the Health Care Criteria for Performance Excellence (www.quality.nist.gov/HealthCare_Criteria.htm). This category examines the effectiveness of the organization's efforts to develop and realize the full potential of its workforce, with a focus on workforce engagement, high performance, aligning compensation and recognition systems to work systems, and establishing learning and development systems.

Unfortunately, many common HR practices, conceived in command–control organizational cultures, are in conflict with the basic principles of CQI (Blackburn & Rosen, 1993; Cicek, et al., 2005; Deming, 1986; Ghorpade & Chen, 1995; Haddock, et al., 1995). Of all HR practices, performance appraisal is perhaps the most significant point of conflict between the principles of CQI and traditional HR practices (Deming, 1986; Haddock, et al., 1995). For example, Deming (1986) cited evaluation of performance, merit rating, and annual performance review—all typical centerpieces of traditional HR management—among the deadly diseases that impede quality improvement. Deming supported ways to manage people based on a philosophy of collaboration, as opposed to one of competition. Moreover, in a study of 14 organizations that had won the Baldrige Award, Blackburn and Rosen (1993) found evidence of a paradigm shift in the HR policies of these organizations, with new HR practices that supported cultures characterized by employee commitment, cooperation, and communication.

Ghorpade and Chen (1995) provide three general prescriptions for improving quality-driven performance appraisal systems. First, within a quality environment, the primary purpose of performance appraisal should be to help the employees improve their performance rather than to monitor and control their actions and behaviors. Second, the modification of the existing performance appraisal systems should be brought about with the active involvement of all those who are affected by the activity. Third, employees

should be judged by absolute rather than relative standards of performance. As discussed in the following sections, both 360-degree feedback and team appraisals support CQI-oriented organizational cultures.

360-Degree Feedback

An estimated 25% of U.S. employers and 90% of Fortune 1000 companies use some form of 360-feedback (Antonio & Park, 2001). In 360-degree feedback, the target of the assessment—a manager or employee—is in the middle of a "circle" composed of multiple raters as opposed to receiving ratings from a single superior. Survey data typically focus on leader behavior issues, such as communication, motivation, and team skills. The 360-degree feedback method is particularly well-suited to appraise managers and cross-functional teams.

The 360-degree feedback method gained in importance due to two major factors: (1) the ineffectiveness of conventional performance-appraisal systems and (2) a gradual shift in management philosophy and practices in organizations from a reliance on hierarchical authority to employee-based expertise and empowerment. However, a review of 600 research studies of 360-feedback found that following the process, one-third of the organizations showed improvement in performance, one-third showed decline in performance, and one-third showed no impact on performance (Atwater & Brett, 2006).

Kuzmits, et al., (2004) had the following concerns about 360-feedback:

- Largely because of a lack of training, managers may not know what to do with 360-feedback or how to act upon the issues covered in the process.

- Many organizations implement 360-feedback without clearly defining the strategic context or mission of the program.

- Feedback provided inappropriately can harm instead of help.

- Gaps often exist between 360-feedback efforts and organizational objectives.

- The quality of feedback data may be affected by the organization's culture. In highly centralized and bureaucratic organizations, for example, raters may be hesitant to provide honest appraisals.

Based on their study, Kuzmits and colleagues provide two major recommendations for more effective 360-feedback implementation. First, they recommend formal training for all involved in the 360-feedback process. The training should focus on 360-feedback purposes and procedures; how to rate behavior and feedback; and how to counsel 360-feedback participants and prepare developmental plans and activities. Second, they suggest that genuine and active participation for all parties involved in the 360-feedback effort is crucial. Significantly, this advice has been heeded and successfully implemented in several situations. For example, Gentry (2006) developed a peer evaluation tool for nurses that constituted 60% of a nurse's total evaluation, with the remaining 40% of the evaluation to be completed by the nurse's manager. In order to create a true peer evaluation, the tool used six registered nurse (RN) peers as evaluators. The author solicited staff-member input into the wording of each performance statement. This was an essential element in the success of the peer evaluation and the longest step. This also helped establish meaning and understanding of the peer review process for everyone involved, ensured consistency among evaluators, and provided staff members with a sense of value and ownership of the project. The performance statements on the form were grouped into eight distinct subcategories. Four subcategories dealt with the nursing process and the other four subcategories dealt with personal performance and character. Before implementing the peer evaluation, the peer-review form was approved by the operating room manager, administrators, and HR personnel in the hospital. Gentry identified confidentiality of the peer evaluation as integral to the success of the program. In addition, the peer review focused on providing constructive feedback for the purpose of improving nursing practice and the profession as a whole rather than on how well nurses were doing.

Another case study of a successful implementation of 360-degree feedback is provided by Pollitt (2004). In this example, the European pharmaceuticals distribution group, Alliance Unichem, used 360-degree feedback among its top managers to drive culture change, support employee development, and increase overall performance. The company employs 30,000 people and serves 81,000 pharmacies in many European countries. Using the latest information technology, 360-degree feedback provided a consistent way of measuring employees across the group. Managers, direct reports, peers, and customers were invited to rate the participants on 100 relevant statements of behaviors. Improving the coaching and feedback skills of managers was considered the key to using performance management to unlock staff potential. The bottom-up approach to redesign was found to deliver significant benefits both in terms of helping to shift perceived ownership of the system from HR to users and in making practical improvements in the performance-management process.

On the effectiveness or ineffectiveness of 360-degree feedback, Kuzmits, et al. note that "Over the decades, the field of management has witnessed numerous innovations in the field of leadership behavior, for example, management by objectives, job enrichment, participative management, self-managed work teams, and quality circles. All have proven successful in many organizations and yet were unsuccessful in others" (2004, p. 325). Implementation is the key to success of most HR interventions, which is greatly dependent upon the internal HR capabilities of health care organizations (Khatri, 2006). Thus, the HR department has to be equipped with skilled and knowledgeable HR staff to be able to effectively implement HR interventions such as 360-degree feedback.

Team Appraisals

Appraising teamwork is a shift in emphasis, as well as a continuing challenge, for appraisal systems. This represents a shift away from the industrial model of work with routine, narrowly defined outputs to a model of work centered on knowledge. Knowledge-based work often requires close cooperation within and between teams in order to stay on top of changes in customer requirements and technologies. This notion is particularly important for health care organizations, whether those organizations care for critically, chronically, or terminally ill patients. In all of these cases, patient care is not the responsibility of one person, but of a team of health care professionals. Indeed, health care work demands continuous learning and social interaction—another set of skills to be included in performance appraisals (Ghorpade & Chen, 1995).

Teams present evaluation challenges to managers and supervisors. Individual evaluations in a team environment can be problematic because they are likely to undermine teamwork and cooperation by stressing individual competitiveness and fault finding (Fallon & McConnell, 2007). They may encourage competitive individuals to circumvent team requirements for individual gain and to fail to provide an open, problem-solving environment necessary for high-performance teams. Individual performance appraisals do not support team-building because they lack a means of identifying the effects of individuals on the group or the group on individuals.

As with individual performance appraisals, team evaluations require criteria and standards. These must be constructed specifically in terms of team performance. Although the emphasis on team performance continues to rise, most reward and recognition systems are focused on individuals (Fallon & McConnell, 2007).

Weitzel (2002) provides an example of implementing a team design in a health care setting successfully. This was done by the members of the department themselves. The members first attended a training program on teams and then used this knowledge to devise ways uniquely suited to their departmental context in order to move away from traditional job design to team design. The team design resulted in the reduction of five management positions to two. The team concept eliminated the corporate ladder that existed in the old structure

and thereby improved the performance of the department. The author commented that "Good people in a great process will overwhelm great people in a bad process" (p. 30).

Davison and Hyland (2002) also found that the palliative care environment is conducive to a team design. For effective team functioning, the work environment needs to have hard, focused, purposeful work requiring diligence, persistence, and commitment. The authors found the above key characteristics of teams and team members present in the palliative care environment. Further, the authors described the organizational capabilities needed for continuous innovation, radical innovations, and continuous incremental improvements by complex teams in such an environment:

- managing knowledge, in terms of its acquisition, creation, and dissemination;
- managing information, including collection, interpretation, and communication;
- interdisciplinary operations;
- collaborative operations;
- managing technologies; and
- managing change and its effects.

Although most of health care is delivered through teams, most health care management systems are premised on the industrial model, with emphasis on measurement of performance and accountability at the individual level. Providing safe and high-quality care requires cooperation across professions and specialties, but health care organizations are well known for silos in their structures that act as strong barriers to communication and information sharing. This major inconsistency between the health care context and its measurement systems results in conflicting demands on health care professionals. For example, Kivimaki, et al. (2001) reported that, of work-related factors, teamwork had the greatest effect on sickness absence in physicians. Physicians working in poorly functioning teams were at 1.8 times greater risk of taking long spells off work than physicians working in well-functioning teams. Risks related to overload, heavy on-call responsibility, poor job control, social circumstances outside the workplace, and health behaviors had smaller effects than stress caused by poor team functioning.

PROBLEMS ENCOUNTERED IN PERFORMANCE APPRAISAL

It is estimated that less than 20% of all employee appraisals are effective in accomplishing their intended purpose (Fallon & McConnell, 2007; Longnecker & McGinnis, 1992). In many health care organizations, managers view performance appraisal as little more than a paper-pushing, file-stuffing activity that is not especially relevant. Some appraisal instruments (appraisal forms and instructions) have become so detailed and complex that the lengthy process becomes another source of dread for the department manager (McConnell, 2003).

Performance appraisal in health care is mandated by organizations and agencies that accredit and regulate health care facilities, such as the Joint Commission. In some instances, mandated evaluation has led to the development of performance appraisal systems that are little more than a formality (Fallon & McConnell, 2007). Such evaluation systems have minimal value as appraisals, and are often seen as merely extra work by those involved. Managers are often uneasy about criticizing employees, especially on a performance appraisal that results in a permanent record for an employee's file, which could affect that person's pay, job future, and long-term career (McConnell, 2003).

Much of the negative attitude toward and misuse of performance appraisals are due to the shortcomings of older appraisal approaches and methods. In what follows, we highlight the problems residing **in personality-based appraisal systems,** comparison-based appraisals, and absolute standard-based appraisals, as well as the hazards of **supervisor-only based appraisals** and fragmented appraisal systems.

Personality-Based Appraisal Systems

Older performance appraisal systems often rely heavily on assessing personality characteristics that yield highly subjective evaluations; they do not focus on how an employee performs relative to an objective standard. With these appraisal systems, managers are required to make judgments they are not qualified to make and cannot easily defend. Such appraisals are as unsettling to employees as they are to managers, and are commonly used in authoritarian management work environments. In such an environment, an evaluator can freely use personal opinions, unsupported judgments, and personal biases on evaluations. Employees who want to keep their jobs have no recourse except to check their anger and return to work. These older performance appraisal systems have not gone away and may still exist in some health care organizations that have a poorly managed HR department.

Comparison-Based Appraisal Methods

Comparison methods are useful in making decisions regarding promotion and selection from within a work unit, and this is their major advantage. They are problematic in that they are time-consuming and useful only for relatively small groups of employees. Also, an employee's performance rating is based on other employees' work, rather than on desired outcomes. Comparisons can lead to judgments about personality rather than job performance. Finally, the ranking process assumes equal distance between employees' ranks, an assumption research shows to be unwarranted (Fisher, et al., 2006).

Absolute Standards-Based Appraisal Methods

Absolute standards of performance appraisal have shortcomings too. For example, the major disadvantage of the use of a weighted (or nonweighted) checklist is that it does not reveal the degree with which a specific behavior occurs, requiring only a mere yes or no judgment. The main disadvantage of the behaviorally anchored rating scale (BARS) is that its development is time-consuming because separate scales are needed for each job. BARS, however, offers objectivity, which is lacking in subjective appraisal methods such as comparative methods and essays. BARS has been used effectively in hospital work units of nurses and ancillary personnel; such successful usage is due to the dimensionality of the BARS scale, which permits identification of separate components of complex job behaviors. BARS also demonstrates a necessary movement toward evaluations that are developmental, rather than merely evaluative. Such developmental evaluations, being behaviorally based, then provide the basis for changes in behavior.

Supervisor-Only Based Appraisals

The typical performance appraisal process involves rating of subordinates by a single supervisor, with the assumption that supervisors are objective in assessing their subordinate. Unfortunately, the performance assessment of employees by their supervisors has been found to suffer from numerous perceptual biases, such as the recency, halo, horn, similar-to-me, and leniency effects. In the *recency effect,* a manager/supervisor completes the employees' evaluation based on recent behaviors only (as opposed to behavior during the entire time period for review). Managers are able to more clearly recall the events of recent behavior. This can result in falsely positive or negative appraisal since doing so fails to take into account performance of an employee over the entire appraisal period. The *halo effect* occurs when a manager/supervisor allows a single positive attribute to affect the entire content of the employee appraisal, leading to a falsely positive evaluation. This bias can also occur when the manager has a friendly relationship outside of the work with the employee. The *horn effect,* which is the opposite of the *halo effect,* occurs when a manager/supervisor allows one negative attribute to affect the entire performance appraisal

of an employee. Personality conflicts between the manager and employee are a common cause of the horn effect. When a manager allows personal conflict to interfere with the overall evaluation of the employee it can result in a falsely negative appraisal of his or her performance. In the *similar-to-me effect,* a manager/supervisor rates an employee higher on his or her performance appraisal because the manager perceives the employee has characteristics similar to her or his own. The opposite can occur when the manager perceives the employee to have differing character traits, resulting in a falsely low evaluation of the employee's performance. When the latter occurs, referred to as the *different-to-me* effect, the employee may not understand the lower rating and this confusion can lead to conflict, diminished productivity, and decreased moral. Many performance appraisals are also ineffective because the manager conducting them is too lenient on his or her employees (*leniency effect*). There are several reasons why a manager might be lenient, including insecurity in his or her own job, a fear of giving "bad" news, and/or a lack of understanding of the appraisal process and the reasons for conducting the appraisal. In some cases, leniency occurs due to organizational policies. Giving an unsatisfactory assessment may require writing a detailed action plan on the part of the manager. In order to avoid writing an action plan, managers may falsely increase an employee rating. Leniency is an important problem to address, because when managers are overly lenient in performance appraisal, the organization no longer has a means to identify low performers.

Fragmented Appraisal Systems

The broad diversity of occupations, along with the variety of technical, professional, and union allegiances in contemporary health care organizations, poses challenges to an effective performance-appraisal process. Medical staff (e.g., physicians), who are central to health care but are not employees of the organization, further complicates performance appraisal and management in health care organizations (Haddock, et al., 1995).

For example, Bryan, Rodgers, and Rosenhauer (2007), in their study of three hospitals (a community hospital, an academic medical center, and a private physician group), found that whereas the HR department was fully involved in managing nonphysician employees, in all three cases physician recruitment issues, to a large extent, were not handled directly by the HR department. Instead, all physician recruitment was done by the CEO with no input from HR except as conduit to manage the accompanying paperwork. Moreover, once a physician was employed, the ongoing evaluation and management of the physician was done by a physician group management team and the CEO, again without any utilization of the HR department. Such practices are common in health care organizations. They create a dysfunction in the health care workforce because they fail to fully integrate physicians, the central actors in the health care delivery process, in the organizational processes and management systems. Moreover, HR practices done by managing physicians do not benefit from the latest advances in human resource management because the people managing them are not conversant with such practices.

Current systems of performance management in the health care sector are unlikely to have a significant influence on improving services (Adcroft & Willis, 2005). Because of the dominance of the clinical culture, management issues in health care organizations have traditionally taken a back seat. Consequently, management practices and systems in health care have lagged behind and remained outdated (Khatri, et al., 2006). Health care organizations continue to implement practices consistent with the industrial model of management, which itself is becoming obsolete. The industrial model focuses on standardization, formalization, and close monitoring of employee behavior. Jobs in the industrial model are defined narrowly and specifically, giving workers little discretion. But health care organizations are knowledge-based services and not amenable to the assumptions of the industrial model. They involve teamwork and cooperation, and rely on the autonomy of health care professionals to deliver higher quality care. Thus, health care

organizations, rather than implementing management practices and systems of 15 to 20 years ago that are premised on the outdated industrial model, should implement more recent management practices that emphasize employee empowerment, cross-functional teams, and flat organizational structures. **Performance management systems** will need to be transformed so that employees that take initiative and are team players get rewarded.

SUMMARY

The appropriate way to appraise performance is to base the evaluation on what an employee does rather than what an employee knows (Fallon & McConnell, 2007). For decades, managers have rated employees on personality or job knowledge. In addition to being subjective, such an assessment provides little or no value for either employee or organizational development. Measuring job knowledge and personality misses the point. What really matters is how knowledge is applied and what results are achieved.

Enough has been learned about performance and its appraisal to say that it is neither appropriate nor fair to base evaluations on the comparison of one individual's performance against another's (McConnell, 2003). Rather, accumulated experience with appraisal systems suggests that the most useful comparison that can be made via appraisal is the comparison of an employee's performance with his or her performance over time, based on clear standards.

Experience with more modern appraisal systems has shown that a low, odd number of gradations work best (McConnell, 2003). Three to five gradations are usually sufficient in assessing performance. For each task on the job description there should be a standard or an expectation of behavior. The employees can then fall into one of three categories: failed to meet the standard, met the standard, or exceeded the standard. These broad gradations do not demand a very high precision in the performance-appraisal process but allow managers to make fair appraisals. If additional precision is required, it is typical to add graduations into the met standard and exceed standard categories.

Deming (1986) and McGregor (1985) believe that performance-appraisal systems should be replaced by leadership and coaching. These authors argue that behaviors cannot meaningfully be modified through a conversation that only takes place annually. Most people want to perform well and succeed. It is the manager's job to make sure employees understand what they need to do to improve performance on an ongoing basis. Performance appraisals can be far more effective tools for improving behavior if they are integrated into an ongoing culture of communications (Rikleen, 2007). Let your workplace be one where regular feedback becomes part of a culture of success. Haddock, et al. (1995) developed an employee-feedback model consistent with this philosophy:

> Performance feedback will be a process of ongoing communication among the employees, customers, suppliers, peers, and supervisors. This feedback will focus on improvements that have been made and, through customer knowledge, will identify further opportunities for continuous improvement. The supervisor will serve as leader, coach, and mentor, creating an environment which fosters individual growth and teamwork. (Haddock, et al., 1995: 145)

There is a current trend away from command-and-control management characterized by hierarchy and authority to a commitment-based management model, with emphasis on employee participation and involvement. Health care organizations are particularly suited to the commitment-based approach (Khatri, et al., 2006). Unfortunately, the majority of health care organizations are still stuck in the industrial model of management, which results in a demoralized, disfranchised health care workforce. We recommend that health care organizations, rather than attempting interventions aimed at individual HR practices, such as 360-degree feedback and self-managed teams, should

look at their broad philosophy of management (such as that demanded by CQI). All these HR practices fit the commitment-based approach quite naturally. Thus, before health care organizations make significant changes in their HR systems, they should first embrace a "Theory Y" philosophy of managing people at the organizational level.

MANAGERIAL GUIDELINES

1. *Know the value of the performance appraisal.* If adopted successfully, the performance-appraisal process can attract and retain highly qualified employees and increase their motivation and performance. A well-implemented system can also develop human resources that synergistically contribute to organizational goals.

2. *Use performance appraisal either in employee development or as an administrative tool.* To promote employee development, set goals, correct wrong behavior, chart career paths, and identify training needs of employees. Administratively, link rewards to performance and assess the efficacy of HRM policies and programs.

3. *Align performance appraisal with organizational goals.* A well-designed HR strategy supported by unifying HRM practices should complement organizational strategy and values to bring out the best in employee job behaviors.

4. *Performance appraisal affects pay-for-performance programs.* If performance can be accurately measured, it can be rewarded accordingly. Correspondingly, terminating low-performing employees can avert or minimize legal liability.

5. *Avoid costly legal mistakes.* Appraisals should support the manager's decisions. Procedures should be adequate and objective. Follow an "organizationally sensible approach" by

balancing salient legal threats with legitimate criteria for organizational performance.

6. *Correctly identify a method best suited for your organization.* Decide on a method based on the competencies your organization desires from employees and the approach that matches your organization's purpose for performance appraisal.

7. *Manage employees with collaboration, not competition, as a fundamental philosophy.* Award-winning organizations have HR practices that support organizational cultures in which employee commitment, cooperation, and communication are hallmarks.

8. *Strive to foster a supportive organizational culture.* Assist employees to enhance their performance instead of monitoring and controlling them. Solicit the input of employees involved in appraised activity. Establish performance on absolute rather than relative standards.

9. *Team appraisals.* Identify the dynamic interaction between individuals on group performance and the group on individual performance.

DISCUSSION QUESTIONS

1. Discuss the strategic role of performance appraisal in managing the health care workforce.
2. What are the common problems encountered in the performance-appraisal process? Suggest ways to overcome them.
3. Explain the conflict between traditional performance-appraisal systems and the TQM philosophy.
4. What are the four core activities of a typical HR department in health care organizations?
5. Do you see any connection of performance appraisal with other major HR roles, such as recruitment and selection, training and development, and compensation and rewards?
6. Why are HR activities typically fragmented in health care organizations?

CASE: MOVING FROM A CULTURE OF BLAME TO A CULTURE OF SAFETY: EASIER SAID THAN DONE

The senior management of a large midwestern nursing home gathered data on its quality of patient care and patient safety. They found that the quality and safety of patient care in the nursing home was deficient. To solve the problem, the managers, with the help of a total quality management expert, implemented a sophisticated continuous quality improvement (CQI) process with structured monthly meetings to review relevant data. Except for the senior nurse manager, other clinical employees did not participate or receive information on the deliberations of the meetings.

While the top managers were very satisfied that the CQI addressed the problem in a systematic and formal manner, the clinical staff employees were very frustrated in their efforts to report medical errors. This was because for every medication error, staff members were assigned one point and disciplined after three points. They could even be terminated as the disciplinary process progressed. The points accumulated over the year were also used to determine the annual salary increases and promotions of the nurses.

Based on the above performance appraisal system, the nursing home reported an improvement in the reduction of medication errors. However, adverse clinical outcomes for patients remained unchanged. To investigate this problem, the top management team hired a new HR consultant.

After promising that all information would be strictly confidential, the consultant was able to convince the clinical staff to talk freely about the problem of patients with adverse outcomes. In fact, the clinical staff admitted not filling out incident reports because of the punitive reporting system and expressed concern about the disconnection between the nursing home's goal of improving medication safety practices and the nursing home's approach to error.

CASE DISCUSSION QUESTIONS

1. How common may be the coexistence of CQI and punitive reporting systems in U.S. nursing homes?
2. What would you do when implementing a CQI process to reduce medical errors?
3. How would you change the incident-reporting and performance-appraisal systems?

REFERENCES

Adcroft, A., & Willis, R. (2005). The (un)intended outcome of public sector performance measurement. *The International Journal of Public Sector Management, 18*(4/5): 386–400.

Antonio, D., & Park, H. (2001). The relationship between rater effect and three sources of 360-degree feedback ratings. *Journal of Management, 27*: 479–495.

Atwater, L., & Brett, J. (2006). 360 degree feedback to managers: Does it result in changes in employee attitudes? *Group & Organization Management, 31*: 578–600.

Beck, S. (1990). Developing a primary nursing performance appraisal tool. *Nursing Management, 21*(1): 36–42.

Blackburn, R., & Rosen, B. (1993). Total quality and human resource management: lessons learned from Baldrige Award-winning companies. *Academy of Management Executive, 7*: 49–66.

Bryan, C., Rodgers, R., & Rosenhauer, E. (2007). *An Evaluation of Human Resource Management Strategies and the Physician-Employee in Various Group Practice Settings.* Working Paper. The Department of Health Management & Informatics, School of Medicine, University of Missouri, Columbia.

Chandra, A., & Frank, Z.D. (2004). Utilization of performance appraisal systems in health care organizations and improvement strategies for supervisors. *The Health Care Manager, 23*(1): 25–30.

Cicek, M.C., Koksal, G., & Ozdemirel, N.E. (2005). A team performance measurement model for continuous improvement. *Total Quality Management, 16*(3): 331–349.

Davison, G., & Hyland, P. (2002). Palliative care teams and organizational capability. *Team Performance Management, 8*(3/4): 60-67.

Deming, W.E. (1986). *Out of the Crisis.* Cambridge, MA: MIT.

Douglas, J., Klein S., & Hunt, D. (1985). *The Strategic Managing of Human Resources.* New York: Wiley.

Dutton, G. (2001). Making reviews more efficient and fair. *Workforce, 80*(4): 76–82.

Fallon, Jr., L.F., & McConnell, C.R. (2007). *Human Resource Management in Health Care: Principles and Practice.* Jones and Bartlett Publishers: Sudbury, MA.

Fisher, C.D., Schoenfeldt, L.F., & Shaw, J.B. (2006). *Human Resource Management* (6th ed.). Houghton Mifflin Company: Boston, MA.

Gentry, M.B. (2006). Registered nurse peer evaluation in the preoperative setting. *AORN Journal, 84*(3): 462–472.

Ghorpade, J., & Chen, M.M. (1995). Creating quality-driven performance appraisal systems. *Academy of Management Executive, 9*(1): 32–41.

Haddock, C.C., Nosky, C., Fargasson, C.A., Jr., & Kurz, R.S. (1995). The impact of CQI on human resources management. *Hospital & Health Services Administration, 40*(1): 138–153.

Ichniowski, C., & Shaw, K. (2003). Beyond incentive pay: Insiders' estimates of the value of complementary human resource management practices. *Journal of Economic Perspectives, 17*(1): 155–180.

Ivancevich, J.M., & Glueck, W.F. (1986). *Foundations of Personnel/Human Resource Management* (3rd ed.). Plano, TX: Business Publications.

Kerr, S. (1995). An academic classic: On the folly of rewarding A, while hoping for B. *Academy of Management Executive, 9*(1), 7–14.

Khatri, N. (2006). Building HR capability in health care organizations. *Health Care Management Review, 31*(1): 45–54.

Khatri, N., Baveja, A., Boren, S., & Mammo, A. (2006). Medical errors and quality of care: From control to commitment. *California Management Review, 48*(3): 115–141.

Kivimaki, M., Sutinen, R., Elovainio, M., Vahtera, J., Rasanen, K., Toyry, S., Ferrie, J.F., Firth-Cozens, J. (2001). Sickness absence in hospital physicians: Two year follow-up study in determinants. *Occupation and Environmental Medicine, 58*: 361–366.

Kuzmits, F.E., Adams, A.J., Sussman, L., & Raho, L.E. (2004). 360-Feedback in health care management: a field study. *The Health Care Manager, 23*(4): 321–328.

Longnecker, C.O., & McGinnis, D.R. (1992). Appraising technical people: Pitfalls and solutions. *Journal of Systems Management, 43*(12): 12–16.

Longnecker, C.O., Sims, H.P., & Gioia, G.A. (1987). Behind the mask: the politics of employee appraisal. *Academy of Management Executive, 1*(30): 183–193.

MacDuffie, J.P. (1995). Human resource bundles and manufacturing performance: organizational logic and flexible production systems in the world auto industry. *Industrial and Labor Relations Review, 48*(2): 197–221.

McConnell, C.R. (2003). *The Health Care Manager's Human Resources Handbook.* Management Concepts: Vienna, VA.

McGregor, D. (1985). *The Human Side of Enterprise.* McGraw-Hill, New York.

Nelson, B. (2000). Are performance appraisals obsolete? *Compensation & Benefits Review, 32*(3): 39–43.

Pollitt, D. (2004). Alliance Unichem uses 360-degree feedback to improve performance. *Human Resource Management International Digest, 12*(10): 27–29.

Rikleen, L.S. (2007). *Time to Reappraise Performance Appraisals.* The Receivables Report, June: 10–11.

Roehling, M.V., & Wright, P.M. (2006). Organizationally sensible versus legal-centric approaches to employment decisions. *Human Resource Management, 45*(4): 605–627.

Timmreck, T.C. (1989). Performance appraisal systems in rural western hospitals. *Health Care Management Review, 14*(2): 31–43.

Tyson, S. (1995). *Human Resource Strategy: Towards a General Theory of Human Resource Management.* Pitman, London.

Weitzel, B. (2002). Moving to a team-based structure in health care. *The Journal for Quality and Participation, 25*(2): 30–34.

CHAPTER 14

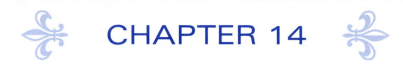

Compensation Principles for the Health Care Environment

Cheryl Locke, BA, Alesia Jones, CCP, MBA, and Katrina Graham, MBA

LEARNING OBJECTIVES

Upon completing this chapter, the reader will be able to:

1. Define and discuss the strategic role of human resources in compensation design for a health care organization.
2. Identify the two general types of compensation and the components of each.
3. Discuss legal and regulatory concerns for a health care organization. Specifically, you will be able to identify the basic provisions of the Fair Labor Standards Act (FLSA) and discuss wage and hour standards.
4. Discuss issues involving pay increases and show how they play a major role in facilitating organizational performance.
5. Define and discuss the major components of any compensation philosophy.
6. Identify the major challenges in compensation at all levels within a health care organization.

KEY TERMS

Compensation Strategy

Competency-Based Pay

Direct Compensation

Compensatory Time Off

Entitlement Culture

Exempt Employees

Indirect Compensation

Market-Based Pay

Nonexempt employees

Pay Mix

Performance-Based Culture

INTRODUCTION

Imagine that you are standing at the hospital bed of your mother or father. You and your parent—in fact, your entire family—are in the hands of the doctor, nurse, health care technician or, more than you might want to acknowledge, support staff. In such moments, we cannot imagine that there is any price too high for the skills and attention of those health care workers. While we hope they are motivated by caring and dedication, they are also motivated by a paycheck. What is the value that we attach to the provision of great, safe, quality health care?

Human resources (HR) professionals generally cite factors such as leadership, personal growth, work/family balance, respect, and communication as drivers of satisfaction. Employee surveys in all types of industries report that the "job itself" and "my manager" are critical to overall workplace satisfaction. As Jac Fitz-enz, referencing Herzberg in the 1950s, states in *The ROI of Human Capital*, fair pay and benefits are a given (Fitz-enz, 2000). In HR circles, we might say that pay and benefits, if not managed well, can be a "dissatisfier." As the changes in the American workforce create new generational and cultural differences, we need to understand what pay and benefits mean to different groups of people. In the face of clinical advancements, the focus on high touch and high tech, workforce shortages, and financial constraints, health care leaders and human resources professionals are constantly challenged to create new and innovative total compensation solutions. The typical solutions will not work for atypical situations. In a sense, then, there are no "textbook answers."

But with an effective **compensation strategy** you can place your organization in a better position to address the challenges that arise from managing the compensation of your workforce.

IMPORTANCE OF COMPENSATION STRATEGY

Determining the compensation strategy of a health care organization can be critical to the organization's overall success. Since health care is a service-related industry, the people who provide the services are oftentimes the primary competitive advantage that you have over your competition. So how you compensate for that advantage is not easy to determine. Total compensation (cash compensation and benefits) represent a large part of most organizations' operating budgets. Therefore, some shifts in strategy can have a significant financial impact.

In determining the compensation strategy for an organization there are five key elements that should be considered: (1) the forms of compensation that will be or can be offered, (2) workforce demographics, (3) the business cycle, (4) the compensation philosophy, and (5) legal and regulatory compliance. All of these elements should be considered in the context of the legal and regulatory requirements related to compensation.

It should be noted that this chapter focuses on the strategic elements of compensation administration. Prior to the administration of a compensation plan there should first be a solid compensation program in place. The development of any compensation program or salary system begins with the assumption that accurate *job descriptions* and *job specifications* (or *minimum qualifications*) are available and updated as needed. The job descriptions then are used for the *job evaluation* and *salary surveys*. These activities are designed to ensure that the pay system is both internally equitable and externally competitive. The data compiled in these two activities are used to design *pay structures*, including *pay grades* and minimum-to-maximum *pay ranges*. After the development of pay structures, individual jobs must be placed in the appropriate pay grades and employees' pay adjusted based on individually determined factors such as length of service and/or performance. Finally, the pay system must be monitored and maintained.

As you would imagine, there are a great number of steps and details involved in design of a pay system or compensation program. Since most of the design work will be handled by the human resources department in the organization, this chapter will not discuss the details of compensation program design. However, key terms have been provided that are involved in compensation plan design.

Not only is compensation plan design a difficult and never-ending work, so too is compensation administration. In order to make the best decisions regarding the financial resources provided for compensation, you must first understand the importance of a compensation strategy. Determining compensation strategy is entrusted work that should not be taken lightly and should be monitored often.

THE FORMS OF COMPENSATION

Compensation programs are made up of two basic components, direct compensation and indirect compensation (see Table 14.1).

Direct Compensation

Direct compensation is all tangible rewards of the working relationship, that is, the sum of base pay plus variable pay (Hall & Liebman, 1998). *Base pay* (all wages and salaries) is the basic compensation that an employee receives. Base pay is typically delivered as a wage or salary. Many organizations use two base pay categories, hourly and salaried. Hourly paid employees are paid for each hour that they work. This includes overtime pay for hours worked in excess of 40 in a work week. Hourly paid employees are oftentimes eligible for differentials that are added to their base pay rate; the most commonly used differential is for working various shifts. The determination of hourly and salaried jobs is based on the Fair Labor Standards Act's definition, which is discussed later in this chapter.

Salaried employees are paid for the job that they do, regardless of the hours it takes to do that job. Most of you will be salaried employees. Typically, salaried employees are eligible for larger variable-pay components in order to recognize the work required of salaried employees. The other element of direct compensation is *variable pay*, which is compensation linked directly to individual, team, or organizational performance. The most common types of variable pay are received as bonuses, incentives, or stock options. Variable pay is often referred to as incentive compensation because it is used as an "incentive" to meet the predefined performance goal (Miceli & Heneman, 2000).

Table 14.1. Forms of Compensation

Direct Compensation	Indirect Compensation
Base Pay	Flexible Benefits
Differential Pay	Income Replacement Programs (i.e., long-term disability)
Short-term incentive	Deferred Pay (retirement programs)
Long-term incentive	Pay for time not worked
Cash Awards	Unpaid Leave

Example One

A manager of radiology earns an annual salary of $85,000 and is eligible for up to 10% of her base pay if the organization meets its financial and patient-satisfaction performance goals. Assuming all goals are met, her earning potential for the year could be $93,500 ($85,000 + 8,500).

Example Two

A medical technologist earns $15.00 per hour on the evening shift, which pays a $1.00 per hour differential. This med tech has typically worked 100 hours of overtime each year. The value of his annual earning potential can vary greatly based on the hours worked, the shift worked, and the amount of overtime worked, but assuming the data presented, he could expect to earn $35,530 based on the following calculations:

1. *Base pay*—$15 × 2,080 hours worked per year (40 hours per week × 52 weeks) = $31,200
2. *Shift differential*—$1 × 2,080 = $2,080
3. *Overtime*—$22.50 (overtime rate = 1½ times base rate) × 100 = $2,250

Indirect Compensation

Pay received in the form of services and benefits is called **indirect compensation.** Some of the most common forms of indirect compensation are health insurance, income replacement programs (life/disability insurance), paid-time off, retirement/pension plans, and educational assistance. Indirect compensation is also a tangible reward of the work relationship because there is a very real cost to the organization for all elements of indirect compensation. However, since employees do not "see" this compensation in their take-home pay they often do not consider it compensation at all. Also, since many organizations offer elements of indirect compensation (namely health insurance and retirement plans) in a cost-sharing method, the employee actually pays something for the service or benefit (Fredericksen & Soden, 1998). For this reason, it is important for the organization

to frequently remind its employees of the value of their total compensation, which is the sum of direct and indirect compensation.

The amount of emphasis that is placed on each of the elements of total compensation creates the **pay mix.** There is no one correct mix of compensation that should be a part of your overall compensation strategy. In fact, many organizations have found that having different pay mixes for various groups of employees best helps them meet their overall organizational goals and objectives. Figure 14.1 shows some different pay mixes that could be used for different employee groups within an organization.

THE WORKFORCE DEMOGRAPHICS

In determining the compensation strategy for your organization, you must consider the characteristics of your workforce. Since the workforce of any service organization is the product the organization offers the marketplace, it is important to consider the make-up and needs of your workforce. This is another area that will change over time, so this element of your strategy needs to be re-assessed frequently. One of the ways to assess the needs of your workforce is through the use of employee surveys, which will be discussed later.

When considering the characteristics of your work force, you should ask yourself the following questions:

- What are the basic demographics of the workforce?
- What benefits does the workforce want or need?
- Can the needs and desires of the workforce be met?

The workforces of many organizations are currently made up of employees who ages range from the early 20s up to the 70s! Historically, the need for more flexibility in scheduling and time off has been more important to employees with young

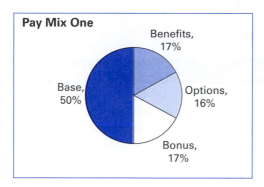

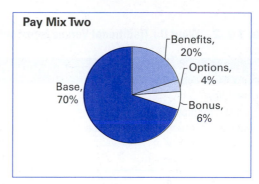

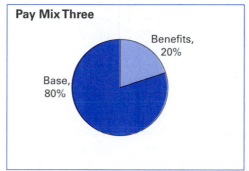

Figure 14.1. **Examples of Different Pay Mix Options**

families. Today more and more employees are finding themselves "sandwiched" between having to take care of their children and their parents. These needs have made the work/life element of the total rewards model an increasingly more important component of the compensation strategy.

The expression "work–life balance" was first used in 1986 in the U.S. to help explain the unhealthy lifestyle choices that many people were making; they were choosing to neglect other important areas of their lives such as family, friends, and hobbies in favor of work-related chores and goals (Greenblatt, 2002).

More and more of the employees entering today's workforce are concerned not just about doing a good job for their employer but also about doing a good job that they enjoy, that makes them feel good about going to work every day, and for some, most importantly, a job that provides them with the flexibility and financial security to do the things they want and need to

do (Greenblatt, 2002). In short, more and more of the employees in today's workforce want work–life balance.

Many studies have been conducted that compare and contrast the typical values of a traditional workforce and the emergent workforce. Table 14.2 is a summary of five key workforce values as defined by Spherion Staffing Group (Harris Interactive, 2005).

Another critical ingredient in determining the compensation strategy for your organization is to assess if you have a culture of entitlement or performance. **Entitlement cultures** and **performance-based cultures** lie on opposite ends of a continuum. Most compensation systems will fall somewhere in the middle of that continuum.

In an entitlement culture you will find automatic increases to all employees every year. Further, most of the employees receive the same or nearly the same percentage increase each year. Employees and managers who subscribe to the entitlement culture

Table 14.2. **What Do Traditional Versus Emergent Employees Value?**

Emergent Employees	VALUES	Traditional Employees
Defined as contribution	LOYALTY	Defined as tenure
Viewed as a vehicle for growth	JOB CHANGE	Viewed as damaging to one's career
Considered employee's responsibility to pursue	CAREER PATH	Considered organization's responsibility to provide
Based on level of performance	ADVANCEMENT	Based on length of service
Rejected as a driver of commitment	JOB SECURITY	Required as a driver of commitment

believe that individuals who have worked another year are *entitled* to a raise in base pay (Mathis & Jackson, 2004). They also believe that incentives programs should always be continued and benefits should be increased regardless of changing industry or economic conditions. Organizations that have an entitlement culture, as it relates to pay, continue their employees' cost increases regardless of employee performance or organizational competitive pressures. External market data is typically monitored in this type of culture but does not necessarily drive compensation strategy decisions unless significant recruitment or retention issues exist for a particular job or positions (e.g., registered nurses or pharmacists).

Hospitals and medical centers have especially struggled with the entitlement orientation of their long-term employees. Today's market pressures on health care organizations and the declining revenues many organizations are experiencing would clearly support a performance-based approach to paying annual increases (Heneman, Greenberger, & Strasser, 1988; Mathis & Jackson, 2004). However, two factors have contributed to the entitlement culture of most organizations: (1) decades of paying automatic increases, called cost-of-living adjustments (COLA) (or merit-pay systems that do not reward based on merit) and (2) collective bargaining agreements that require automatic step increases.

In organizations where unions are present, pay and benefits are the most commonly negotiated aspects of the contract, although not the only issues up for bargaining. In some settings, various segments of the employee population may be organized. What surfaces at the bargaining table from either side is a function of what groups of employees are in the bargaining unit. Nurses and health care technical staff are likely to have different issues than environmental aides (housekeeping), or support staff.

Nonetheless, health care unions have successfully surfaced staffing ratios, scheduling, patient safety, and workplace safety as critical issues for consideration. In the absence of real solutions to those issues, additional compensation has frequently been offered as the panacea. Sometimes when there are other solutions to such issues, union leadership is either not receptive or not trusting. Some unions, though, have been more straightforward and have a stated goal of a living wage. Within the realm of health care, every pay and benefit program can be surfaced at the bargaining table. Having a compensation philosophy for the entire organization is wise, since agreements made at the bargaining table generally impact all other decisions throughout the organization. Since many unions resist performance-based compensation, it is critical to understand how across-the-board compensation and benefit changes will affect the validity of other performance-based programs. This is often the area in which the entitlement culture and performance-based culture suffer real clashes.

Where a performance-based culture exists, organizations do not guarantee additional or increased compensation for simply completing another year of service with the organization. Instead, pay and incentives reflect performance differences among employees. Employees who perform well receive larger compensation increases and those who do not perform satisfactorily see little or no increase in base pay. Bonus compensation may be paid on the basis of individual, team, or organizational performance.

Whether you are operating in an organization with a pay culture of entitlement or one that is based on performance will have an impact on the overall compensation strategy you design.

THE BUSINESS CYCLE

Compensation decisions must be viewed strategically. Since so many organizational funds are spent on compensation-related activities, it is critical for top management and HR professionals to match compensation practices with what the organization is trying to accomplish (see Figure 14.2). Consider the following examples. The compensation program for a new physician practice will probably be different from that of a mature, more established clinic. If a new practice wanted to accelerate its growth, it may offer a competitive base pay, higher-than-average incentives, and a modest benefits package. In such a situation, you may also find lucrative

retention bonuses in order to attract talented workers who can quickly contribute to the success of the practice. Conversely, for a large, stable clinic with a well-established patient-referral base, a more structured (or higher) base pay and benefits program may exist and incentives will typically be lower.

Determining where the organization is in the business cycle is an important component of developing an effective compensation strategy. Once the overall organization reaches the stability point then the cycle should be accessed within segments of the organization. For example, the neurology service line may be in a high growth cycle while the women and infants service line may be in a decline growth cycle. This information, along with knowing where you want the organization to go, will greatly impact the decisions that are made when determining the compensation philosophy.

THE COMPENSATION PHILOSOPHY

Even though health care organizations might wish to pay the top wages and salaries relative to their competition, that might not be possible

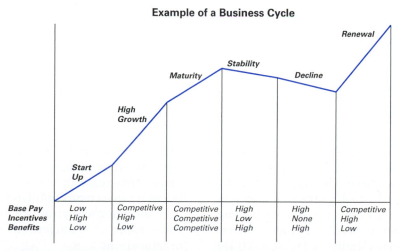

Figure 14.2. Example of a Business Cycle

because of the significant pressure that health care organizations face to control their costs. Three basic approaches to health care compensation include **market-based pay, competency-based pay,** and team-based pay. An overview of each approach follows.

Market-Based Pay

Some health care organizations establish specific policies around where they wish to be positioned in the labor market. Oftentimes, this position relative to the labor market is the only element of some organization's compensation philosophy *and* their compensation strategy. Market position is an important element; it is these authors' hope that from what you have read up to this point, you realize that there is much more to establishing a compensation strategy.

Position in the market is usually defined as one of the following market positions: (1) leading the market, (2) matching the market, or (3) lagging behind the market. Data from salary surveys reveal that the actual dollar difference between positions is generally from 15 to 25%.

Most employers choose to position themselves in the *match-the-market* position, which is in the middle of the market (median), based on the survey data of other employers' compensation plans. Choosing this level attempts to balance employer cost pressures and the need to attract and retain employees by providing a standard level of compensation.

An employer using a *lag-the-market* approach might choose to pay below market compensation for several reasons. The employer might be experiencing a shortage of funds and be unable to pay more and still meet objectives. It is important to note that the organization's ability to pay is most often the determining factor for which this approach is used. This approach is also used when an abundance of workers is available, particularly those with lower skills—a lag-the-market approach can be used to attract sufficient workers at lower costs (Mathis & Jackson, 2004).

Not surprisingly, there are downsides to this approach to the market. Sometimes it will cause the voluntary turnover to be greater if employees realize that they can get higher wages at other organizations. Also, when the labor market supply tightens, then attracting and retaining workers becomes more difficult. When organizations shift from a lag position to a match position in order to improve recruitment efforts, they should be careful not to create, or proliferate, salary compression between existing staff and new hires. Salary compression is the existence of very narrow pay differentials among jobs as a result of wages for jobs filled from the outside increasing faster than the internal staff's wages. This typically happens with entry-level jobs but can exist within any job or job groups.

A *lead-the-market* approach uses an aggressive pay-above-the-market emphasis. This strategy generally enables an organization to attract and retain sufficient workers with the required capabilities and to be more selective when hiring. However, because it is a higher-cost approach, organizations often look for ways to increase the productivity of employees receiving above-market wages (Mathis & Jackson, 2004).

In many cases, depending on the availability of workers with certain skills (e.g., pharmacists, certified nurse anesthetists), organizations may adopt a strategy to utilize a lead approach for those positions, yet pay at lag or match positions for less-hard-to-fill positions. This approach entails a "market-driven" philosophy (see Table 14.3).

In a purely market-driven philosophy, data from the external market is used to base the pay for most if not all positions. External market data should be used to validate the internal pay structure (the relationship that jobs have to each other within the organization) and support the organizations' business objectives. Pure market pricing carried to the extreme ignores internal alignment completely. It basically states that the compensation decisions of organizations' competitors determine the pay within that organization.

Table 14.3. Probable Relationships Between External Pay Policies and Objectives

Policy	Compensation Objectives			
	Ability to Attract	Ability to Retain	Contain Labor Costs	Reduce Pay Dissatisfaction
Pay above the market (lead)	+	+	?	+
Pay with the market (match)	=	=	=	=
Pay below the market (lag)	−	?	+	−

SOURCE: Adapted from Milkovich and Newman (2005).

Competency-Based Pay

The design of most compensation programs rewards employees for carrying out their tasks, duties, and responsibilities. The job requirements and responsibilities determine which employees have higher base rates. Employees receive more for doing jobs that require a greater variety of tasks, more knowledge and skills, greater physical effort, or more demanding working conditions (Brown, Sturman, & Simmering, 2003). However, some health care organizations are emphasizing competencies rather than tasks—competencies such as the ability to perform a particular clinical procedure or the attainment of a clinical credential such as a certified emergency room nurse. A number of organizations are paying employees for the competencies they demonstrate rather than just for the specific task performed. Paying for competencies rewards employees who exhibit more versatility and continue to develop their competencies.

In knowledge-based pay (KBP) or skill-based pay (SBP) systems, employees start at a base level of pay and receive increases as they learn to do other jobs or gain other skills and therefore become more valuable to the employer (Brown, et al., 2003). For example, in an RN clinical ladder program, RNs will have the opportunity to move up two or more pay levels based on their ability to demonstrate higher levels of clinical competency. Table 14.4 depicts the pay structure of a clinical nursing ladder program.

Table 14.4. Example Depicting the Pay Structure of a Clinical Nursing Ladder Program

Position	Grade	Range (Hourly)	
		Minimum	Maximum
Clinical Nurse I	10	$28.00	$42.00
Clinical Nurse II	11	$31.00	$46.00
Clinical Nurse III	12	$34.00	$50.00

The success of competency plans requires managerial commitment to a philosophy different from those traditionally found in organizations. This approach places more emphasis on training employees and supervisors. Due to the extensive commitment to training and the need to monitor the competencies of employees that competency-based programs require, they are more likely to be implemented in larger health care organizations. Also, workflow must be adapted to all workers to move from job to job as needed. Additionally, clinical ladder programs have been used effectively for other health care professions such as medical technologist and pharmacy techs.

When a health care organization moves to a competency-based system, considerable time must be spent identifying the required competencies for the various jobs. Progression of employees must be possible, and they must be paid appropriately for all of their competencies. Any limitations in the numbers of people who can acquire more competencies (for pay) should be clearly identified. Training in the appropriate competencies is particularly critical. Also, a competency-based system needs to acknowledge or certify employees as they acquire certain competencies and then to verify the maintenance of those competencies. In summary, the use of a competency-based system requires significant investment of management time and commitment.

Individual Versus Team Rewards

As health care organizations have shifted to using work teams, they face the logical concern of how to develop compensation programs that build on the team concept. At issue is how to compensate the individual whose performance may also be evaluated on the basis of team achievement. Paying all members of the team the same amount, even though they demonstrate differing competencies and levels of performance, obviously creates equity concerns for employees (McClurg, 2001).

Many organizations use team rewards as variable pay added to base pay. Variable pay rewards for teams are most frequently distributed annually as a specified dollar amount, not as a percentage of base pay. Delivering pay in this way helps to create a greater sense of equity among the team, since the reward is typically the same for all team members. Rather than substituting for base-pay programs, team-based rewards appear to be useful in rewarding a team beyond the satisfactory level of performance.

Perception of Fair Pay

Another area that must be considered while developing the compensation philosophy for an organization is the perception of fairness around pay. Most people in health care organizations work in order to gain rewards for their efforts. Except in a volunteer capacity, people expect to receive what they feel is fair and tangible compensation

for their efforts. Whether base pay, variable pay, or benefits, the extent to which employees perceive compensation to be fair often affects their performance and how they view their jobs and employers (Brown, et al., 2003).

Employee-satisfaction surveys show that compensation is not the primary driver of satisfaction for employees. In fact, as mentioned above, employee satisfaction surveys typically indicate that the drivers of employee satisfaction are the job itself and leadership, specifically, an individual's immediate supervisor. There are other factors that are in some way related to the job itself and supervision, such as growth, opportunity, learning, communication, and finding purpose in one's work. Other factors that surface involve meaningful human interaction, such as relationships with co-workers and customers. So where is pay and benefits in this picture? As mentioned, fair pay and benefits are considered by employees to be a given. At least, that is what Herzberg and others have believed since the 1950s. Of course, though, the whole notion of work has changed over the last nearly 60 years. The question is whether we can still assume that the current and emerging workforce views its job satisfaction in the same way.

The 2006/2007 WorkUSA™ Survey Report conducted by Watson Wyatt asserts that top performers leave an organization because of pay more than anything else, or at least that is what the workers state. The report states that employees may be placing greater emphasis on pay because of recent decreases in other benefits, including pension plans and health care coverage; an indication that the "employment deal" is clearly in flux (Watson Wyatt Worldwide, 2006/2007). Combine that view with the projections about how long new entrants into the workforce want to work and how often they are expected to change jobs, we may see a significant shift in the drivers of satisfaction in the future, and we should prepare for it now. Organizations that have embraced the total rewards approach may be nimble enough for the inevitable. Before you finalize the compensation philosophy for an organization, it is important to "hear" what your employees value.

LEGAL AND REGULATORY CONCERNS

In managing compensation systems, health care organizations must comply with a myriad of federal, state, and local regulations and reporting requirements. Important areas addressed by the laws include minimum wage standards and hours of work. The following discussion examines the laws and regulations affecting base compensation.

Fair Labor Standards Act (FLSA)

The major federal law affecting compensation is the Fair Labor Standards Act (FLSA), which was passed in 1938. Amended several times to raise minimum wage rates and expand employers covered, the FLSA affects both private and public sector employers. Compliance with FLSA provisions is enforced by the Wage and Hour Division of the U. S. Department of Labor. To meet FLSA requirements, health care employers must keep accurate time records and maintain these records for three years. Compliance investigations from the Wage and Hour Division follow up complaints filed by individuals who believe they have not received the overtime payments due them. Also, certain industries that historically have had a large number of wage and hour violations can be targeted by the Wage and Hour Division, and firms in those industries can be investigated.

Complaints regarding FLSA violations are the fastest growing area of human resource-related complaints. Penalties for wage and hour violations often include awards of back pay for affected current and former employees for up to two years. For example, a large medical center had allowed the nursing supervisors to arbitrarily pay overtime wages to some regularly scheduled charge nurses, who had been classified as **exempt employees.** This was done to encourage these charge nurses to pick up additional shifts. Some of the charge nurses who had not been recipients of the overtime

pay complained to the Wage and Hour Division. Upon investigation, the division determined that the payment of indiscriminate overtime wages to otherwise exempt employees nullified their exempt status, and the Division subsequently negotiated a large back-pay award for the charge nurses.

Changes in FLSA Regulations

Many HR professionals argued that the nearly 70-year-old law created great difficulties for employers trying to follow all the requirements of the law. For instance, it has been difficult to use the older regulations when examining jobs such as physician assistant, clinic office manager, or biomedical engineer that did not exist in 1938 or that have changed significantly since then.

The Department of Labor has now revised various sections of the FLSA and its regulations governing who must be paid overtime. These changes took effect on August 23, 2004. The provisions of both the original act and subsequent revisions focus on the following major areas: (1) establishing a minimum wage; (2) discouraging inappropriate wage practices for child labor; and (3) encouraging limits on the number of hours employees work per week, through overtime provisions (exempt and nonexempt statuses).

Minimum Wage

The FLSA sets a minimum wage to be paid to the broad spectrum of covered employees. The actual minimum wage can be changed only by congressional action. A lower minimum wage is set for "tipped" employees, such as restaurant workers, but their compensation must equal or exceed the minimum wage when average tips are included. Minimum wage levels continue to spark significant political discussions and legislative maneuvering. The U.S. Federal Minimum Wage became $5.15 in September 1997. Ten years later, Congress approved an increase in the minimum wage from $5.15 per hour to $7.75 per hour by July 24, 2009. This will be implemented in three steps of 55 cents each year, beginning on July 24, 2007 (U.S. Dept of Labor, 2008a).

There also is a debate about the use of a living wage versus the minimum wage. A living wage is one that is supposed to meet the basic needs of a worker's family. In the United States, the living wage typically aligns with the amount needed for a family of four to be supported by one worker so that family income is above the officially identified "poverty" level. Currently in the United States, at about $8.20 an hour, the living-wage level is significantly higher than the minimum wage. Although many employees working in health care organizations earn significantly above the federal minimum wage and the livable wage, many do not, especially front-line staff working in extended-care facilities.

Without waiting for U.S. federal laws to change, over 80 cities have passed local living-wage laws. Those favoring living-wage laws stress that even the lowest-skilled workers need to earn wages above the poverty level. Those opposed to living-wage laws point out that many of the lowest-paid workers are single, which makes the "family of four" test inappropriate. Obviously, there are ethical, economic, and employment implications on both sides of this issue.

Child Labor Provisions

The child labor provisions of the FLSA set the minimum age for employment with unlimited hours at 16 years. For hazardous occupations, the minimum is 18 years of age. Individuals 14–15 years old may work outside school hours with certain limitations. Many employers require age certificates for employees because the FLSA makes the employer responsible for determining an individual's age. A representative of a state labor department, a state education department, or a local school district generally issues such certificates (U.S. Dept of Labor, 2008a).

Exempt and Nonexempt Statuses

Under the FLSA, employees are classified as exempt or nonexempt. Exempt employees hold positions classified as executive, administrative, professional, or outside sales, for which employers are not required to pay overtime. Exempt employees are paid for the job that they do, not the hours that they work. As health care executives you will be exempt employees and will likely work more than 40 hours in many of your work weeks. **Nonexempt employees** are paid for the hours that they work and therefore must be paid overtime under the Fair Labor Standards Act (U.S. Dept of Labor, 2008a).

As noted above, in 2004 the FLSA regulations changed the terminology used to identify whether or not a job qualifies for exempt status. The categories of exempt jobs are

- Executive
- Administrative
- Professional
- Computer employees
- Outside sales

The regulations identify factors related to salaried pay levels per week, discretionary authority, and other criteria that must exist for jobs to be categorized as exempt. In base-pay programs, employers often categorize jobs into groupings that tie the FLSA status and the method of payment together. Employers are required to pay overtime for hourly jobs in order to comply with the FLSA. Employees in positions classified as salaried nonexempt are covered by the overtime provisions of the FLSA and therefore must be paid overtime. Salaried nonexempt positions sometimes include secretarial, clerical, and salaried blue-collar positions.

The FLSA does not require employers to pay overtime for salaried exempt jobs, although many health care organizations have implemented policies to pay a flat rate for extensive hours of overtime. For instance, hospitals may pay first-line supervisors extra using a special rate for hours worked over 50 a week during periods of high census or low staffing. A number of salaried exempt professionals in various information technology jobs also receive additional compensation for working extensive hours.

Overtime Provisions

The FLSA establishes overtime pay requirements. Its provisions set overtime pay at one and one-half times the regular pay rate for all hours over 40 a week, except for employees who are not covered by the FLSA. Overtime provisions do not apply to farm workers, who also have a lower minimum-wage schedule.

The workweek is defined as a consecutive period of 168 hours (24 hours × 7 days) and does not have to be a calendar week. If they wish to do so, hospitals and nursing homes are allowed to use a 14-day period instead of a 7-day week, as long as overtime is paid for hours worked beyond 8 in a day or 80 in a 14-day period (U.S. Dept of Labor, 2008a).

The most difficult part of the act is distinguishing who is and is not exempt. Some recent costly settlements have prompted more white-collar workers to sue for overtime pay.

Compensatory Time Off

Often called comp-time, **compensatory time off** is hours given to an employee in lieu of payment for extra time worked. Unless it is given to non-exempt employees at the rate of one and one-half times the number of hours over 40 that are worked in a week, comp-time is illegal in the private sector. Also, comp-time cannot be carried over from one pay period to another. The only major exception to these provisions is for public sector employees, such as fire and police employees, and a limited number of other workers (U.S. Dept. of Labor, 2008b).

Independent Contractor Regulations

The growing use of contingent workers by many health care organizations has focused attention on another group of legal regulations—those identifying the criteria that independent contractors must meet. Classifying someone as an independent contractor rather than an employee offers three advantages for the employer. First, the employer does not have to pay Social Security, unemployment, or workers' compensation costs. These additional payroll levies may add 10% or more to the costs of hiring the individual as an employee. Second, if the person is classified as an employee and is doing a job considered nonexempt under the federal FLSA, then the employer may be responsible for overtime pay at the rate of time-and-a-half for any week in which the person works more than 40 hours. Third, if the person is working enough hours to be eligible for organizational benefits, including pension eligibility, then the organization may be responsible for providing benefits consistent with its plan requirements. With the escalating cost of employee benefits, this is a key reason many employers consider using independent contractors. Most other federal and state entities rely on the criteria for independent contractor status identified by the Internal Revenue Service (IRS).

Equal Pay and Pay Equity

Various legislative efforts address the issue of wage discrimination on the basis of gender. The Equal Pay Act of 1963 applies to both men and women and prohibits using different wage scales for men and women performing substantially the same jobs. Pay differences can be justified on the basis of merit (better performance), seniority (longer service), quantity or quality of work, or factors other than gender. Similar pay must be given for jobs requiring equal skills, equal effort, or equal responsibility of jobs done under similar working conditions.

Pay equity is an issue different from equal pay for equal work. Pay equity is the concept (similar to comparable worth) that the pay for all jobs requiring comparable knowledge, skills, and abilities should be the same even if job duties and market rates differ significantly. States with such laws for public sector jobs include Hawaii, Iowa, Maine, Michigan, Minnesota, Montana, Ohio, Oregon, Washington, and Wisconsin. However, simply showing the existence of pay differences for jobs that are different has not been sufficient to prove discrimination in court in most cases.

State and Local Laws

Many states and municipalities have enacted modified versions of federal compensation laws. If a state has a higher minimum wage than that set under the Fair Labor Standards Act, the higher figure becomes the required minimum wage. As an example, Alaska, Minnesota, California, and Florida have basic minimum wage requirements that are higher than the federal minimum wage.

National Labor Relations Act (NLRA)

The National Labor Relations Act (NLRA), which is also known as the Wagner Act, is a federal law established in 1935 that protects the rights of most private sector workers to organize labor unions, to engage in collective bargaining, and to take part in strikes and other forms of concerted activity in support of their demands. Later in this chapter, we will discuss labor unions and the impact of this law on today's workforce.

Garnishment Laws

Garnishment of an employee's wages occurs when a creditor obtains a court order that directs an employer to set aside a portion of one employee's wages to pay a debt owed to a creditor. Regulations passed as part of the Consumer Credit Protection Act established limitations on the amount of wages that can be garnished and restricted the right of employers to discharge employees whose pay is subject to a single garnishment order. All 50 states have laws applying to wage garnishments.

PRACTICAL APPLICATION

All of the concepts previously discussed are parts of the "technical' application" of compensation in the Health care environment. This final section focuses

on the "practical" application of those concepts. As senior leaders in your organizations, you may encounter situations that do not match what you have learned in class or read in your textbooks. While the legal requirements should always be met, most of the other elements of compensation administration will vary by organization. Many of those variances will be a result of the key elements discussed earlier: the forms of compensation that will be or can be offered, the workforce demographics, the business cycle, and the compensation philosophy of the organization.

We will next discuss ways to best manage the following typical compensation related issues:

1. Communicating your compensation plan
2. Managing individual employee compensation
3. Managing compensation during staffing shortages
4. The expectation of high tech versus high touch
5. Executive Compensation

What Should You Communicate About Your Compensation Plan?

Compensation communicates. It signals what is important to your organization and what is not important. A major communication concern is the degree of openness that health care organizations have regarding their pay systems. Pay information kept secret in "closed" systems includes how much others make, what raises others have received, and even what pay grades and ranges exist in the organization. Some organizations have policies that prohibit employees from discussing their pay with other employees, and violations of these policies can lead to disciplinary action. However, several court decisions have ruled that these policies violate the NLRA. If employees who violate these "secrecy" policies are disciplined, the employers can be liable for back pay, damages, and other consequences.

Many health care organizations are opening up their pay systems by providing employees with more information on compensation policies, distributing a general description of the compensation system, and indicating where an individual's pay is within a salary range. Such information allows employees to make more accurate equity comparisons. For instance, an academic medical center in the South posts all of its open positions with corresponding pay grades and ranges on its Web site. This allows full access to pay information to both its own employees as well as potential applicants for its open positions. While it is never appropriate for employees to discuss individual salaries, having a more open pay system has been found to have positive effects on employee retention and organizational effectiveness.

Two appropriate reasons to practice open communications are (1) to show that the pay practices are both fair and defensible. One of the most challenging tasks for an organization is to communicate to its employees that the compensation program is fair and defensible; and (2) to address any issues of increased scrutiny. Currently, most employees have access to a computer, trade publications, and friends at other organizations—therefore, pay decisions are more carefully scrutinized than in the past. With a policy of open communication, the methodology and survey sources can be relayed and understood by the employee population; fear of the compensation program being unfair can be minimized; and employees can understand why their jobs are priced the way they are and what they need to do to advance in their careers.

On the flipside, in some organizations it could be more appropriate to practice closed communications. For those organizations, some of the reasons that they would not communicate pay rates are

1. The pay philosophy might be difficult for employees to understand or agree with. If the organization targets the 25th percentile, it might not want to communicate this information. Typically, when an organization targets a percentile below the 50th (or lagging behind the market) it is using other total rewards components to enhance the overall total rewards package; however, this could be potentially difficult to communicate to employees.

2. Historically, this information has been held "close to the vest," and to open communications requires buy-in from upper management. There are instances where upper management does not believe this information should be public (it could be a competitive advantage for the organization).

3. With all of the salary survey information being easily accessible for all employees (Internet, trade publications, etc.), the credibility of survey vendors may come into question by the employees. Employees might question why one survey source was used over another. Employees may not understand what makes a survey valid and reliable.

4. It might generate more confusion among employees. If the communication is not clear and concise, more questions concerning the compensation program could arise (Kovac, 2005).

The culture and overall philosophy on internal employee communications will be paramount to the decision of how to best communicate your compensation plan and resulting decisions. Regardless of which type of communication option that is used—open or closed—remember, compensation itself communicates.

Managing Individual Employee Compensation

Most of the time spent on compensation-related activities is typically spent on managing individual employee pay. One of the biggest advantages to having pay ranges is that they give flexibility by

Effective corporate communication linked to better financial performance

According to a recent study conducted by Watson Wyatt Worldwide, companies with effective internal communications, including compensation communications, have a 19.4% higher market premium and deliver 57% higher shareholder return compared to organizations with less effective internal communications. The 2005/2006 Communication ROI Study also found strong correlation between company communications and its employee engagement and retention levels. Investing in internal communications also provides other organizational benefits such as improved employee engagement and retention. According to the study, companies that communicate effectively are 4.5 times more likely to report a high level of employee engagement and are 20% more likely to report lower turnover rates than firms that communicate less effectively.

This study was conducted with companies across all industry sectors, and health care organizations, which made up 23.8% of the survey participants, and tended to rank among the least effective communicators. Although respondents came from various industry sectors, the findings revealed some interesting commonalities among the highly effective companies. These firms were particularly effective in treating managers as a key audience; regularly providing communication counsel to senior management; having a communication program in place and a documented internal communication strategy; and openly communicating with employees, sharing business plans and goals as well as providing information about matters that affect them.

SOURCE: Workspan, Published on May 22, 2006 (Watson Wyatt Worldwide, 2006)

---

allowing individual employees to progress within a pay grade without having to be moved to a new grade each time they receive a raise. A pay range also allows managers to reward better-performing employees while maintaining the integrity of the pay system.

Regardless of how well-constructed a pay structure is, there usually are a few individuals whose pay is lower than the minimum or higher than the maximum. These situations occur most frequently when organizations have had an informal pay system develop into a new, more formalized one or when unclear guidelines exist regarding managing pay within the pay system.

Red-Circled Employees

A red-circled employee is an incumbent who is paid above the range set for the job. For example, assume that an employee's current pay is $12.00 per hour but the pay range for that grade is $6.94 to $10.06. Over time, management would attempt to bring the employee's rate into grade.

Several approaches can be used to bring a red-circled employee's pay into line. Although the fastest way would be to cut the employee's pay, that approach is not recommended and is seldom used. Instead, the employee's pay may be frozen until the pay range can be adjusted upward to get the employee's pay rate back into the grade (Carson & Carson, 2007). Another approach is to give the employee a small lump-sum payment but not adjust the pay rate when others are given raises; this is referred to as a red-circled bonus (Mathis & Jackson, 2004).

Green-Circled Employees

An individual whose pay is below the range is a green-circled employee. Promotion is a major cause of this situation. Generally, it is recommended that the green-circled employee receive pay increases to get him or her to the pay-grade minimum fairly rapidly. Frequent increases should be considered if the increase to minimum would be substantial (Mathis & Jackson, 2004).

Pay Compression

One major problem many health care employers face is pay compression, which occurs when the pay differences among individuals with different levels of experience and performance becomes small. Pay compression occurs for a number of reasons, but the major one involves situations in which labor market pay levels increase more rapidly than current employees' pay adjustments. Such situations are prevalent in many health care occupational areas, such as registered nurses.

In response to competitive market shortages of particular job skills, managers occasionally may deviate from the priced grades to hire people with skills that are scarce. For example, suppose the worth of a radiological special procedures technician's job is evaluated at $48,000 to $58,000 annual salary in a hospital, but qualified individuals are in short supply and other employers are paying annual salaries of $70,000. The hospital must pay the higher rate to attract new technicians. Suppose also that several technicians who have been with the hospital for several years started at $48,000 and have received 4% increases to their rates each year. These current employees will still be making less than the salaries paid to attract new technicians from outside with less experience, causing a significant pay compression issue between the current employees and the new hires.

There is no easy fix to compression problems, at least for health care organizations that do not have an endless source of funds for salary adjustments (Mathis & Jackson, 2004). As indicated in the example given above, in order to attract talent to the organization it will take paying them more than the existing staff. Management can decide not to fill the open position in order to not create a compression problem, but typically that is not an option. Therefore, when a person is

hired at $70,000 onto a team where the average salary is $56,153 ($48,000 times four years of 4% increases), it would take almost $14,000 per person to correct the compression problem! Let's assume there are only five other employees who are in the radiological special procedures technician job; that would be an annual cost of $69,234 just to correct the compression for that job classification. That is almost the cost to hire another person. Now consider what the cost implications would be if there were 50 employees in the classification! This illustrates why compression problems are not as easy as it may seem to correct or avoid.

The source of many compression issues stems from health care organization attempts to maintain external equity and sustain a competitive market position. External equity considers the rates paid by other organizations in determining a competitive position for an organization's compensation program. Maintaining external equity is extremely important for health care employers in order to effectively compete for workers, especially in consideration of the shortage of skilled health care workers today. If a health care employer does not provide compensation that employees view as equitable compared to other organizations, that employer is more likely to experience higher turnover. Other drawbacks include greater difficulty in recruiting qualified and high-demand individuals. Also, by not being competitive, the employer is more likely to attract and retain individuals with less knowledge, skills, and abilities, resulting in lower overall organizational performance. The use of pay surveys is how organizations track external equity. But external equity must be married to internal equity in order to most effectively manage a compensation system. Focusing too much on one element of equity at the expense of the other can have costly and long-term adverse consequences.

Issues Involving Pay Increases

Decisions about pay increases often are critical ones in the relationships among employees, their managers, and the health care organization.

Individuals express expectations about their pay and about how much increase is fair, especially in comparison with the increases received by other employees. There are several ways to determine pay increases.

Pay Adjustment Matrix

Many health care employers profess to have a pay system based on performance. But relying on performance appraisal information for making a pay adjustment assumes that the appraisals are accurate and done well, which is not always the case. Consequently, a system for integrating appraisals and pay changes must be developed and applied equally. Often, this integration is done through the development of a pay-adjustment matrix, or salary-guide chart. Using pay-adjustment matrices, adjustments are based in part on personal performance and in part on position in the salary range, as shown in Table 14.5 (Mathis & Jackson, 2004).

Such charts can facilitate an employee's upward movement in an organization, which depends on the person's performance, as rated in an appraisal, and on the person's position in the pay range, which has some relationship to experience as well. Notice that as employees move up the pay range, they must exhibit higher performance to obtain the same percentage raise as those lower in the range performing at the "meets performance expectations" level. This approach is taken because the firm is paying above the market midpoint ($36,000 in this example) but receiving only satisfactory performance rather than above-expectations performance. Charts can be constructed to reflect the specific pay-for-performance policy and philosophy in an organization.

Seniority

Seniority, or time spent in the organization or on a particular job, can be used as the basis for pay increases. Many employers have policies that require a person to be employed for a certain length of time before being eligible for pay increases. Pay adjustments based on seniority often are set as automatic steps once a person has been employed the required length of time, although performance must be at least satisfactory in many nonunion systems.

Step systems, which use pay increases based solely on the attainment of a designated period of employment (typically 2,080 hours), continue to be a popular method of awarding pay increases in health care organizations, especially in states where there is significant unionization of health care employees. Each step represents the pay adjustment for employees as they attain one full-time equivalent year of employment (2,080 hours).

Cost-of-Living Adjustments (COLA)

A common pay-raise practice is the use of a standard raise or cost-of-living adjustment (COLA). Giving all employees a standard percentage increase enables them to maintain the same real wages in a period of economic inflation. Often, these adjustments are tied to changes in the consumer price index (CPI) or some other general economic measure. However, numerous studies have revealed that the CPI overstates the actual cost of living.

Table 14.5. Pay-Adjustment Matrix

Performance Rating	Q1 $28,000 to $32,000	Q2 $32,001 to $36,000	Q3 $36,001 to $40,000	Q4 $40,001 to $44,000	Over Max. > $44,001
Exceeds Expectations	5.0	4.0	3.0	2.0	1.0 (in lump sum)
Meets Expectations	4.0	3.0	2.0	1.0	
Does Not Meet Expectations					

Unfortunately, some health care employers give across-the-board raises and call them merit raises, which they are not. If all employees get the same increase, it is legitimately viewed as an across-the-board adjustment that has little to do with good performance. For this reason, employers should reserve the term "merit" for any amount above the standard raise and they should state clearly which amount is for performance and which amount is the COLA adjustment.

Lump-Sum Increases

A compensation practice that has gained popularity among some health care organizations is a lump-sum bonus in lieu of an incremental increase to an employee's base pay. As an example, employees who receive a pay increase, either for merit or seniority, may receive a lump sum increase in the amount of their regular monthly or weekly paycheck. For instance, an employee who makes $15.00 per hour and then receives a 3% increase will move to $15.45 per hour.

In contrast, a lump-sum increase (LSI) is a one-time payment of all or part of a yearly pay increase. The pure LSI approach does not increase the base pay. Therefore, in this example the person's base pay remains at $15.00 per hour. If an LSI of 3% is granted, then the person receives $936.00 (45¢ per hour for 2,080 working hours in a year.) However, the base rate remains at $15.00 per hour, which slows down the progression of the base wages. It also allows for the amount of the "lump" to be varied, without having to continually raise the base rate. Some organizations place a limit on how much of a merit increase can be taken as a lump-sum payment. Other organizations may split the lump sum into two checks, each representing one-half of the year's pay raise.

Pay-for-Performance

Another ongoing question regarding compensation is the impact that pay has on employee productivity. Numerous critics, led by Alfie Kohn, argue that incentives are wrong both from a moral and a practical standpoint. The moral argument suggests that incentives are flawed because they involve one person controlling another (Kohn, 1999). The counterargument to this notes that employment is a reciprocal arrangement. Especially in low periods of unemployment, workers can choose whether they want to work under compensation systems with strong pay-for-performance linkages (as in the case of incentive systems). We know that employees are not totally risk averse. There are circumstances in which they will prefer an incentive component to compensation rather than a totally fixed salary. Generally, if the incentive depends on individual performance, employees find the company more attractive. Team-based incentives, in contrast, are less attractive. Kohn also suggests that incentive systems can actually harm productivity, a decidedly negative practical outcome.

There are countless studies on pay-for-performance systems, but the conclusions on whether they work are mixed. Many of the studies are based on isolated situations or individuals. In the real world, people interact with each other and know who is performing and who is not, and they react according to this knowledge when rewards are allocated. Without any link to performance, the less-motivated employees will eventually recognize that harder work is not necessary. It quickly becomes evident that some workers are being paid the same for doing less. Think, for example, of the last time you completed a group project. Were you happy with the team member who did less but received the same grade? Did you think it fairer when you had a teacher who asked for evaluations of all group members' performances and used these data to assign individualized grades (rewards tied to performance)? The same situation arises in health care and makes the question "Should we tie rewards to performance?" at least a question worthy of further review within the context of achieving organizational objectives.

Managing Compensation During Staffing Shortages

In many health care organizations, 24/7 staffing is required. This is a reason why managing the number of employees and/or the hours they work is one of the most common challenges that managers in the health care industry face. The challenge is even more taxing when staffing shortages make it difficult to provide adequate coverage without breaking the bank!

Staffing Levels

The use of various staffing relationships is becoming a popular way to manage staffing levels. Many health care employers have established diverse relationships with different groups of employees. The two primary groups are commonly referred to as core employees, with whom a long-term relationship is desired, and contingent workers, whose employment agreements may cover only short, specific time periods. Rather than expand or contract the core workforce, many employers achieve flexibility and control labor costs by expanding or contracting the contingent workforce. When employees within the contingent workforce are used, the fixed portion of the organization's labor costs becomes smaller and the variable portion larger. This variable portion can be expanded or contracted more easily than the core.

Many hospitals use diverse sources for nurses, and the costs vary with the type of contingent workers used. Regular-status, pool, registry, and traveler nurses are paid differently, and the variable cost increases for each type of nurse are listed accordingly. Some nurses have benefits from the employing hospital (regular-status nurses), while others have benefits from the contracting agencies (registry and traveler nurses), and still others must purchase their own benefits (pool nurses). The tradeoffs in managing cost include balancing patient loads, nurse-to-patient ratios, costs of alternative sources, and quality of care.

The Expectation of High Tech Versus High Touch

In medical centers across the United States, there is an increasing need to focus on health care staff as having two sets of skills that in the past were viewed as opposing ends of the spectrum. Now, health care organizations want their staff to be both high touch and high tech. Especially within our academic

medical centers with their teaching and research components, it is critical to have staff that can grasp and apply new techniques and modalities of treatment. Consumers, though, have spoken loudly with their feet by opting for care in smaller, community-based settings in order to receive the human, caring touch long assumed to be the draw for those organizations. All of these health care organizations have come to realize that they will need to attract and retain staff that can and will combine those skills. Patients and their families expect well-trained RNs, nursing assistants, health care technicians, and physicians who can, and will, also hold their hand. Neither set of skills can be assumed, though both will require consideration on the compensation front.

Executive Compensation

Executive compensation in health care organizations is typically treated much differently than nonexecutive pay. Executive compensation typically includes multiple components, whereas nonexecutive compensation may only include pay and benefits. The common components of executive compensation are salaries, annual bonuses, long-term incentives, supplemental benefits, and perquisites.

Executive Salaries

Salaries of executives vary by type of job, size of organization, region of the country, and industry segment. On average, salaries make up about 40 to 60% of the typical top executive's annual compensation total.

Executive Bonus and Incentive Plans

Executive performance may be difficult to evaluate, but incentive and bonus compensation must reflect some performance measures if they are to be meaningful. Bonuses for executives can be determined in several ways. A discretionary system whereby bonuses are awarded based on the judgments of the chief executive officer and the board of directors is one way. However, the absence of formal, measurable targets detracts significantly from this approach. Also, as noted above, incentives can be tied to specific measures, such as effectively managing costs, improving patient satisfaction, or meeting revenue targets. More complex systems create incentive pools and thresholds above which payments are computed. Whatever method is used, it is important to describe it so that executives trying to earn incentives and bonuses understand the plan: otherwise, the incentive effect will be diminished.

As an example, a major medical center ties annual bonuses for senior managers to both operating cost reductions and employee retention. The bonuses have amounted to as much as 25% of each senior manager's base salary.

Performance Incentives: Long-Term Versus Short-Term

Performance-based incentives attempt to tie executives' compensation to the long-term growth and success of the organization. However, whether the emphasis is really on the long term or merely represents a series of short-term rewards is controversial. Short-term rewards based on quarterly or annual performance may not result in the kind of long-run-oriented decisions necessary for the organization to continue to do well.

Benefits for Executives

As with benefits for nonexecutive employees, executive benefits may take several forms, including traditional retirement plans, health insurance, and vacations. However, executive benefits may include some items that other employees do not receive. For example, executive health plans without co-payments and without limitations on deductibles or physician choice are popular among small and middle-sized organizations. Organization-owned life insurance on the life of the executive is popular and pays both the executive's estate and the company in the event of death. Trusts of various kinds may be designed by the organization to help the executive deal with estate tax-planning issues. Deferred compensation offers another possible means of helping executives with tax liabilities caused by incentive compensation plans.

Executive Perquisites

In addition to the regular benefits received by all employees, executives often receive benefits called perquisites. Perquisites (perks) are special executive benefits—usually noncash items. Perks help tie executives to organizations and demonstrate their importance to their companies. Many executives value the status enhancement of perks because these visible symbols of status allow executives to be seen as very important persons (VIPs) both inside and outside their organizations.

Current Nature of Health Care Executive Compensation

Health care executives—typically those in the top two levels of an organization, such as CEOs, administrators, presidents, or vice presidents—are paid very well. Increasingly, executives in the highest-ranking positions may also be physicians, complicating the compensation decisions.

In most health care organizations, the board of directors sets policy (Beekun, Stedham, & Young, 1998). For publicly traded companies covered by federal regulatory agencies such as the Securities and Exchange Commission (SEC), in particular those covered by Sarbanes-Oxley, the board must approve executive compensation packages. Nonprofit organizations are subject to IRS regulations as a condition for maintaining their tax exempt status. Health care organizations are required to file annual Form 990 statements with the IRS, identifying the total compensation of the highly compensated. These regulations make it prudent for nonprofit boards as the "authorizing body" to establish compensation committees, which set policy and provide oversight of executive compensation for reasonableness. It is the board's responsibility to review and approve the compensation for top-level executives (Beekun, et al., 1998). Failure to perform this duty places the organization, its board members, and, to some degree, the executives themselves at risk of sanctions from the IRS.

The compensation committee of the board of directors usually is a subgroup of the board

Hospital tax-exempt status and executive compensation

Tax-exempt hospitals are becoming increasingly aware that they may be the focus of a broadening IRS enforcement initiative examining executive compensation practices. The IRS has announced that the initiative is aimed at organizations that pay excessive compensation and benefits to their officers and other insiders. The IRS has indicated that their efforts are designed to identify and halt abuses by tax-exempt organizations. Areas of critical concern may be paying executives more than $1 million per year and offering excessive benefit transactions, including such items as car leases, spousal travel, tickets to sporting events, and other similar perquisites. The IRS can impose penalties and fines for excess-benefit transactions under IRC 4958. These penalties are known as *intermediate sanctions* since they fall short of revoking the organization's nonprofit status. Beyond the fines, the imposition of intermediate sanctions places the organization and its board members under greater scrutiny.

Most tax-exempt hospitals are very sensitive to their responsibilities with regard to paying reasonable executive salaries. In the event of an IRS executive compensation review, tax-exempt hospitals must be able to document the reasonableness of their executive compensation based on sound compensation practices, appropriate market analyses, and assessment of their executives' performance levels.

composed of directors who are not officers of the firm. Compensation committees generally make recommendations to the board of directors on overall pay policies, salaries for top officers, supplemental compensation such as bonuses, and additional perquisites for executives.

Determining "Reasonableness" of Executive Compensation

The reasonableness of executive compensation is often justified by comparison to compensation market surveys, but these surveys usually provide a range of compensation data that requires interpretation. Various questions have been suggested for determining if executive pay is "reasonable," including the following:

- Would another organization hire this person as an executive?

- How does the compensation for the executive compare with that for executives in similar organizations in the industry?

- Are the pay and benefits for the executive consistent with those for other employees in the organization?

Boards must address the need to continually link organizational performance with variable pay rewards for executives and other employees (Beekun, et al., 1998). There is certainly more controversy about executive compensation in other industries, but health care boards of directors must also be mindful of the reasonableness of executive pay and benefits.

One approach utilized by board compensation committees is to contract with a recognized executive compensation consultant firm. The firm should be contracted directly by the board and not the health care executives whose compensation is the subject of the review. The board should give the firm its direction and establish the appropriate methodology for the firm to assess current compensation and benefits plans, identify comparable organizations and executives in the market, evaluate compensation surveys and Form 990 statements, and make recommendations to the compensation committee. The report to the committee forms the foundation for a rebuttable presumption of reasonableness. The report documents the decision-making process so that compensation decisions for executives are not only reasonable and defensible but also competitive in the market.

SUMMARY

Many philosophies, strategies, and approaches to compensation management exist today. Health care compensation issues are increasingly arising, and it will be the informed HR professional who will be best equipped to handle evolving employee needs. This chapter should have helped to shape the reader's perspective on how organization strategies, the internal environment, and the external environment ultimately affect compensation strategy. From compensation for nurses and technologists to managers and health care executives, compensation packages run the gambit and are designed to meet not only the needs of the employee but to also meet regulatory and legal standards. The goal for every HR professional should be to develop a strategy that means success to your organization.

MANAGEMENT GUIDELINES

1. *Determine the compensation strategy for the health care organization.* The compensation strategy should be developed by considering (1) the forms of compensation that can be offered, (2) workforce demographics, (3) the business cycle, (4) the organization's compensation philosophy and, (5) legal and regulatory compliance.

2. *Frequently remind employees of the value of their total compensation.* The sum of direct and indirect compensation is total compensation. Indirect compensation is a tangible reward of the work relationship that serves as a very real cost to the organization. However, since indirect compensation is not included in take-home pay, most employees do not consider it as compensation.

3. *Clarify the organization's compensation philosophy.* Health care organizations may desire to pay top wages and salaries relative to their competitors; however, it may not be feasible to do so due to cost-containment pressures. Approaches to compensation philosophy include market-based pay, competency-based pay, and team-based pay.

4. *Maintain compliance with all federal, state, and local regulations.* Numerous laws and regulations surround issues of compensation. Chief among these are minimum wage and hours of work standards.

5. *Determine if you should adopt open- or closed-communication policies regarding the organization's compensation plan.* Providing employees with more information on compensation policies, compensation systems, and salary ranges allows them to make more informed equity comparisons. Alternatively, if the pay philosophy is difficult to understand or agree with, a closed-communication approach to the organization's compensation plan may be more appropriate.

DISCUSSION QUESTIONS

1. Contrast the compensation philosophies of entitlement and pay-for-performance.
2. Market competitiveness has a strong impact on compensation. Discuss the strategies employed by health care organizations to compete in the market.
3. FLSA employee classifications are federally mandated for health care organizations. Discuss the attributes included in this chapter.
4. Name and describe three factors affecting pay increases.

REFERENCES

Beekun, R.I., Stedham, Y., & Young, G.J. (1998). Board characteristics, managerial controls and corporate strategy: A study of U.S. hospitals. *Journal of Management, 24*(1): 3–19.

Brown, M.P., Sturman, M.C., & Simmering, M.J. (2003). Compensation policy and organizational performance: The efficiency, operational, and financial implications of pay levels and pay structure. *Academy of Management Journal, 46*(6): 752–762.

Carson, P.P., & Carson, K.D. (2007). Demystifying demotion: A look at the psychological and economic consequences on the demotee. *Business Horizons, 50*(6): 455–466.

Fitz-enz, J. (2000). *The ROI of Human Capital: Measuring Economic Value of Employee Performance.* AMACOM Books.

Fredericksen, P.J., & Soden, D.L. (1998). Employee attitudes toward benefit packaging: The job sector dilemma. *Review of Public Personnel Administration, 18*(3): 23–41.

Greenblatt, E.D.Y. (2002). Work/life balance: Wisdom or whining. *Organizational Dynamics, 31*(2): 177–193.

Hall, B.J., & Liebman, J.B. (1998). Are CEOS really paid like bureaucrats? *Quarterly Journal of Economics, 113*(3): 653–691.

Harris Interactive. (2005). Emergent Employers More Attuned to Employee Retention Drivers, *Emerging Workforce Fast Facts:* Spherion Corporation.

Heneman, R.L., Greenberger, D.B., & Strasser, S. (1988). The relationship between pay-for-performance perceptions and pay satisfaction. *Personnel Psychology, 41*(4): 745–759.

Kohn, A. (1993). *Punished by Rewards: The Trouble with Gold Stars, Incentive Plans, A's, Praise, and Other Bribes.* Boston: Houghton Mifflin Company.

Kovac, J.C. (2005). Salary Communication, *WorldAtWork.*

Mathis, R.L., & Jackson, J.H. (2004). *Human Resource Management* (10th ed.). Australia: Thomson/South-Western.

McClurg, L.N. (2001). Team rewards: How far have we come? *Human Resource Management, 40*(1): 73–86.

Miceli, M.P., & Heneman, R.L. (2000). Contextual determinants of variable pay plan design: A proposed research framework. *Human Resource Management Review, 10*(3): 289–305.

Milkovich, G.T., & Newman, J. M. (2005). *Compensation* (9th ed.). Plano: Business Publications.

U.S. Dept of Labor. (2008a). *Compliance Assistance— Fair Labor Standards Act (FLSA),* Vol. 2008. Washington: U.S. Dept of Labor.

U.S. Dept of Labor. (2008b). *Wage and Hour Division (WHD),* Vol. 2008. Washington: U.S. Dept of Labor.

Watson Wyatt Worldwide. (2006). Effective corporate communication linked to better financial performance, *WorkUSA Survey Report.* Toronto.

Watson Wyatt Worldwide. (2006/2007). Aligning rewards with the changing employment deal. *Strategic Rewards Report.*

CHAPTER 15

Labor Relations

Leonard H. Friedman, PhD, MPH

LEARNING OBJECTIVES

Upon completing this chapter, the reader will be able to:

1. Understand the issues surrounding union activities among employees.

2. Chronicle the rise of unionization within the health care industry and what future events or trends might arise; view management as a catalyst in the unionization equation; and understand how management actions are perceived by the ordinary employee.

3. Develop strategies to create and sustain productive relationships between unions and management.

4. Link the concept of an antiunion environment to other management functions and explain the effects of this relationship.

KEY TERMS

Employee Attitude Surveys

Employee Relations Program

Fair Grievance Procedure

Just Cause

Management Rights

Nonunion Policy

INTRODUCTION

The concept of strategic labor management relations is concerned with the application and maintenance of positive labor relations within the organization. Regardless of what one might think about the presence of organized labor unions, these organizations are here and will not disappear any time in the near future. This chapter serves as a guide to the practitioner in developing effective labor relation strategies with the objective of creating a relationship between management and labor that is positive and mutually beneficial.

This chapter assumes that employees are in an organized labor environment and is written from the perspective of management's need to understand the total framework and process of negotiating and administering contracts with a union. It was developed in the belief that good acumen of both cognitive and behavioral requirements can lead to a relationship that minimizes the adversarial factors and enhances the probability of mutual trust and respect. Many strategic decisions must be made during the negotiation process, either for an initial contract or for a replacement contract. Also, administering the contract fairly and consistently requires a high level of attention from management to yield a productive and positive labor management relationship.

With more than 9 million workers, the health care industry represents one of the largest workforce population groups in the United States. As of 2006, there were approximately 800,000 unionized health professionals (including nurses and physical therapists) and another 312,000 unionized health care support workers (including home health aides, medical transcriptionists, and others) (Evans, 2007). The health care industry also represents one of the largest pools of non-union employees, and, therefore, is a prime target for union organizers. This situation is particularly true in times of economic stress, when management decisions must be made concerning the employment status of many employees, both professional and nonprofessional. The 1991 National Labor Relations Board regulation, upheld by the U.S. Supreme Court, increased the number of allowable bargaining units within the hospital environment from three to eight. This is a change that resulted in an increasing number of unionization attempts in the health care industry. The net effect of the growth of organized labor activities across all health care delivery organizations has forced management to learn to deal more effectively with both currently organized workers and those seeking union representation.

DEVELOPING AN EMPLOYEE-RELATIONS PHILOSOPHY AND STRATEGY

Management strategies, specifically those regarding desired relationships to labor organizations, should be formulated as part of overall policy development. This strategy formulation must, of course, take into consideration the geographic, demographic, and historical factors pertinent to the setting. For example, an organization that is located in an area where unionization is prevalent may find it extremely difficult to prevent unionization of groups of its employees. Nonetheless, it is management's responsibility to develop and communicate to its employees the organization's employee relations philosophy.

The organization's employee relations philosophy should be developed on the basis of its objectives regarding such factors as communication with employees, **management rights,** and union preferences. If an organization is not currently unionized, management should consider the array of environmental and organizational issues in the process of determining its policy relating to unions. Specifically, management should consider the available strategic options for developing and maintaining a positive employee relations climate.

One option is to adopt a **nonunion policy** and to begin to implement a proactive management program that significantly reduces or eliminates the need for workers to seek union representation. This option is explored in detail in this chapter. A second option is for management to implement essentially the same program without communicating a formal nonunion policy, depending on its analysis of circumstances and objectives. Regardless of the strategic option chosen, it is essential for management to do the necessary analysis and adopt an appropriate **employee relations program** focused on maintaining good communication and positive relations.

MAINTAINING NONUNION STATUS

Maintaining nonunion status depends largely on what managers do to prevent the need for a union. This view is based on the philosophy that unionization is preventable if management is doing enough of the "right things." When management actions do not support a positive employee relations climate, workers may find it necessary to seek external help; in some situations, workers deserve help from union representation.

This argument may be supported further by noting that union organizers typically do not attempt to organize an employee group until workers themselves have sought union assistance. Union certification elections seem to suggest that employees really are voting for or against management instead of for or against a particular union. Based on these premises, this chapter seeks to help health care managers by identifying issues important to good personnel relations and the maintenance of nonunion status. *Avoidance* of a union election is preferable to *winning an election* (Goodfellow, 1991).

To provide a sound basis for prevention of unnecessary problems, it is essential to understand the historical perspective of the underlying issues, including employee perceptions of the need for unionization. The purpose of this chapter, therefore, is accomplished through a review of labor law history and trends, an overview of the fundamental causes of friction between management and labor, a summary of reasons health care employees give for joining unions, an analysis of criteria used by union organizers to evaluate health care institutions, and, finally, specific recommendations for establishing a preventive management program and for maintaining nonunion status. Because knowledge of the legal framework is essential to any manager who desires to avoid foolish mistakes in the implementation of a well-conceived program, it is appropriate to review labor law history and trends first.

LABOR LAW HISTORY AND TRENDS

The National Labor Relations Act (NRLA) is the foundation for the labor laws of the United States. The NLRA, or so-called Wagner Act, was adopted in 1935 and has been amended by the Taft-Hartley Act of 1947, the Landrum-Griffin Act of 1959, and Public Law 93-360 (the Health Care Amendments) in 1974.

The Wagner Act authorized the formation of the National Labor Relations Board (NLRB) to administer the provisions of the Act. The Wagner Act encompassed all institutions that had an impact on interstate commerce. The status of nonprofit health care institutions was left to the interpretation of the courts. Proprietary institutions and nursing homes were considered within the jurisdiction of the Act. Under terms of the Act, federal, state, and municipal hospitals were specifically exempted from legislating jurisdiction.

Under the protection of the Wagner Act, unions flourished in industries of virtually all types, creating a host of problems regarding the regulation of union-management relations. Industries had to contend with many jurisdictional strikes caused by disputes between competing unions. The Wagner Act proved inadequate in curbing these and other abuses of the bargaining process. Therefore, in 1947, Congress passed the Labor Management Relations (Taft-Hartley) Act.

The Taft-Hartley Act amended the Wagner Act by listing specific unfair labor practices. In addition, it specifically exempted nonprofit health care institutions from coverage under the Act. The status of other types of health care institutions did not change.

In 1959, the Taft-Hartley Act was amended by the Labor-Management Reporting and Disclosure (Landrum-Griffin) Act. Among its many provisions, this Act requires employers, including voluntary nonprofit health care facilities, to submit a report to the U.S. Secretary of Labor detailing the nature of any financial transactions and/or arrangements that are intended to improve or retard the unionization process (Rakich, 1973).

Until 1967, the courts determined on a case-by-case basis which proprietary health care institutions and nursing homes had an impact on interstate commerce and thus were subject to the NLRA. As a result of several court cases, in 1967, the NLRB determined that proprietary health care institutions with annual gross revenues of at least $250,000 and nursing homes, regardless of ownership, with annual gross revenues of at least $100,000 were covered by the Act.

With voluntary hospitals constituting the largest sector of the health care industry, it was only a matter of time until they, too, fell under federal legislation. Their shift in status occurred in 1974, when Congress passed Public Law 93-360 to amend the Labor Relations Act. These amendments, which extended the coverage of the labor laws to include all health care institutions under nonpublic ownership and control, defined a health care institution as any "hospital, convalescent hospital, health maintenance organization, health clinic, nursing home, extended care facility, or other institution devoted to the care of sick, infirm, or aged persons" (Public Law 93-360). This legislation specifically addressed the health care industry and, as such, provided special considerations due to the nature of patient care concerns. These considerations included requirement of a 10-day advance strike or picketing notification, longer periods of intention to modify existing agreements, and mandatory mediation (Zimmerman & King, 1990).

Since the 1974 Amendment, the NLRB has used various methods to establish the number and scope of bargaining units. Initially a community-of-interest (resulting in narrow units) was utilized. Then a disparity-of-interest (resulting in wide groupings) was the model employed, and recently the NLRB has determined that eight units are appropriate for health care facilities (Gullett & Kroll, 1990). An April 1991, Supreme Court ruling (*AHA v. the National Labor Relations Board, No. 90-97__U.S.__*[April 23, 1991]) upheld the NLRB determination, appealed to the U.S. Supreme Court by the American Hospital Association, that expanded the number of allowable bargaining units within the hospital environment to eight specified groups. These eight groups are physicians; registered nurses; all professionals except physicians and nurses; all guards; all nonprofessional service workers except technical, skilled maintenance, business office clerical employees, and guards; technical workers; maintenance personnel; and clerical employees. Because union organizing activities are more successful with smaller bargaining units (as this creates a more homogenous voting unit with more work-related commonalities), this criterion is viewed as a major victory for organized labor (Goodfellow, 1991; Gullett & Kroll, 1990; Hepner & Zinner, 1991; Stickler, 1990, 1991; Zimmerman & King, 1990). This decision has had far-ranging labor management implications for the health care manager.

The legislative background and prospects certainly suggests that it is difficult for health care managers seeking to stay nonunion. For a realistic perspective on maintaining nonunion status, management should have a good understanding of the fundamental causes of labor problems. Reasons for labor–management friction are summarized next.

CAUSES OF LABOR–MANAGEMENT PROBLEMS

Fundamental differences between the goals and objectives of management and labor create friction that cannot be totally explained in terms of desires for higher wages, shorter working hours, or better working conditions. Two fundamental causes of such friction are the issue of management rights and the issue of efficiency versus human value. Management will always assert its right to prescribe certain modes of action or levels of desired productivity to justify its existence or that of the organization. Yet labor unions question whether management should have complete power over the work force. This is a point of conflict. Organized labor attempts to shift the locus of control by seeking to obtain a voice for employees about working conditions and terms of employment.

The question of management's right to govern is paralleled by the question of human value versus efficiency. If management is to achieve its stated goals and objectives, it must maintain efficiency through increased productivity and cost containment. However, the union seeks to improve its members' standards of living. Neither side may be totally right or totally wrong in its demands, and unfortunate circumstances often trigger open conflict. For example, management that wishes to improve the existing fringe benefits package for employees may be prevented from doing so by pressures to contain costs. Evidence of this type of conflict in health services organizations is mounting almost daily, especially as new crises (e.g., cost increases of commercial health insurance, malpractice insurance rate hikes, continued third-party cost containment efforts, and restrictive reimbursement policies) arise and cause even greater cost constraints on management.

With an understanding of the fundamental causes of labor problems, administration can begin developing its philosophy for a preventive management program by reviewing research on employee reasons for joining unions. This research provides insight into employee relations and subsequent unionization activities. The analysis that follows summarizes findings from a selected number of such studies.

Why Employees Join Unions

The desire to unionize is thought to be centered on three issues—wages, employees' dissatisfaction with work benefits, and employees' perceptions about the organization as a place to work that could reflect perceptions about management or the employer. However, other factors have contributed to increased union activity in the health care industry. During the past four decades, social turmoil has precipitated Civil Rights legislation and stimulated changes in the attitudes and social consciences of many individuals. The idea of being represented by a union is not considered as unprofessional as it once was (Fennell, 1987; Fenner, 1991; Hepner & Zinner, 1991; Zimmerman & King, 1990). The health care industry is now feeling the effects of this turmoil, and passage of Public Law 93-360 served only to release the pent-up emotions of the industry's workers and union leaders. Recent labor reform efforts are further evidence of labor's continuing struggle to swing the pendulum in its favor.

In a study pertaining to why employees want unions, Goodfellow (1991) found the following three errors made by hospital administrators that lead to employee unionization:

1. Acceptance of the notion that low wages and poor fringe benefits cause most employee dissatisfaction. (This is fallacy, because the real reason for unionization is related to whether the employees perceive management treatment as being fair and respectful.)

2. The assumption that interviewing of supervisors is a true barometer of employee feelings. (The supervisors may not be trained in the identification of employee morale or may feel threatened by the revelation of morale problems within their departments.)

3. Ignorance of what is troubling the employees. (This is a function of not listening to the employees' understanding of the situation and not allowing communication to flow from the bottom to the top. Employees may feel that administration is indifferent to their welfare and unconcerned with their work environment.)

In another study examining why nurses choose to join labor unions, it was discovered that health care reform, staffing levels, and a perceived lack of a voice in hospital decision making were key influences on this decision (Darr, Schraeder, & Friedman, 2002). It should be noted that nowhere in this study are the issues of salary or benefits mentioned.

Table 15.1 shows that nonunion members report higher overall job satisfaction, more interesting work, increased task freedom, more pleasant surroundings, increased chances of job promotions, and increased ability to influence work decisions. Union workers reported greater feelings of job security and increased satisfaction with pay level.

Although the rationale for union-seeking activities by workers varies, Table 15.2 analyzes 10 articles to determine commonalities in the attitudes of workers who desire union representation. The results suggest that work conditions, grievances, poor communications, personnel policies, quality of supervision, and job security are the most important considerations in why employees seek union representation. Issues concerned with wages, fringe benefits, shift differentials, and other human dignity factors are somewhat less important factors in those who consider unionization. This finding should convince the health care manager that employees are apparently looking for nonpay-related conditions of work.

What the Union Organizer Looks For

Employees usually try to resolve their problems internally before seeking outside help. Typically, union organizers appear on the scene only if they have been invited by the workers. In other words, if a union organizer is involved, it is likely that relationships between workers and management

Table 15.1. The Correlation Between Job Satisfaction and Voting for Union Representation[a]

	Correlation with Vote[a]
1. Are you satisfied or not satisfied with your wages?	−0.40
2. Do supervisors in this company play favorites or do they treat all employees alike?	−0.34
3. Are you satisfied or not satisfied with the type of work you are doing?	−0.14
4. Do your supervisors show appreciation when you do a good job or do they just take it for granted?	−0.30
5. Are you satisfied or not satisfied with your fringe benefits, such as pensions, vacations, holiday pay, insurance, and sick leave?	−0.31
6. Do you think there is a good chance or not much chance for you to get promoted in this company?	−0.30
7. Are you satisfied or not satisfied with the job security at this company?	−0.42
8. Taking everything into consideration, would you say you were satisfied or not satisfied with this company as a place to work?	−0.36

[a]$p < 0.1$; $r = 0.08$; $N = 1004$

SOURCE: Reprinted, by permission of publisher, from ORGANIZATIONAL DYNAMICS, Spring/1980 © 1980. American Management Association, New York. All rights reserved.

[a]The negative correlations indicate that employees who were satisfied tended to vote against union representation.

Table 15.2. Reasons Health Care Employees Join Unions: Derived from a Sampling of Studies in 10 Publications

Issue	Publication									
	1[a]	2[b]	3[c]	4[d]	5[e]	6[f]	7[g]	8[h]	9[i]	10[j]
Poor communication	X	X	X	X	X	X	X	X	X	X
Personnel policies	X	X	X	X	X	X	X	X	X	X
Supervision	X	X	X	X	X	X	X	X	X	X
Fringe benefits	X	X			X	X				X
Work conditions	X	X		X		X			X	
Grievances		X	X	X				X	X	
Job security	X	X		X	X	X	X	X	X	X
Human dignity		X	X	X			X	X	X	
Shift differentials	X	X		X	X					
Wages	X				X	X	X			

[a] Becker and Rowe (1989)
[b] Fennell (1987)
[c] Fenner (1991)
[d] Goodfellow (1991)
[e] Hepner and Zinner (1991)
[f] Hoffman (1989)
[g] Meng (1990)
[h] Powills (1989)
[i] Stickler (1991)
[j] Stickler (1990)

have degraded to a level that a union is viewed as the only way to address perceived inequities (Eubanks, 1990a; Imberman, 1989; Powills, 1989).

There is no blueprint the health care manager can use to determine how a union organizer will evaluate a given situation. The method of evaluation depends on the organizing team sent into the area and its previous experience or success. Tactics may vary considerably, depending on the contacts from employees and management's response to the situation. However, the organizer may concentrate in certain areas, including the following.

Employee Loyalty by Work Shift

Normally, the first shift is the most loyal to the organization, the second shift less loyal than the first, and the third shift the least loyal. This probably is because new employees usually start on the second or third shift. They see top management rarely or never, and the supervisory force is usually smaller. Thus, there is no one who can provide consistent HR information (e.g., answering employee questions about personnel policies or benefits). These employees tend to feel overlooked and forgotten. They are more susceptible to the pleas of the union organizer, who usually is available on the later shifts (Goodfellow, 1991).

Female-Male Employee Ratio

Women historically have been less interested in unions than have men. In the past, many women worked to supplement the family income, but this has changed rapidly. Today, women are prevalent in the workforce and frequently earn a primary or major part of the family income. Pay inequities are being addressed by unions as the number of female-related health care occupations increases (Fennell, 1987). This increase in the number and scope of health care occupations has opened additional avenues to union organizers in their efforts to establish a health care beachhead.

Nursing personnel, a majority of whom are women, are increasingly recognizing the need to organize to improve their status. Numerous professional organizations, such as the American Nurses Association and the American Society of Medical Technologists, are attempting to upgrade and negotiate conditions of employment for their memberships. Unions have capitalized on the issue of gender-based pay inequities at the bargaining tables and through legislative and legal actions (Fennell, 1987).

Work Environment and Job Safety

Employees expect management to provide clean and safe working environments. If the health care institution allows the work environment to deteriorate, employees may think that the institution does not care much about them (Goodfellow, 1991). Work place hazards and related fears about such issues as AIDS and hepatitis B will be cultivated by union organizers as major organizing issues (Becker & Rowe, 1989; Fennell, 1987).

Wage Rates

Traditionally, the health care employee has subsidized health care institutions with low wages. This is an injustice to the employee, who must compete daily in the retail market for goods and services. In addition, the institution must have fair and regular wage differentials. Failure to update these differentials will cause a compression effect between the new employees' base pay and the tenured employees' level. Additional avenues of employment of various health care professionals (e.g., alternative care facilities, insurance companies, and general industry) has further affected the need for the health care industry to reward its employees adequately (Goodfellow, 1991; Stickler, 1991).

Incentive Pay

In areas in which an incentive pay program has been implemented, employees may complain that some of the performance expectations are too high. High expectations obviously breed dissatisfaction if management does not respond by reexamining these pay thresholds periodically. Wage differentials as a means of incentive pay must remain competitive and should not be adjusted arbitrarily (Goodfellow, 1991).

Overtime Practices

Problems arise when overtime is scheduled without the employee's consent. Management assumes that the worker will not object to the extra hours spent because of the overtime pay, but this often is not a valid assumption. Overtime can be very disruptive to the employee's family life and leisure time. The union organizer will exploit this point of dissatisfaction and force management to hire additional workers. Inequities in the distribution of overtime represent another aspect of this problem (Goodfellow, 1991). Mandatory overtime requirements of health personnel in shortage professions, such as registered nurses, has lead to increased pro-union feelings (Becker & Rowe, 1989).

Seniority/Job Security

Although management may prefer to recognize the skills and health of a worker in assigning a new job, it must not overlook the employee's view of seniority (Goodfellow, 1991; Hepner & Zinner, 1991). Seniority, to the employee, is job security. If management takes the time-honored seniority concept away completely, it is asking for employee dissatisfaction and unionization, particularly in geographic areas where unionization already is well-entrenched (Fennell, 1987). Cost containment efforts precipitated by changes in the reimbursement system and mandates from third-party payers have further added to the employees' feelings of job insecurity (Becker & Rowe, 1989).

Promotion Policy

When a new job becomes available or an employee leaves, present personnel should be given an opportunity to apply for the position. A good job-posting policy can be extremely helpful. Health care institutions also should have education and training programs available to assist employees' vertical or lateral career movements (Goodfellow, 1991).

Fringe Benefits

Research has revealed that in many cases management underrates the value of fringe benefits to the employee. Also, as employers continue to increase the benefits portion of total compensation, the benefits package is likely to increase in relative importance to employees (Hoffman, 1989). This is particularly true today, given the ever-increasing costs of health insurance. With the news media and the next-door neighbors discussing the benefits of union representation, it is foolish for health care management to neglect to establish a good benefits program and to explain adequately to employees the benefits offered by the institution. A mechanism of providing this benefit information is through the employee benefits fair. This allows management to graphically display the value of the benefits package to the employees and to secure employee feedback on desired new benefits. With the development of various benefits packages resulting from cafeteria-style benefits programs, the benefits fair is an ideal management concept.

Discipline and Grievance Procedures

If the institution does not provide employees with written rules covering what is not allowed and what is and to what degree, some supervisors may abuse their authority to reprimand. The grievance procedure serves as a safety valve for employees to release their frustrations about supervisors or other major problems (Fenner, 1991; Hoffman, 1989). Management should develop and implement an internal procedure that employees will use instead of resorting to an outside agency to settle disputes. Management also should review the procedures periodically to make sure they are serving the worker's needs. Employees who have the opportunity to address their complaints or concerns about working conditions through the grievance procedure are less likely to feel the need for unionization (Becker & Rowe, 1989; Eubanks, 1990).

Multi-Unit Systems

As the American health care system undergoes reorganizations, mergers, and acquisitions, the hospital workplace has experienced dramatic changes. Increased centralized decision making, information systems developed to minimize costs and overheads, and increased employee production standards have all added to employee stresses. These factors are being viewed by organized labor as prime issues toward increased unionization potentials within the health care industry. Multi-unit systems are facing the prospects of multifacility bargaining units (Fries, 1986; Zimmerman & King, 1990). This condition, coupled with the narrowing in the definition of bargaining units, should alert hospital administrators within the multi-unit system of increased unionization activity.

A PROACTIVE MANAGEMENT PROGRAM

Assessing an institution's employee relations climate and implementing a program to prevent unionization is a process for which a myriad of management responses are possible. Each institution must carefully design a strategy that is both practical and suited to its situation. Recognizing the significant relationship between the reasons given by employees for joining unions and what a union organizer looks for, there is substantial reason to believe that the primary causes of unionization include "communication problems" and the perception by employees of "unfair treatment."

Therefore, a proactive management program should be designed with a primary emphasis on improving in an honest and fair manner. This emphasis is detailed in several ways in the following recommendations for establishing a proactive management program. These recommendations are an outgrowth of previously described employee-related issues and could serve as the general framework within which each management team builds its own strategy.

Nonunion Policy

If a health care institution intends to be nonunion, it should give careful consideration to the development and publication of such a policy. Good labor counsel should be consulted to assist in the development of an up-front nonunion policy and to advise the best alternatives for communicating the policy to all who wish to work at the institution. All prospective employees should be informed in the screening process and given written evidence of the institutional position regarding unionization, along with other significant policies. The prospective employee then has the choice of whether to work for a nonunion institution. This, in itself, should be an indication of fair treatment. Management also should consider publishing the nonunion policy in the employee handbook for reference during orientation and other worker group meetings. This policy should include the following key resolutions (Rutkowski & Rutkowski, 1984):

1. Commitment of the administration to provide equitable treatment to all employees in their wages, benefits, hours, and conditions of employment

2. Commitment of adequate funds and time to provide all managers with the information that they need to be effective in employee relations and knowledgeable in ways of avoiding unionization

3. Commitment of administrators to the philosophy that each employee is important as an individual vital to the optimal functioning of the entire hospital team

4. Commitment to oppose efforts of outside organizations to unionize employees

Personnel Selection

Management must have effective policies and procedures regarding selection of new employees. Prevention of labor-management problems begins with the proper matching of personnel to specific jobs. A good wage and salary program, including job analyses, job descriptions (with performance objectives), and job evaluation, is essential. If good procedures are used for selecting on the basis of both the individual's qualifications and the requirements of a specific job, the result is likely to be a better fit for the institution and the employee. Concurrently, the institution is likely to avoid many communication and morale problems. A fair wage and salary system provides at least a basis for establishing an objective employee evaluation system.

Employee Attitude Assessment

Employee attitude surveys, when conducted properly, can provide valuable management information at nominal costs. The method chosen should be simple to implement and should elicit concise employee responses. The result should be an accurate assessment of the topics surveyed, clearly differentiating between positive and negative attitudes.

Attitude surveying should be done on a planned, periodic basis so that employees perceive continual concern for their needs and management keeps abreast of fluctuations in worker attitudes. If this procedure is combined with efforts to obtain upward communication through formal and informal channels at all levels of the institution, the result should be a positive change in employees' attitudes and the development of management systems for dealing with personnel problems before they become sore spots. After attitudes have been assessed and problems identified, management should be ready to take corrective action, including an appropriate training program. Probably the single most important part of the attitude measurement analysis process is communication with the employees about the following:

- Purpose of the survey
- How data will be analyzed and used

- Confidentiality of individual responses
- Feedback concerning findings
- What changes, if any, employees can expect as a result of survey findings

Management should be careful not to make promises that cannot be fulfilled, but should make a strong effort to do whatever is possible to improve employee relations. In summary, when management asks employees to take valuable time to participate in a survey, it is extremely important for employees to feel that the administration values their input and is doing what it can to meet their needs.

Employee Training

Administration should examine its role and responsibilities in training employees as a function of management, rather than as a staff function. If this self-examination indicates that management is assuming little, if any, responsibility for employee training, such abdication is very likely to be related directly to workers' perceptions of poor treatment. For employees to perceive fair, honest, or decent treatment, top-level management must make the commitment to assume responsibility for training and must transmit it down through all levels to first-line supervisors. This is necessary, for example, before management can develop an adequate performance appraisal and reward system that employees will consider equitable.

After management has made the commitment to assume its training responsibility, it must determine what type of training program to implement. The following questions may provide evaluative insight into employee needs:

1. Are employee functions and responsibilities agreed on and clear?
2. Do employees have the ability (e.g., technical training and experience) to do what is expected?
3. Do job descriptions contain specific performance objectives?
4. Do employees know what performance standards are being used to evaluate their work?
5. Is there a positive relationship between employee performance and reward?

Management implementation of an appropriate training program should have positive effects on employee attitudes and productivity and should be a major asset in eradicating the dead-end job syndrome.

Employee Value Systems

Management should recognize the different types of value systems that exist among various employee groups in both professional and nonprofessional categories. Research has identified as many as seven different employee value systems, varying from tribalistic to existentialist (Hughes, 1976). Some examples of responses to the myriad of value systems and needs include flexible work scheduling, earned-time programs, methods of job enrichment, and a cafeteria-style approach to fringe benefits. Management must develop a variety of imaginative ways to respond to the needs of multiple employee families.

First-Line Supervisors

Management must recognize the importance of first-line supervisors in preventing serious labor problems. Supervisors become management's first line of defense against unionization by determining how policies are implemented, serving as liaisons between top-level management and employees, and being strong nonunion advocates (Eubanks, 1990a). If these supervisors do not have good management skills, the institution is inviting unionization. Frequently, a problem with first-line supervisors is manifested by the number of grievances filed involving situations that are either about or under the direct control of such persons. Management should evaluate the effectiveness of first-line supervisors' employee-relations skills carefully and regularly. When deficiencies are found, management should either assist the supervisor through training or terminate the person, depending on his or her past record and potential.

Performance Appraisal

The institution should establish a performance appraisal policy that reflects management's desire to develop employees to their optimal potential.

If management behavior indicates anything else, workers are likely to perceive treatment by supervisors as poor or unfair. To be effective in improving morale and productivity of all employees, performance appraisal must be done honestly and on a regular basis.

Management's avoidance of an honest appraisal of the nonproductive employee simply demonstrates to all workers that the reward is inequitable or that the laggards receive the same rewards as those who are productive. This can be interpreted logically by productive employees as evidence that the nonproductive actually are rewarded more than the productive in relation to their effort. If this attitude prevails, management is very likely to "teach" employees to move toward mediocrity and union thinking. The implementation of a good performance-appraisal system depends largely on the management skills of the first-line supervisors. In other words, the appraisal system used is not nearly as important as the people (i.e., managers) who implement it. Even the best system is as weak as the people who operate it.

Disciplinary Policies and Procedures

Management must take great care in applying disciplinary policies and procedures consistently. Consistent and fair application normally can prevent unnecessary employee-relations problems and grievances. One basic principle is that management should have **"just cause"** for imposing discipline. The definition may vary from case to case, but several basic tests can be applied to determine whether "just cause" exists for disciplining employees. These basic tests include the following:

1. Was the disciplinary rule reasonably related to efficient and safe operations?

2. Were the employees properly warned of potential consequences of violating the rule?

3. Did management conduct a fair investigation before applying the discipline?

4. Did the investigation produce substantial evidence of guilt?

5. Were the policies and procedures implemented consistently and without discrimination?

6. If a penalty resulted, was it related to the seriousness of the event as well as the past record of the employee? (i.e., did the punishment fit the crime?)

Some form of grievance procedure should be viewed as a part of any prevention program because employees should be able to complain about perceived problems formally without fear of subjective reprisal. Although any grievance procedure is open to problems of interpretation and application, some basic factors can be applied equally in evaluating the system from the employees' perspective. These factors include the following:

1. All employees should be able to understand the mechanics of filing a grievance and should know where they can go to ask questions about any step of the system. Thus, the procedure should be written.

2. When employees file grievances, they expect prompt action. Promptness is one of the most important aspects of a grievance settlement, and failure to resolve the problem with reasonable speed is likely to lead to adverse feelings.

3. The first-line supervisor typically is the first step in a grievance procedure. When that individual is perceived to be the problem, however, employees must know they can access the grievance machinery without going through the first-line supervisor. However, the employees should take every reasonable step to solve the problem with the immediate supervisor before going to someone else with the grievance.

When employees realize that a **fair grievance procedure** is available and when management is doing what it can to prevent unnecessary problems, the result should be a decreased number of complaints, fair and objective processing of those that are filed, and an employee feeling that management is concerned about employee needs.

Wages

The health care institution should be very careful to stay competitive with regard to wages and should compare its rates at least annually to similar institutions in the same geographical area. Frequently, wage-survey data can be found that apply to the local area, but if this is not the case, management should conduct its own survey. Even a sample survey of representative jobs will help to keep the institution abreast of trend information. Of course, certain shortage points will have to be dealt with on a case-by-case basis and possibly more frequently than every year. Competitive wages are a necessary condition in any preventive management program, but it should not be concluded that being competitive in wages is sufficient for maintaining nonunion status.

As has been indicated, wages are only one of the many factors that may enter into employees' decisions to seek union help. Health care is no longer as far behind other industries in wages as it once was, and, indeed, wages are probably not the major motivating factor for a significant portion of employees in a given institution. Although there may not be a great deal that management can conclude definitely from research regarding wages as a motivating factor, the folly of relying totally on competitive wages to prevent unionization can be illustrated best by review of wage structures in institutions that have had union elections recently.

In summary, the absence of competitive wage levels (particularly in times of continuing inflation) is a potentially severe problem, but the presence of good wage levels is not sufficient, in itself, to prevent unionization. This is particularly true in multidimensioned institutions that employ a diverse group of employees with a variety of value systems.

MANAGEMENT STRATEGY FOR REACTIONS DURING UNION-ORGANIZING CAMPAIGNS

Even if many "proactive" steps have been implemented, managers should not be so naive as to believe that a union organization attempt cannot happen. An extremely important part of a preventive management program is to have a well-planned strategy for reacting if such an attempt does occur. One important attribute to keep in mind is that employers have rights, as do unions, and the rights of management must be upheld. In a particularly interesting case, Sutter Health in Northern California was awarded a $17 million judgment against a union hoping to organize nurses at their hospitals. A postcard was sent to more than 11,000 patients and prospective patients of Sutter Health's maternity unit warning that new parents might be "bringing home more than your baby," thanks to reports that the hospital's laundry contractor "does not ensure that 'clean' linens are free of blood, feces, and harmful pathogens." These postcards were sent out allegedly as part of a campaign to gain corporate concessions in a union negotiation (Dreiling, 2006).

Brett's (1980) two-point conceptualization of employee reactions during a union organizing campaign holds the following important implications for both employers and unions:

1. An employer's antiunion campaign that attempts to persuade employees by emphasizing economic control over them and using fear tactics is unlikely to be successful.

2. The employer's most effective antiunion campaign stresses the desire to remain nonunion; provides factual information pertaining to working conditions, benefits, and so forth; and indicates that a labor organization cannot guarantee the conditions that will exist under union representation.

SUMMARY

Maintaining nonunion status is a desirable goal. Whether it will be achieved is related directly to the behavioral dedication of management in demonstrating its concern for meeting employees' needs fairly and equitably. Although the material in this chapter is not all-inclusive and does not offer a formula to guarantee nonunion status, it is suggestive of the management practices necessary to prevent communication problems and to avoid employees' perceptions of unfair treatment.

The unionization process is highly situational and in some locations may be essentially inevitable. Nevertheless, a positive nonunion philosophy and a preventive management program usually should obviate the need for a labor organization. When employees do not perceive a need for union assistance, the probability is slim that they will elect to begin paying union dues.

MANAGERIAL GUIDELINES

1. It is important for health care managers to recognize that even with cooperative relationships between labor unions and health care organizations, conflicts will still exist. The long-term solution is communication and integration. While an integrative solution is difficult to develop, it provides a win-win answer to both parties without compromising the other side's needs.

2. Health care managers can learn the lessons of labor–management relationships from various case studies in the health care field, as well as other industries, such as the auto industry. The lessons can be adapted to fit the specific circumstances a particular health care organization may be facing when attempting to develop a cooperative strategy.

3. Before developing a labor–management strategy or policy, management must conduct thorough analyses of the external environment and internal circumstances. These analyses will assist management in selecting an appropriate employee-relations program, which can result in positive outcomes in the relationship.

4. Management can maintain a proactive role in this relationship by implementing a nonunion policy. In other words, if management does the right things to begin with, then unionization can be preventable. In order to achieve this, management must be transparent, unbiased, accessible, supportive, fair, and trustworthy. Actions and decisions must serve not only the best interests of the organization, but also the best interests of the employees.

5. Management must recognize the particular needs of different groups of employees. Many approaches can be used to gauge the attitudes, needs, and performance of employees. Management must ensure that it hears the voice of employees on which appropriate actions are based. Also, management should not make promises that cannot be delivered or fulfilled, but should make a strong effort in maintaining a positive relationship with the employees.

DISCUSSION QUESTIONS

1. Develop a management strategy to deal with perceived union sentiments among the professional nursing staff in one of the critical care units in a hospital. This plan should address activities to be considered and whom to involve in the development of this plan.

2. Discuss the future trends of hospital unionization efforts and how the hospital should be prepared to confront these issues. What departments are the most vulnerable to union attack and what can the organization do to manage these areas?

3. Relate the concept of a union-free work environment to professionalism, and describe how professionals can accept the concept of unionization. What might you do as a senior health care executive to address this professional inconsistency?

4. Poll the health care providers in your area to determine the prevalence of unionization and what they think about future union potentials. Map a strategy that might incorporate these issues.

REFERENCES

AHA v. the National Labor Relations Board, No 90-97. (April 23, 1991).

Becker, W.L., & Rowe, A.M. (1989). Update on union organizing in health care. *Review of Federation of American Health Systems, 22*(5): 11–2, 14–6.

Brett, J.M. (1980). Why employees want unions. *Organizational Dynamics, 8*(4), 47–59.

Darr, K., Schraeder, M., & Friedman, L. (2002). Collective bargaining in the nursing profession: Salient issues and recent developments in healthcare reform. *Hospital Topics, 80*(3): 21–25.

Dreiling, G.L. (2006). Fighting fire with fire. *ABA Journal, 92*(12): 18.

Eubanks, P. (1990a). Avoiding unions: Supervisors are the first line of defense. *Hospitals, 64*(22): 40, 42.

Eubanks, P. (1990b). Employee grievance policy: Don't discourage complaints. *Hospitals, 64*(24): 36–37.

Evans, M. (2007). SEIU's power player. *Modern Healthcare, 37*(6): 10.

Fennell, K.S. (1987). The unionization of the health care industry: General trends and emerging issues.

Journal of Health in Human Resource Administration, 10(1): 66–81.

Fenner, K.M. (1991). Unionization: Boon or bane? *Journal of Nursing Administration, 21*(6): 7–8.

Goodfellow, M. (1991). Study shows ways to win, avoid union elections. *Healthcare Financial Management, 45*(9): 48, 50, 52.

Gullet, C.R., & Kroll, M.J. (1990). Rule making and the National Labor Relations Board: Implications for the health care industry. *Health Care Management Review, 15*(2): 61–65.

Hepner, J.O., & Zinner, S.E. (1991). Nurses and the new NLRB rules. *Health Progress, 72*(8): 20–22.

Hoffman, H.L. (1989). Personnel practices can help discourage unionization. *Healthcare Financial Management, 43*(9): 48, 50, 52.

Hughes, C.L. (1976). *Making Unions Unnecessary.* New York: Enterprise Publications.

Imberman, W. (1989). Rx: Strike prevention in hospitals. *Hospital and Health Services Administration, 34*(2): 195–211.

Meng, R. (1990). The relationship between unions and job satisfaction. *Applied Economics, 22*(12): 1635–1648.

Powills, S. (1989). Hospitals learn to deal with unionization. *Hospitals, 63*(13): 44–49.

Rakich, J.S. (1973). Hospital unionization: Causes and effects. *Hospital Administration, 18*(1): 7–18.

Rutkowski, A.D., & Rutkowski, B.L. (1984). *Labor Relations in Hospitals.* Rockville, MD: Aspen.

Stickler, K.B. (1990). Union organizing will be divisive and costly. *Hospitals, 64*(13): 68–70.

Zimmerman, D.A., & King, G.R. (1990). Union elections and the NLRB. *Health Progress, 71*(1): 96–101.

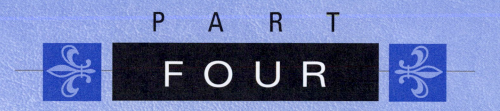

Professionals in Organizations and Future Challenges

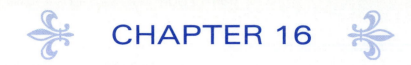

CHAPTER 16

Physicians and Health Care Organizations: Achieving Aligned Performance

William F. Jessee, MD, FACMPE

LEARNING OBJECTIVES

Upon completion of this chapter, you will be able to:

1. Describe the environmental factors that affect the economic performance of medical practices and discuss the impact of those factors on physicians' relationships with health care organizations.

2. Define three distinct populations of physicians, describe how they differ, and discuss specific approaches to creating better economic alignment between the physicians in each population and the hospital(s) with which they are associated.

3. Describe how physicians' roles in hospitals and in medical groups differ, and discuss approaches to achieving aligned performance between physicians and each of those two types of health care organizations.

4. Describe and discuss six specific principles for achieving aligned performance between physicians and health care organizations.

KEY TERMS

Hospital-Dependent Physicians

Hospital-Independent Physicians

Hospital-Neutral Physicians

Hospitalist

Management Services Organization (MSO)

Medicare Conversion Factor

Physician-Hospital Organization (PHO)

Relative Value Units (RVUs)

Three-Legged Stool

INTRODUCTION

Regardless of the type of organization in which they work, one of the major challenges facing health care administrators is that of working effectively with the physicians who practice in that organization. While physicians are key to the production of revenue in virtually every health care organization, they are usually outside the normal employment relationships of others in that organization. In addition, all physicians—whether employed or not—are driven by professional ideals of clinical autonomy and independent decision-making that may make it difficult to integrate them into the culture of a larger organization.

The economic importance of physicians to the health care organizations in which they practice is obvious. For hospitals, physicians are the source of hospital admissions as well as the initiators of ancillary services. A 2004 survey of hospital chief financial officers (Merritt, Hawkins and Associates, 2004) found that the annual hospital revenue generated per FTE (full-time equivalent) physician ranged from a high of almost $3 million per year (for orthopedic surgeons) to a low of $860,000 per year (for pediatricians) (see Figure 16.1). And

Specialty	Revenue (in dollars)
Orthopedic surgery	2,992,022
Cardiology	2,646,039
General surgery	2,446,987
Neurosurgery	2,406,275
Internal medicine	2,100,124
Family practice	2,000,329
Obstetrics/Gynecology	1,903,919
Gastroenterology	1,735,338
Urology	1,317,415
Pediatrics	860,600

Figure 16.1. Annual Hospital Revenues Produced per FTE Physician for Selected Specialties, 2004

for medical practices, physicians are often the sole source of revenue production for the practice. They must not only generate sufficient income to compensate themselves but must also support the salaries of clinical and nonclinical support staff, as well as the other operating expenses of the practice.

Accordingly, the importance of physicians as vital human resources in health care organizations of all types cannot be overstated. It is critical that every health care manager or executive—regardless of the setting in which he or she works—has a good understanding of the forces that drive physician behavior in health care organizations and of how to effectively work with physicians to accomplish the organization's goals. This chapter examines the historical relationships between physicians and health care organizations; how those relationships have changed in recent times; and what administrators can do to create better economic alignment and cultural integration of physicians into the health care organizations in which they practice.

TRADITIONAL ROLES OF PHYSICIANS IN HEALTH CARE ORGANIZATIONS

A 1977 text, widely used in health care administration education at the time, described the role of physicians in hospitals as follows:

> The physician is traditionally described as a guest in the hospital and its primary customer. Except when a physician chooses to run a hospital for profit, he has no personal responsibility to see that the hospital is available to provide care for his patients. The physician uses the hospital as his workshop. . . .
>
> Whenever a physician admits a patient to the hospital, he is free to order whatever tests or treatments he deems necessary. Thus he basically determines the amount of services used and consequent costs of individual

patients' care. . . . Physicians have every reason to want the best possible institutional setting in which to practice medicine, especially when it is provided at no personal cost to them. (Enright & Jonas, 1977)

In the mid-1970s, the vast majority of physicians viewed themselves as independent professionals whose primary place of business was generally the office in which they provided ambulatory care. Surgical specialists, of course, were very dependent on hospitals as a place to treat their patients, but still saw their own offices as their primary workplace. Family physicians and medical specialists routinely cared for patients in their offices and continued to care for those patients if they required hospitalization. Most physicians, regardless of specialty, spent part of each day in one or more hospitals, as well as seeing patients in their offices.

These primarily office-based physicians were generally the owners of their practice. Some (those in solo practice) were structured as sole proprietorships, while others were partnerships. A few larger groups had evolved into professional corporations, and some few large multispecialty groups were structured as tax-exempt foundations, with the physicians employed by the foundation. But the vast majority of practices were small, for-profit enterprises owned by the physicians who practiced there.

These physician owners saw themselves as independent, autonomous professionals. That autonomy was reflected both in their clinical activities and in the business activities of their practices. Even in group practices, the prevailing culture was one in which physicians joined the group in order to enjoy clinical autonomy while leaving the business of managing the practice to the administrative staff. Concepts of shared responsibility for patient care, physician involvement in quality and efficiency improvement, and physician accountability to anyone other than the individual patient had not yet begun to emerge.

With that culture and mindset, it is easy to understand why the clinical activities of physicians in the hospital were viewed by most physicians as beyond the scope of responsibility (or even

understanding) of the hospital's management and governance. This was reinforced by the classic **"three-legged stool"** model of hospital operations in which management, governance, and medical staff were viewed as relatively separate and equal components. Under that model, codified in hospital accreditation standards from the (then) Joint Commission on Accreditation of Hospitals (JCAH) (Joint Commission on Accreditation of Hospitals, 1975), management was responsible for hotel functions, the medical staff had an autonomous role in overseeing clinical care, and governance was more focused on fundraising than on oversight of management and the medical staff. In fact, as late as 1985, the perspective on the role of the hospital human resources department with respect to physicians was as follows:

It is noteworthy that although the functions and scope of the human resources department have grown significantly in recent years, medical staff relations remain outside its authority and are the domain of the HSO [health services organization] governing body and the CEO. When private practice physicians are involved, there is some logic to this because . . . the physician is usually not employed and is controlled by the organization only as required in medical staff bylaws and by the specific clinical privileges granted. However, when physicians are salaried (residents, program directors, or some facility-based specialists such as pathologists and radiologists), they take on more of the characteristics of an employee and may be included in the organization's employee benefit program. Even in these cases, it is rare to see any involvement of the human resources department in wage administration or maintaining personnel files involving physicians. The organization does not view them as typical employees. (Rakich, Longest, & Darr, 1985)

Administrators who tried to exercise control over members of their medical staff often found that to be a career-limiting decision. Physicians could retaliate against administrative controls by moving their business to another hospital or demanding that the governing board replace the administrator. Unfortunately, conflicts between physicians and administrators rarely were in the economic interest of either the hospital or the involved physician, and often became significant sources of community-wide controversy.

What Has Changed?

The environment that physicians face today is radically different from that of a quarter-century earlier. For one thing, physician groups have become much more common, and the average size of those groups has grown. In 2005, only 32% of physicians were in solo or two-physician practices (Cook, 2007), compared with 68% in 1975 (Goodman, Bennett, & Odem, 1977).

This change in practice arrangements has been driven by a variety of forces, some economic, some technological, and others cultural. The economic pressures on physician practices, particularly small ones, have increased steadily over the last decade.

One bellwether of this change has been the Medicare payment rate for physicians. From 2001 to 2008, the **Medicare conversion factor** (i.e., the dollar amount which, when multiplied by the number of **relative value units (RVUs)** associated with a particular service, determines the fee paid by Medicare to the physician) did not increase at all (Federal Register, 2000–2007). Over that same period of time, the Consumer Price Index (CPI) rose more than 24% (Bureau of Labor Statistics, 2008), and the median operating cost of a multispecialty medical group practice escalated by 43.1% (Gans, 2008) (see Figure 16.2). Since most private health insurers also index their payments to the Medicare rates, those payment rates have, in many cases, declined as well. A 2007 survey of payment rates for particular physician services found that the average private-payer reimbursement for routine office visits declined from $102.69 in 2004 to $73.48 in 2007 (Grace, 2007). The economic dilemma faced by medical practices is obvious: flat or declining revenues in the face of steeply rising operating expenses.

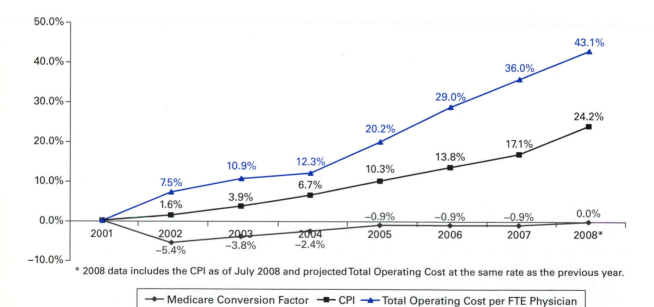

Figure 16.2. Medicare Physician Fee Schedule Conversion Factor; Consumer Price Index (CPI); and Multispecialty Medical Group Practice Operating Cost as a Percentage of Gross Revenues, 2001–2008. Resources.

So how do medical practices survive? For the most part, the answer lies in increases in the volume of patients treated or in the numbers of services provided, or both. Many primary care physicians have expanded their office work hours or have otherwise increased their patient volume to compensate for the flat payment rates. Procedural specialists have added a variety of ancillary services to their practices in order to increase the numbers of procedures that they can provide per patient. In addition, many practices have made much more extensive use of mid-level practitioners to increase the number of RVUs that they produce. Figure 16.3 illustrates the trend of rising RVUs over the period from 1999–2006.

Technological changes in the way care is provided have also profoundly affected physician practice patterns. For example, cancer treatment, formerly provided on an inpatient basis in hospitals, has progressed to the point where the vast majority of care is provided in ambulatory settings. In response, physicians have expanded their office capabilities or constructed purpose-built outpatient treatment centers to provide this care. Insurance payment policies have encouraged this migration away from hospitals by offering incentives for ambulatory treatment. At the same time, these incentives have made it possible for medical oncologists to bill for drugs, facility fees, and other ancillary services, in addition to billing for their professional

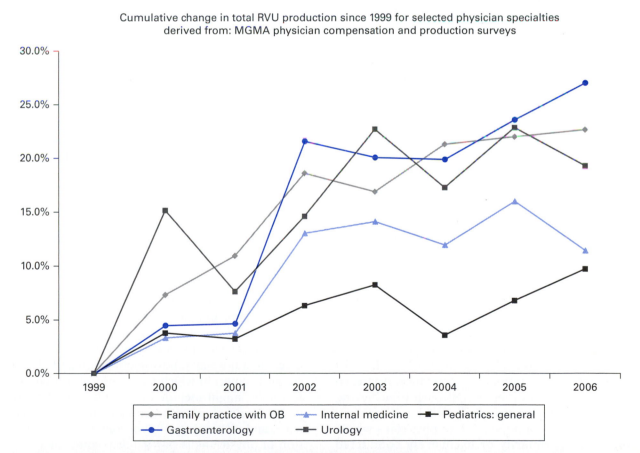

Cumulative change in total RVU production since 1999 for selected physician specialties derived from: MGMA physician compensation and production surveys

Figure 16.3. Trend of Rising RVUs Over the Period from 1999–2006

services. Largely because of this shift in site of service, oncologists have been able to more than compensate for the lack of growth in payment for their professional services. As evidence of this change, consider that the median compensation for general internists grew by 86% over the 20-year period from 1986 to 2006. During that same time, the median compensation of hematologist-oncologists grew by 199% (Medical Group Management Association, 2007). Similar changes in compensation have occurred in many other specialties where technological changes have allowed physicians to provide services in their offices that were formerly provided in hospitals.

These environmental changes have also profoundly altered the role of physicians in hospitals, and the relationships between physicians and hospitals. For example, Medicare data for 2003 show that almost 38% of physicians no longer do any work in a hospital (Fisher, et al., 2006). Rather, they have chosen to make their practices exclusively office-based and to refer to another physician any of their patients who may require inpatient treatment. The emergence of the hospitalist as a distinct medical specialist, devoted exclusively to the care of hospital inpatients with no office-based practice, has made this shift easier.

THREE DISTINCT PHYSICIAN POPULATIONS IN HOSPITALS

To best understand the relationships between physicians and hospitals, particularly in urban areas with a number of competing hospitals, it is necessary to consider three distinct physician populations. Each of these groups is important to the ability of the hospital to achieve a high level of financial and operational performance. And each group requires a different approach to achieving strategic alignment with the hospital.

First, there is a population of physicians whose practice is primarily or exclusively conducted within the walls of a single hospital. This group includes the traditional hospital-based specialties (such as pathology, radiology, anesthesiology, and emergency medicine); the newer hospital-based specialists (**hospitalists,** intensivists, and neonatologists); and a variety of physicians who are either employed or under contract to provide medical director services to various hospital departments or units (for example, the ICU medical director). In addition, a growing number of physicians in a variety of specialties are now employed by a hospital, or by another entity that is wholly owned by a hospital. Many of these physicians are in primary care specialties, and they have become hospital employees either by selling their formerly independent practice to the hospital or by entering into a direct employment relationship. Increasingly, physicians in other specialties also are becoming hospital employees because of hospital strategic initiatives, hospital needs for specialist emergency coverage, economic pressures on physicians in private practice, or some combination of these forces. The economic fate of all these physicians is deeply enmeshed with that of the hospital. Accordingly, they have a strong interest in the hospital's economic success, and hence are likely to be actively involved in hospital initiatives designed to improve safety and quality, reduce waste, and enhance patient satisfaction. This group may be termed **"hospital-dependent" physicians.**

A second population consists of physicians who spend a substantial amount of their professional time caring for hospital inpatients, but who also have extensive office-based practices. Often, these physicians will have privileges at several hospitals, but will generally concentrate most of their admissions in one. A number of specialties are common to this group, and all of them are characterized by a substantial degree of economic dependence on their office-based practices, as well as a need for access to a hospital (and sometimes an ambulatory surgical center) in which they perform procedures. Examples might include orthopedics, cardiology, otolaryngology, gastroenterology, pulmonary medicine, and obstetrics and gynecology. This population of physicians is particularly concerned with the efficiency with which their time at the hospital is used, since much of their income depends upon their availability to see patients in their office. They may be particularly difficult to convince to take hospital emergency calls without compensation, since having to leave their office to see a patient in the hospital can both reduce their income and produce significant problems with patient dissatisfaction. It is also difficult to get them to commit significant amounts of time for such activities as medical staff governance, peer review, and quality assurance, since every hour they volunteer for those activities is an hour unavailable to them for income production or family time. Finally, this is a group of physicians whose "loyalty" to the hospital is particularly tenuous. Since a significant proportion of their income is generated through their office practices, and since they often have privileges at more than one hospital, they may be quick to voice their displeasure with events that they dislike at their principal hospital and to threaten to move their patients to a competitor. This group may be referred to as **"hospital-independent" physicians.**

The third distinct population consists of those physicians who rarely if ever provide care to hospital inpatients. It includes a steadily increasing proportion of primary care physicians (internists, family physicians, and pediatricians), as well as a number of other specialties (dermatology, psychiatry, allergy, occupational medicine, etc.). While these physicians will usually have privileges at a hospital (frequently required in order to participate in various health insurance plans), those privileges will usually be in the "courtesy" or "consulting" category, rather than as members of the "active" staff. Accordingly, they are seen relatively rarely at the hospital and have little or no significant involvement in medical staff governance, peer review, or quality assurance activities. For these office-based physicians, the hospital has little relevance to them or to their practices. As noted earlier, Medicare data indicate that as many as 38% of physicians fall into this group. This group, whose economic fate is largely unaffected by the performance of the hospital, may be called **"hospital-neutral" physicians.**

Each of these three populations demands a different management approach. The hospital-dependent physicians are the group whose professional and economic objectives are most aligned with the interests of the hospital. These physicians generally care deeply about the organization in which they work and are often the champions for patient safety and quality assurance initiatives. Because they are usually salaried, they are less concerned about the impact on their compensation of time devoted to hospital administrative activities. Since they generally are not dependent upon physician referrals, they are also less likely to be the subjects of economic retribution if they take action against a physician whose performance is subpar. As with members of the senior hospital administrative staff, this physician group offers a unique opportunity to align the organization's compensation philosophy with specific performance objectives. For example, salaried physicians can receive incentive compensation for meeting defined objectives in such areas as patient satisfaction, safety, and quality of care. Similarly, physicians who are independent contractors can have incentive clauses built into their agreements. For example, a medical group that is contracted to provide medical director services for the hospital's intensive care units can have a contractual provision for a significant bonus payment if the rate of ventilator-associated pneumonias in those intensive care units is held below a specified target figure. With the growing transparency of hospital clinical performance data, the ability to align physician compensation with hospital performance objectives has become a tremendously valuable management tool.

The "hospital-independent" physician population presents a variety of challenges. The primary objective of these physicians is the business success of their own practices, and while the hospital may be an important factor in that success, it is definitely in a secondary role. These physicians are also the group that is most likely to become hospital competitors as they strive to develop new revenue streams in response to the continued downward pressures on their own fees. It is common for physicians in this group to add ancillary services such as imaging and other diagnostic testing to their practice, thereby attracting revenues to their practice that were previously going to hospitals. The entrepreneurial spirit is strong among this group, and they may become investors in ambulatory surgery centers, specialty hospitals, and other specialized treatment facilities that compete directly with general hospitals. In addition, this group is not hesitant to threaten to move their business elsewhere—and sometimes will carry through on the threat—if the hospital makes decisions that they feel infringe on their professional autonomy or adversely affect their practice.

The same entrepreneurial spirit that may pose problems for the hospital should these physicians choose to become competitors may also offer unique opportunities for the creation of "win-win" business partnerships. For example, joint ventures between the hospital and physicians from this population to build ambulatory surgery centers, endoscopy centers, imaging centers, medical office buildings, and other similar enterprises are becoming increasingly common. Care must be taken in structuring these ventures, however, to avoid both economic and legal problems. If a joint venture is created with a selected group of physicians, there may well be a backlash from other physicians who see themselves as disadvantaged by their exclusion. Further, the complex web of laws and regulations governing such ventures makes good legal advice on their creation essential.

While the "hospital-neutral" physician population may consider the hospital to be irrelevant to them and their practice, this physician group is hardly irrelevant to the hospital. In particular, the primary care physicians are the source of the lion's share of the hospital's admissions. While these physicians do not themselves direct their patients to a specific hospital, their referral patterns—usually to physicians in the "hospital-independent" group—are the critical determinant of where the patient is to be hospitalized. Accordingly, they can exert a significant economic influence on the hospital through those referral patterns.

Because their relationship to the hospital is so indirect, this group can be very difficult to actively engage. There is little reason for them to volunteer their time for hospital activities that they see as having no real relationship to their office-based practices. At the same time, they want to be kept in the communications loop and to have their voices heard in important hospital strategic decisions that may affect their patients.

Strategies that may be particularly useful in achieving alignment with this physician population are those that can help them increase the efficiency (i.e., lower operating costs) of their practices. Examples might include the provision of practice management services through a hospital-owned **management services organization (MSO);** access to hospital purchasing contracts which offer favorable pricing; and assistance with electronic health records implementation in their offices.

Rural Hospitals Are Different . . .

A number of features make the relationships between physicians and hospitals quite different in rural communities. First, there is rarely more than a single hospital in a rural community. Accordingly, the physicians in that community are very dependent upon the continued economic health of that hospital if they wish to continue to live and practice in that community. Second, practice patterns among rural physicians are very different from those of their urban counterparts. For example, most primary care physicians in rural areas continue to admit and follow their own patients when hospitalization is required, rather than referring them as do their urban colleagues. The array of specialists available in many of these communities is also much more limited than in urban areas, resulting in an outflow of patients requiring more specialized care. Finally, physicians who become dissatisfied with the hospital do not have the option of moving their business elsewhere. They can, however, choose to relocate out of the community—a very potent threat in areas that are already medically underserved.

For all these reasons, the mutual dependency of physicians and hospitals is much more extensive in rural communities and extends to essentially all the physicians in these communities. Accordingly, the segmented strategies appropriate for creating alignment in an urban or suburban environment are not as well suited to rural areas.

In rural areas, it is especially true that "physicians are the hospital's competitors, partners, collaborators, customers and employees, all at the same time" (Molpus, 2006, p. 24). This heightens the importance of building relationships between physicians and administrative leaders that are characterized by mutual trust and open and frequent communication. The experience of a newly hired rural Oklahoma hospital CEO with his chief of medical staff is illustrative:

> When interviewing for his job, he noted that the chief of the medical staff was 'downright hostile.' When he got the job, the relationship remained chilly. [He] finally pulled the physician leader aside and asked what the problem was. 'He told me that working with the hospital was like running against a 40 mile-an-hour Oklahoma wind.' So [the administrator] asked if he could join the physician's daily lunchtime runs to feel what that 'against the wind' experience was like. 'For the first month, he just vented,' [the administrator] says. But eventually the two developed a dialogue and a level of cooperation. Today, instead of division, the hospital has 100 percent participation in meetings for annual strategic planning . . . . (Molpus, 2006, pp. 24–25)

As with many aspects of health care administration, relationships and communication are critical to attaining aligned incentives between rural hospitals and their physicians. And those relationships require constant attention and reinvention. In the words of a physician who is also a hospital CEO:

> Entropy is a rule of nature—if energy is not put into systems, they fall apart. Relationships require constant attention, care and feeding, and hospital-physician relations are no exception to that rule. Do not assume that because something is working today it will work tomorrow. (Byrne, 2007)

WHAT ABOUT MEDICAL GROUPS?

As noted earlier, the majority of physicians are now in group practices of three or more physicians, and the evidence seems to indicate that group sizes are growing. This is, in part, a consequence of the increasingly difficult economic environment. Larger groups have more leverage in negotiating payment rates with insurers and can also realize economies of scale that are not available to solo or two-physician practices.

The proportion of these groups employing professional practice administrators is significant and growing. The administrative leader of a medical group, regardless of its size or specialty composition, faces a different set of physician management challenges than those faced by their hospital counterparts.

Although the number of physicians in group practices has grown tremendously since the mid-1970s, and the average size of those groups has also grown, their legal form has not changed significantly. Most are structured as professional corporations (PCs) or partnerships and are owned by the physicians who practice in the group. That factor alone makes these organizations sharply different from hospitals: the physicians are not just providers of clinical services, but are in fact the owners of the business. Accordingly, the administrative leader of the group practice is usually an employee who serves at the pleasure of the physician owners.

Medical Group Management Association (MGMA) data for 2006 indicate that 55% of the members of this professional association for medical group managers have a master's degree or higher (Webster, 2008). This reflects the growing professionalization of practice managers and also reflects the growing size and complexity of group medical practices.

Physicians join medical groups for a variety of reasons, but one of the most common is to be able to practice their profession somewhat autonomously, without having to be concerned with the business aspects of the practice. At the same time, however, they expect their administrative staff to optimize the practice's revenues and minimize its expenses such that the income of the physician owners is increased. In addition, physicians often find that the ready access to colleagues who can provide a second opinion on complex cases, the ability to share call and emergency coverage responsibilities with others, and the collegial culture within most group practices are attractive benefits of that organizational form.

However, the rapidly escalating economic pressures on medical practices are forcing physicians in medical groups to reexamine the relationship between the individual physician and the group. As the downward pressures on fees have increased, "productivity" has become critical to revenue generation. Physicians are pressed by their administrators (and their co-owners, as well) to see more patients per unit of time, work longer hours, and generate more charges per patient in order to compensate for lowered payment rates. To incentivize such productivity, most group practices now compensate their physicians using some formula that is based on their production, as measured by total relative value units (RVUs) or gross charges generated. This means that an effective administrator in a medical group must not only prod the physicians to be productive, but must design scheduling, patient intake, patient flow, medical recordkeeping, and other systems to minimize physician downtime and maximize patient throughput.

Those same economic pressures mean that physicians can no longer focus solely on their clinical responsibilities and ignore the business operations of their practice. Nor can they ignore the quality and safety of care provided by their colleagues. Today, shared accountability has become the watchword, and physicians in group practices must be active partners with their administrative staff in evaluating proposed insurance contracts, monitoring the practice's financial performance, evaluating individual physician financial performance, reviewing and improving patient care quality and

satisfaction, and in a variety of other tasks related to consumer and payer demands.

Some large medical groups have formalized the mutual expectations of the individual physician and of the organization in the form of a written "compact." At Virginia Mason Medical Center in Seattle, a large multispecialty group practice with its own hospital and clinics, the "old" compact between physicians and the organization was unwritten. But physicians understood that the basics were: "I'll take care of my patients, and the group will run the business"; clinical autonomy; work-style autonomy; and loose governance. The new compact, first implemented in 2003 (Figure 16.4), is much more detailed and spells out clearly the expectations of both parties. They include shared accountability for the financial performance of the organization and for the care received by patients. Every physician at Virginia Mason is expected to agree to the compact as a condition of joining the group and of continuing to be a part of it.

Another unique physician management challenge facing administrators in medical group practices is the changing demographics of the physician population. Medicine has historically been a male-dominated profession. But by 2004, 25.2% of the physician workforce was women, and 41% of residents-in-training were women. Estimates are that, by 2010, about 40% of practicing physicians will be women (Kotulak, 2005). In addition, some 36% of physicians in 2007 were over the age of 55. And of physicians over the age of 50, 33% said they would retire immediately if they could afford to (Salsberg, 2007). These facts mean that the active physician population is rapidly becoming younger, and female.

The implications of this change for medical groups are profound. Both younger physicians and women place much higher priority on flexible scheduling of their time and availability of time for pursuits other than medicine than did their older colleagues. For example, 71% of physicians younger than 50 report that time for family/personal life is "very important" to them (Salsberg, 2007). Broken down by gender, 66% of men under age 50 and 82% of women under age 50 rated time for family/personal life to be

Organization's Responsibilities

Foster Excellence

- Recruit and retain superior physicians and staff
- Support career development and professional satisfaction
- Acknowledge contributions to patient care and the organization
- Create opportunities to participate in or support research

Listen and Communicate

- Share information regarding strategic intent, organizational priorities and business decisions
- Offer opportunities for constructive dialogue
- Provide regular, written evaluation and feedback

Educate

- Support and facilitate teaching, GME and CME
- Provide information and tools necessary to improve practice

Reward

- Provide clear compensation with internal and market consistency, aligned with organizational goals
- Create an environment that supports teams and individuals

Lead

Manage and lead organization with integrity and accountability

Physician's Responsibilities

Focus on Patients

- Practice state of the art, quality medicine
- Encourage patient involvement in care and treatment decisions
- Achieve and maintain optimal patient access
- Insist on seamless service

Collaborate on Care Delivery

- Include staff, physicians, and management on team
- Treat all members with respect
- Demonstrate the highest levels of ethical and professional conduct
- Behave in a manner consistent with group goals
- Participate in or support teaching

Listen and Communicate

- Communicate clinical information in clear, timely manner
- Request information, resources needed to provide care consistent with VM goals
- Provide and accept feedback

Take Ownership

- Implement VM-accepted clinical standards of care
- Participate in and support group decisions
- Focus on the economic aspects of our practice

Change

- Embrace innovation and continuous improvement
- Participate in necessary organizational change

© Virginia Mason Medical Center, 2009.

Figure 16.4. **The Virginia Mason Medical Center Physician Compact**

CREDIT: Used with permission of Virginia Mason Medical Center. Further distribution prohibited.

"very important." And among physicians with children, 2% of men practice part time compared with 24% of women (Salsberg, 2007). What this means for the practice is that these younger, increasingly female physicians are not as "productive" as their older counterparts—resulting in a need for additional physicians to meet patient demands. With no significant influx of new physicians on the horizon, the management challenge this poses is obvious.

WHAT DOES THE FUTURE HOLD?

It seems clear that achieving aligned incentives between physicians and health care organizations will be even more important in the future than it is today. Market forces are pushing both physicians and health care organizations toward greater integration. While hard data are difficult to obtain, most industry watchers are convinced that hospital and health system acquisition of physician practices, and employment of physicians, is on the up-swing (Center for Healthcare Governance, 2007). Mechanisms for achieving hospital–physician integration range from such loose connections as hospital support for a physician IPA or creation of a **physician-hospital organization (PHO);** through the provision of MSO services to physician groups; to clinical integration through shared medical record information systems; to full integration through a captive medical group, often using a foundation organizational model (Center for Healthcare Governance, 2007).

Public policy initiatives seem to be encouraging this trend towards integration. The Medicare Payment Advisory Commission (MedPAC) began, in 2007, to explore the potential for "combining providers into accountable health systems that would be rated on the quality and efficiency of their care and paying them accordingly" (Ream, 2008). The concept would involve direct Medicare contracts with integrated delivery systems, large medical groups or other entities with the size and capacity to accept financial risk for caring for a defined population of Medicare beneficiaries. The accountable system's revenues would be based on predetermined measures of quality and efficiency, and the distribution of those revenues among hospitals, physicians, and others would be determined internally by the system, rather than by Medicare. Clearly, this approach would require close alignment of economic incentives among all the parties in such a system.

An interim step in this direction is the creation of so-called "bundled payments" for specific inpatient services. Under this approach, a payer would pay a hospital a fixed, pre-negotiated amount for all services associated with an inpatient episode of care— for example, for a coronary artery bypass graft. The hospital would then be responsible for determining what proportion of that bundled payment amount was to be paid to the surgeon, anesthesiologist, radiologist, and others associated with that episode of care, and what amount would be retained by

the hospital. Here again, the incentives to achieve economic alignment between the hospital and its physicians, and to assure a shared commitment to quality, safety and efficiency, are obvious.

SUMMARY

The ability to understand, relate to, and work with physicians is a critical success factor for any health care executive. To achieve strategic alignment between a health care organization and the physicians associated with that organization, the following managerial guidelines can serve as key points. Applying these guidelines can help health care organizations succeed in working with physicians. The ultimate beneficiaries of achieving alignment between physicians and health care organizations are the patients and communities that those physicians and organizations both exist to serve.

MANAGERIAL GUIDELINES

1. *Learn as much as possible about the economics of physician practices.* Understanding how physicians are paid, the key factors affecting their practice operating expenses, reimbursement trends of both public and private payers, and so on, is critical knowledge for understanding what motivates physician actions.

2. *Understand that there may be significantly different economic motives among different groups of physicians.* Different physicians (and different practices) may have very different economic motives, depending on specialty, form of practice, practice ownership, age and gender, and a variety of other factors. Gaining a thorough knowledge of what motivates different individuals and subgroups is essential to creating alignment with the health care organization.

3. *Look for opportunities to create initiatives that are "win-win" for both physicians and the health care organization.* Many of these initiatives may be joint venture business opportunities. But they can also include such things as information technology support, campaigns to improve patient satisfaction, joint efforts to influence legislation, and so on.

4. *When launching joint ventures with selected physicians, anticipate and proactively manage opposition from physicians who are not involved in that venture.* It will prove impossible to involve every physician who may wish to participate in a particular joint venture opportunity with the health care organization. Accordingly, understanding who may be disappointed or opposed, and opening up an early dialog with those individuals, can be valuable in minimizing backlash. Often, a simple reassurance that there will be other opportunities to be involved in other such ventures in the future may be sufficient to avoid significant repercussions from a decision to go forward with other individuals or groups.

5. *Communicate to excess.* Nothing breeds suspicion and distrust more quickly than lack of information. Err on the side of overcommunicating with physicians about the organization's plans, activities, and results. Include not only those physicians and practices that are directly affected but also those physicians who may have a more casual or infrequent relationship with the health care organization. Transparency can be a bridge to trust.

6. *Develop relationships with administrative leaders of physician groups.* The executives who manage physician groups can be powerful allies—or potent opponents—in working with the physicians in that practice. Communicating directly with them and involving them in planning and strategy development that will impact their physicians can be an invaluable step in gaining their support.

DISCUSSION QUESTIONS

1. How does clinical autonomy play a role in the physician–health care organization relationship?

2. What does the term "three-legged stool" mean in the health care context? And what are the components of this model?

3. Discuss the factors that have influenced the changes in physician practice arrangements over the last three decades and the impact of these changes.

4. Discuss three different populations of physicians associated with hospitals and possible managerial approaches to aligning the interests of each of those populations with the interests of the hospital.

5. What are the main reasons that physicians decide to join a medical group practice?

REFERENCES

Bureau of Labor Statistics. *Consumer Price Index,* accessed on January 27, 2008, from http://www.nclis.gov.

Byrne, F. (2007). Aligning physician-hospital relations: an integrated approach. *Healthcare Executive,* 22(4): 9–12, July/August.

Center for Healthcare Governance. (2007). *Hospital—Physician Clinical Integration.* Chicago: American Hospital Association.

Cook, R. (2007). Finances driving physicians out of solo practice. *American Medical News,* Sept. 10.

Enright, M., & Jonas, S. (1977). Hospitals. In S. Jonas (ed.), *Health Care Delivery in the United States* (p. 191). New York: Springer Publishing Company.

Federal Register, 2000–2007.

Fisher, E., Staiger, D., Bynum, J., & Gottlieb, D. (2006). Creating accountable care organizations: the extended hospital medical staff. *Health Affairs* (Web Exclusive), accessed 5 December, 2006, from http://content.healthaffairs.org.

Gans, D. (Nov. 26, 2007). Personal communication.

Goodman, L., Bennett, E., & Odem, R. (1977) Current status of group medical practice in the United States. *Public Health Rep,* 92: 430–433.

Grace, S. (2008). Fee schedule survey: 2007 results. *Physicians Practice, 18* (1): 22–23, January.

Joint Commission on Accreditation of Hospitals. (1975). *Accreditation Manual for Hospitals.* Chicago: Joint Commission on Accreditation of Hospitals.

Kotulak, R. (2005). Increase in Women Doctors Changing the Face of Medicine. *Chicago Tribune,* January 12, accessed January 28, 2005, from www.chicagotribune.com/features/health/chi-0501120279jan12,1,4042416.story.

Medical Group Management Association. (2007). *Physician Compensation and Production Surveys, 1986–2006.* Englewood, CO: Medical Group Management Association, 1987–2007.

Merritt, Hawkins and Associates. (2004). *Physician Inpatient / Outpatient Revenue Survey.* Accessed January 25, 2008, from http://www.merritthawkins.com.

Molpus, J. (2006). Dr. Partner. *Health Leaders,* October, pp. 24–25.

Rakich, J., Longest, B., & Darr, K. (1985). *Managing Health Services Organizations* (2nd ed.) (p. 428). Philadelphia: W. B. Saunders Company, 1985.

Ream, K. (2008). Washington watch: MedPAC recommends 2008 payments, prepares to report to Congress. American Academy of Emergency Medicine, accessed January 28, 2008, from http://www.medscape.com.

Salsberg, E. (2007). The state of the physician workforce: trends, developments and lessons. Presentation to the Advisory Committee on Group Practice, American Medical Association, Honolulu, HI, November 4, 2007.

Webster, K. (2008). Personal Communication, January 25.

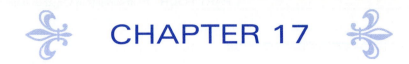

CHAPTER 17

Future Challenges in Human Resources Management

S. Robert Hernandez, DrPH and Stephen J. O'Connor, PhD, FACHE

LEARNING OBJECTIVES

Upon completing this chapter, the reader will be able to:

1. Identify and discuss key environmental trends that can affect human resources in health care organizations.

2. Understand the benefits of diversity and cross-cultural initiatives to health care organizations, especially as it relates to a diverse workforce and patient population.

3. Explain how the concept of pay-for-performance is intended to promote improvements in the quality, efficiency, and cost effectiveness of health care.

4. Identify barriers to implementing, and realizing the potential, of pay-for-performance programs.

INTRODUCTION

Dramatic changes are occurring in the United States health care environment. Kaluzny and Shortell (2006) identify these changes as happening across a broad spectrum of areas, including demographic composition of the population and changing disease patterns, societal norms and values, shifts in the focus of health care technology, and financing pressures. These and other changes affect future approaches to human resources management.

Demography and Disease Patterns

The number of older Americans is expected to increase significantly in the coming years. The number of citizens 65 or older will more than double, from approximately 40 million in 2010 to over 87 million by 2050. More drastically, the oldest of the old (those 85 and older) will triple from 6 million to over 20 million during the same time span (U.S. Bureau of the Census, 2004). Since the elderly use medical care more than any other age group except infants (Burt, McCaig, & Rechtsteiner, 2007), the aging population will contribute to increased demand on medical care in coming years. We saw an increase in outpatient demand in physician office visits, hospital outpatient and emergency department visits from the mid-1990s to 2005 of 36% (Burt, et al., 2007). We can expect even more increases in demand with the graying of the population.

Chronic conditions are also expected to increase in the future. The mean percentage of persons told they had diabetes in 2001 was 6.6 for all age groups, but was more than double that amount for those 65 to 74, at 15.8%. That same year, 25.7% of the general population reported being told they were hypertensive, but 52.3% of those 65 to 74 reported that condition. Reports of high cholesterol also increased with age, as 30.4% of all persons reported being told they had high blood cholesterol while 45.4% of those 65 to 74 reported such

information (Center for Disease Control, 2003). The aging population will stress our ability to manage the anticipated increase in chronic diseases.

The nation's population is extremely diverse. U.S. Census Bureau estimates place the total population at 301.6 million in July of 2007, with 45.5 million Hispanics, 40.7 million blacks, and 15.2 million Asians (U.S. Census Bureau, 2008). We can expect racial and ethnic diversity to increase during this century with the continued migration to the United States. In 2006, U.S. immigrants numbered 37.5 million, which was the largest number ever recorded and represented 12% of the population (Ohlemacher, 2007). The largest two groups in the United States are 11.5 million from Mexico and 10 million from Asia. Some studies suggest there is lower access to and usage of health care by immigrants (Brown, et al., 1998). As the immigrant population grows, more individuals may remain outside the mainstream of health services delivery.

Societal Norms and Values

Societal norms and values have played a significant role in defining the type of health care delivery system our country has. Individualism characterizes our system, with significant value placed on consumer choice, which has resulted in a system that views health care as a commodity sold in the marketplace rather than as a social responsibility. With health care seen as a marketable product, some argue that the relationship between health services and wealth is strengthened and the relationship between health services and need is weakened (Arbuckle, 2000).

The current change in political leadership in the United States (with the election of Barack Obama in 2009) suggests that health care will reemerge as a topic for public scrutiny. During the last national debate on health care and health care reform, it was noted that we are unlike other Western countries in that we treat health care as a market commodity (editorial NEJM, 1993). Future debate may call this norm into question as our population ages, new expensive treatment options emerge, and significant demand is placed on our delivery system. While as a society we have valued equality of access, patient safety, and accountability, these values have not been the primary drivers of our delivery system. Increasing demand and cost pressures may force us toward significant reforms as fewer Americans are able to afford health care services. Greater pressure for evidence-based health care decisions is expected to increase under these conditions.

The availability of the Internet and the rapid expansion of information have provided the general public and patients with tremendous access to knowledge about medical conditions and treatment procedures. Physicians and other caregivers can no longer completely control decisions about medical treatments. The patient plays a greater role in the choice of treatment protocols, and patient preferences will increasingly modify the role of professionals in the delivery of health care.

Health Care Technology Focus

Advances in health care technology are expected to place increased emphasis on better prediction and early management of illness and debility. Earlier detection of illness states offers the potential for earlier interventions, which provides greater opportunity for better outcomes. It also means that future illness states might be predicted before they occur. For example, genetic screening offers the potential for identifying individuals at risk for illness and the development of monitoring and prevention protocols for their conditions. It also raises ethical issues concerning patient information that might be inappropriately used in employment decisions or to deny some forms of insurance.

Financing Pressures

The increases in demand for services, technological advances, and scarcity of professionals will cause cost pressures to rise. Purchasers will increasingly seek methods to ensure that cost-effective services are provided in a quality manner. Pressures will continue for development of rewards for providers who can produce positive clinical outcomes for patients, such as pay-for-performance, which will be discussed later.

Financial pressures, increases in technology, shortages of professionals, and the increasing role of the patient in determining treatment options will affect professional roles. Physicians will no longer monopolize information and must expect more participation by patients in decision making. With a looming nursing shortage and reduced financial resources, professional nursing must play a greater role in management and supervision of the lower-skilled assistant personnel who must be hired to perform more routine care practices. The very nature of the roles professionals play in health care delivery will be modified during the coming years because of these pressures.

Shortage of Health Care Professionals in Critical Areas

Health care workforce shortages are expected to persist for many years. The reasons for this are many and include the previously discussed increase in numbers of the elderly that will make greater utilization demands on health care. At the same time, retirements from health care occupations will continue to accelerate. The net result of this will be increased demand for more health care professionals and workers to fill the many available job slots. Meeting this demand will be difficult and will require government policies that facilitate growth in a high quality health care labor pool along with organizational human resource initiatives that support effective recruitment and retention of health care workers.

Diversity and Cross-Cultural Training

As the health care workforce grows in diversity (including the international recruitment of health care workers), and as the U.S. population expands and becomes increasingly diversified, the need for improved diversity and cross-cultural and linguistic training has never been greater. The benefits of such initiatives by health care organizations are wide ranging and include (1) increased market share for services, (2) reduced staff turnover,

(3) increased patient trust (Brach & Fraser, 2000; Chyna, 2001), (4) better quality of care, (5) a greater labor pool from which to attract scarce workers, (6) lower labor costs, and (7) more effective team functioning (Dreachslin, 1996). Thus, cultural awareness issues are extremely important from a human resources perspective because successful cross-cultural and diversity training efforts are essential to employment, and, consequently, to patient encounters and outcomes. Moreover, cultural issues can directly influence employee recruitment and retention efforts, productivity, communication, and collaborative efforts, as well as legal responsibility. Cultural issues can also affect patient experiences with the health care organization and its employees. These issues can be related to religious beliefs and customs, communication preferences, dietary requirements, reactions to pain, gender and family roles, interactions with authority, and how death is confronted.

As a direct response to cultural and language concerns, the U.S. Department of Health and Human Services, Office of Minority Health (2001) developed 14 national standards for culturally and linguistically appropriate services (CLAS) in health care. These are referred to as the "CLAS standards" and were developed in order to make certain that patients receive quality care in a culturally and linguistically appropriate manner (see Figure 17.1). The standards are arranged according to the following groupings: Culturally Competent Care (Standards 1-3), Language Access Services (Standards 4-7), and Organizational Supports for Cultural Competency (Standards 8-14). These groupings differ according to the level of compliance that is required: mandates, guidelines, and recommendations. CLAS mandates are requirements for all recipients of federal funds and include CLAS Standards 4, 5, 6, and 7. CLAS guidelines are recommended by the Office of Minority Health to be required by national accrediting bodies and include CLAS Standards 1, 2, 3, 8, 9, 10, 11, 12, and 13. CLAS recommendations are presented for voluntary implementation by health care organizations and include CLAS Standard 14.

The implications of cultural concern for human resource departments are enormous. Human resources must ready a workforce that reflects the patient population being served. It must also train that workforce to become culturally literate in order to respond in a suitable fashion to different cultural situations. Creating human resource policies that codify cultural and linguistic requirements for a health care organization's workforce is one method for establishing a minimum level of competence in this area.

A study by the Joint Commission, entitled *Hospitals, Language, and Culture: A Snapshot of the Nation* (Wilson-Stronk & Galvez, 2007), examined how sixty U. S. hospitals deliver services to culturally and linguistically diverse consumers. The study found that few of the hospitals examined had developed official policies relating to hospital staff cultural and linguistic competency. The study also asked hospitals to specify which types of human resources programs (new-employee orientation, ongoing training, and competency assessment) focused on culturally and linguistically appropriate services and to whom these programs were directed. The results indicated that new-employee orientation sessions addressed these issues more frequently than ongoing training or competency assessments and that nonphysician clinical staff and senior management were more likely to be the recipients of these programs. Physicians were the least likely to receive this training in new-employee orientation (32%) or ongoing training (20%).

Cultural Awareness and Foreign Health Care Workers

The number of workers available to fill key jobs in U.S. health care organizations has been insufficient in recent years (Harvey, Hartnell, & Novicevis, 2004), with shortages in the nursing profession being particularly acute (Brush, Sochalski, & Berger, 2004). As such, many organizations have sought to address this issue by seeking to recruit foreign health care workers, especially nurses. While nurse immigration to the United States is not a new occurrence, recent rates of inflow have been unprecedented.

Standard 1. Health care organizations should ensure that patients/consumers receive from all staff members effective, understandable, and respectful care that is provided in a manner compatible with their cultural health beliefs and practices and preferred language.

Standard 2. Health care organizations should implement strategies to recruit, retain, and promote at all levels of the organization a diverse staff and leadership that are representative of the demographic characteristics of the service area.

Standard 3. Health care organizations should ensure that staff at all levels and across all disciplines receive ongoing education and training in culturally and linguistically appropriate service delivery.

Standard 4. Health care organizations must offer and provide language assistance services, including bilingual staff and interpreter services, at no cost to each patient/consumer with limited English proficiency at all points of contact, in a timely manner at all hours of operation.

Standard 5. Health care organizations must provide to patients/consumers in their preferred language both verbal offers and written notices informing them of their right to receive language assistance services.

Standard 6. Health care organizations must assure the competence of language assistance provided to limited English proficient patients/consumers by interpreters and bilingual staff. Family and friends should not be used to provide interpreter services (except on request of the patient/consumer).

Standard 7. Health care organizations must make available easily understood patient-related materials and post signage in the languages of the commonly encountered groups and/or groups represented in the service area.

Standard 8. Health care organizations should develop, implement, and promote a written strategic plan that outlines clear goals, policies, operational plans, and management accountability/oversight mechanisms to provide culturally and linguistically appropriate services.

Standard 9. Health care organizations should conduct initial and ongoing organizational self-assessments of CLAS-related activities and are encouraged to integrate cultural and linguistic competence-related measures into their internal audits, performance improvement programs, patient satisfaction assessments, and outcomes-based evaluations.

Standard 10. Health care organizations should ensure that data on the individual patient's/consumer's race, ethnicity, and spoken and written language are collected in health records, integrated into the organization's management information systems, and periodically updated.

Standard 11. Health care organizations should maintain a current demographic, cultural, and epidemiological profile of the community as well as a needs assessment to accurately plan for and implement services that respond to the cultural and linguistic characteristics of the service area.

Standard 12. Health care organizations should develop participatory, collaborative partnerships with communities and utilize a variety of formal and informal mechanisms to facilitate community and patient/consumer involvement in designing and implementing CLAS-related activities.

Standard 13. Health care organizations should ensure that conflict and grievance resolution processes are culturally and linguistically sensitive and capable of identifying, preventing, and resolving cross-cultural conflicts or complaints by patients/consumers.

Standard 14. Health care organizations are encouraged to regularly make available to the public information about their progress and successful innovations in implementing the CLAS standards and to provide public notice in their communities about the availability of this information.

Figure 17.1. National Standards for CLAS in Health Care

SOURCE: National Standards for Culturally and Linguistically Appropriate Services in Health Care (March 2001). Washington, DC: U.S. Department of Health and Human Services, Office of Minority Health.

This has resulted in new concerns related to human resource recruitment strategies and the use of recruitment agencies. Furthermore, from a broader policy perspective there are concerns related to quality, health care workforce planning, and ethics in recruiting.

As the types of patients utilizing health care organizations exhibit greater cultural and linguistic diversity, many perceive the immigration, or inpatriation, of overseas health care workers, and the diversity they bring to the workplace, as being of net benefit to organizations and patients and communities alike (Troy, Wyness, & McAuliffe, 2007). Conversely, patients may perceive that they will be the recipients of lower quality services from immigrant clinicians who can be paid a lower wage. This has been referred to as the "liability of foreignness" (Guisinger, 2002; Mezias, 2002). Either way, the current inflow of foreign health care workers will continue. It is, therefore, necessary to ensure that such inpatriation is conducted carefully so that workers feel integrated, comfortable, confident, and supported. If not, they may feel that they have been "set up" by the organization and begin to look for employment elsewhere.

Entering into a foreign workplace can be a very difficult process. In addition to feelings of social isolation and loneliness (Konno, 2006), others experience culture shock, anxiety, and communication issues (Daniel & Chamberlain, 2001). Strategies to aid in the adjustment process include culturally appropriate orientation programs, training, support services, human resource policies, and adequate prospects for personal and career growth. Moreover, support programs for the organization's domestic workers can be equally important in developing cultural and linguistic learning capacity for the organization. Harvey, et al. (2004) note that such programs can "educate healthcare workers about the foreign healthcare workers' home countries, communication styles (especially if foreign workers are coming from culturally distant countries) and celebration norms of foreign holidays (e.g., Cinco de Mayo)."

Patients can also be the recipients of culturally suitable education activities. Such programs can leverage patients' ability to better access and navigate the health care organizational environment, as well as make them more able participants in their care process (Institute of Medicine, 2003).

Pay-for-Performance

How does one get individual employees and organizations to work more productively, efficiently, and effectively? The motivational literature is replete with theories, studies, and methods regarding how to go about doing this. One long-advocated approach is to tie financial incentives (compensation) to the achievement of specific organizational goals. Employing financial inducements to stimulate individual or organizational action is not a new phenomenon by any means and, in fact, has been used since antiquity (Peach & Wren, 1992). Usually these schemes have sought to promote greater efficiencies and work intensity. For example, Frederick Taylor (1923), the "father of scientific management," is best known for his lifelong, compulsive search for more *efficient* work methods in Pennsylvania steel mills—methods that harnessed a worker's desire for economic gain to organizational work activities. Likewise, gain-sharing approaches, which take more of a cost-saving focus, have long been used by hospitals (Young & Conrad, 2007) to encourage *efficiencies* among physicians and other employees. Recently however, incentive-based methods that seek to achieve more than enhanced efficiencies have been observed in many business sectors globally. It has become especially widespread within the U.S. health care system, where individual providers such as physicians and hospitals earn pay incentives for meeting or surpassing specified quality objectives (Young & Conrad, 2007). This phenomenon has been referred to as "pay-for-performance" (P4P).

Pay-for-performance programs are intended to encourage improvements in quality, efficiency, and cost effectiveness by giving financial rewards and incentives to health care providers. However, the major emphasis of these programs is on quality of care (Young & Conrad, 2007). The effects of financial incentives on medical practice can be effective in improving adherence to practice guidelines, meeting general health goals, and in reducing health care resource use (Chaix-Couturier, et al., 2000). Others have found individual physician productivity to be closely tied to financial incentives (Conrad, et al., 2002; Gaynor & Pauly, 1990); however, as the size of a physician group increases, the power of financial inducements appears to weaken (Conrad, et al., 2002). Although most P4P programs are currently directed toward physicians (Ferman, 2004a), hospitals, hospital executives (Rollins, 2004), and even consumers (Galvin, 2003) are beginning to be rewarded for achieving quality objectives in such programs.

In P4P, providers are typically evaluated on the degree to which they meet clinical standards embodied within structural, process, or outcome measures, including patient satisfaction. Still, process standards for chronic conditions are where the promise of P4P is greatest, and where most of the emphasis has been to date. Only recently, evidence-based medicine has advanced to the point where widely agreed-upon standards or guidelines have been developed that correspond to better outcomes.

A simple example of a standard or guideline is the administration of aspirin to every patient (without contraindications) presenting with cardiac arrest. For a hospital emergency department, a clinical protocol could be written detailing when aspirin should or should not be given. Corrigan and Ryan (2004) maintain that the guidelines are similar to the "checklist a pilot goes through when taking off and landing. Airlines know that the landing gear has to be deployed on 100 percent of the flights, not just 80 or 90 percent" (p. 89).

Why Pay-for-Performance Now?

More than 150 P4P quality initiatives are presently operational or in developmental stages. A few of the better-known P4P initiatives include the Integrated Health Care Association (IHI), Bridges to Excellence, and the Centers for Medicare and Medicaid Services' Premier Hospital Quality Incentive Demonstration Project. These programs have become popular partly because of the continued growth in health care expenditures. Large employers face huge and increasing health expenditures, thus they have the impetus and the power to bring about change (Galvin & Milstein, 2002). Large employers also do not see a return to more intensive versions of managed care as the panacea to solving this problem, especially given that insurers are not seen as having the ability to truly manage care and costs effectively (Robinson, 2001b).

The second reason P4P programs have become so popular is the extensive and increasing occurrence of chronic diseases in the United States. As noted earlier, approximately one-third of the U.S. population has at least one chronic disease, the associated costs of which exceed 20% of total U.S. personal health expenditures (Druss, et al., 2002). In older Americans, chronic diseases are even more widespread and costly. Among Medicare beneficiaries, for example, those with four or more chronic conditions are "99 times more likely to experience one or more potentially preventable hospitalizations than those without a chronic condition" (Wolff, Starfield, & Anderson, 2002).

Although chronic diseases are widespread, costly, and debilitating, they are not managed well. This situation continues to persist because the health system is so heavily oriented toward acute care delivery. According to Wolff, et al. (2002) many expensive hospitalizations could be avoided with better care and with better integrated and coordinated primary care. Even with the employment of strategies such as continuous quality improvement (CQI), evidence-based medicine, and disease management guidelines to deal with chronic conditions, the result has still been irregular and minor improvements in quality.

The third, and perhaps most important, reason for the interest in P4P programs concerns the continued provision of inappropriate care to the American people as manifest by the large and unwanted variation in the use and application of evidence-based clinical practice guidelines (Fisher, et al., 2003a, 2003b; Wennberg, 1984, 2004; Wennberg & Gittelsohn, 1982) and in needless medical errors (Institute of Medicine, 1999, 2001). According to Wennberg (2004), unwanted variation is an omnipresent characteristic of the U.S. health care landscape.

Pay-for-performance programs are a response to the failure to improve quality of care delivery that is commensurate with the scientific evidence. Various strategies such as continuing medical education, patient education, and academic detailing have been unsuccessful. Despite these efforts, adherence to these guidelines is still not being fully accomplished. This has been a key driver behind the P4P initiatives.

Barriers to Implementing P4P

Physicians

Generally, clinical practice guidelines have been very carefully and scrupulously developed. They enjoy broad expert agreement and have been proven effective in saving lives and improving quality. The problem is that translating the guidelines into practice and getting physician compliance with them is difficult to achieve. Below are some barriers to implementing practice guideline adherence by physicians and, where practical, suggestions for addressing these barriers.

First, physicians are typically not paid for those extra steps taken to meet a guideline. Expectancy theory (Vroom, 1964) can help to explain this barrier and offer a possible solution. Expectancy theory views people as rational decision makers who expend effort on those tasks that will result in preferred rewards. The theory also assumes that people are clear about what rewards they want and how their work performance will lead to the rewards that they value. For example, a physician taking care of a diabetic patient may know that he or she can help to keep the patient's disease under control by following detailed diabetic practice guidelines, for example, getting the patient to test his or her blood sugar levels and monitoring the patient by requiring frequent laboratory tests, podiatric referrals, and glaucoma screenings. In other words, the physician knows that his or her efforts will lead to good performance. However, if the physician receives the identical payment for not

implementing the guidelines, expectancy theory suggests that he or she has less reason to be fully motivated in carefully applying those guidelines. Pay-for-performance initiatives try to obviate this problem by providing desired rewards (financial and nonfinancial) for good performance.

A second barrier to translating practice guidelines into practice has to do with patient compliance and follow-up. Even if a physician is rewarded for adhering to a practice guideline, he or she may know that the effort will be for naught if the patient does not also comply with the treatment plan. Is the patient's diet, amount of exercise, or socioeconomic situation—all which can impact a patient's health—the responsibility of the physician? Likewise, even if the patient is motivated to comply, a lack of personal and community health infrastructure may not be supportive of the physician's efforts.

A lack of patient compliance and/or health infrastructure can act as an unwanted outcome that can serve to suppress physician performance. Bridges to Excellence and some other P4P models design patient incentives and bonuses into their programs by motivating consumer-patients to be more able and effective treatment team members. A motivated consumer-patient is an important, albeit underutilized, element for improving quality. However, as Galvin (2002) has noted, "consumers will have to be activated to seek more efficient, higher quality care."

A third barrier to implementing P4P is a possible perceived loss of professional autonomy. Physicians may see accountability to practice guidelines, ostensibly representing the best in current clinical knowledge, as being foisted on them by nonphysicians and as interfering with their independent judgment and professional autonomy. The traditional physician professional socialization process instills strong norms regarding quality, patient-centered care, and freedom from outside interference in the physician–patient relationship. In spite of this, physicians that disparage the use of financial incentives as a way to shape their behavior "need to come to grips with the pathologies and weaknesses of [professional socialization] mechanisms for achieving the same objectives, or admit that they do not share the objectives being pursued" (Robinson, 2001a, p. 167).

A fourth barrier involves the identification and prioritization of the performance areas being evaluated. What specifically will physicians be held accountable for? What if the performance standard is not met? Will reimbursement be reduced? Will poor performers be publicly exposed? Raising these types of questions can create fear on the part of providers and can serve as the greatest impediment to implementing P4P programs (Corrigan & Ryan, 2004). It also is at odds with Demings' (1986) key point in his model of total quality management—the importance of driving out fear in making any quality scheme work.

Case mix and risk adjustment issues represent yet a fifth barrier. Physicians carrying a high number of patients with chronic conditions, for example, may perceive that they are at a disadvantage vis-à-vis other physicians. This obstacle could be overcome through risk assessment and the risk adjustment of financial incentives such that physicians or physician groups carrying heavier medical burdens would be recognized for doing so.

Hospitals

The Centers for Medicare and Medicaid Services' Premier Hospital Demonstration P4P experiment has also been criticized for focusing on whether or not specific treatments or protocols are delivered to a patient as opposed to considering if patients actually benefit from such treatments (Abelson, 2007, NYT). Furthermore, public reporting of hospital results may be a greater motivator to improvement than any additional bonus pay.

Other Employees

Chapter 14 (Compensation Management) noted that some employees view pay as an entitlement and do not view it as being related to their job performance or lack thereof. This attitude will serve as a strong barrier to P4P programs initiated with employees. Financial incentives can cause employees to become excessively concerned with what they need to do to reap monetary rewards, at the expense of attending to other activities and behaviors that are also required by the organization (Beer & Cannon, 2004). Moreover, P4P can have a damaging influence on important personal factors such as self-esteem, personal motivation, creativity, and teamwork behaviors (Amabile, 1988; Beer & Katz, 2003; Kohn, 1993; Meyer, 1975).

To overcome these concerns, some have suggested that pay-for-performance initiatives be directed toward teams as opposed to individuals. Beer and Cannon (2004) examined such a team-based P4P initiative within Hewlett-Packard's San Diego division. This approach was to encourage employees to become better team players and to become more concerned with team performance (e.g., operational improvements, productivity, quality). In addition, it was hoped that the teams would develop themselves into adaptive and continuous learners such that this goal could be achieved. The program was discontinued because managers deduced that the team-based P4P system neither stimulated employees to exert greater work effort nor to increase their learning. The reasons for this included aggravation from outside factors that had an effect on their work, such as mechanical breakdowns and shipment delays, but were beyond control of the team. Strong-performing teams did not allow low-performing individuals to join them. As the interchange of people among teams declined, so did organizational learning. Finally, greater pay levels led to higher living standards. However, if the higher pay level could not be sustained, workers became frustrated and irate. Additional research and innovative management approaches are needed if P4P methods are to be implemented successfully with other health care workers.

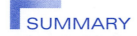

█ SUMMARY

Major changes are occurring in the demography of the U.S. population, with our citizens living longer and with significant increases in diversity among patients and health care providers.

We might anticipate shifts in societal norms and the potential for imminent change in the political climate. Advances in health care technology, financing pressures, shortages of numerous types of health professionals, and the need for sensitivity to diversity issues will place significant pressures on human resource management professionals to rethink the workplace environment for the health care workforce of the future. Guidelines for provision of culturally and linguistically appropriate services were reviewed. Pay-for-performance approaches have been suggested for health care delivery in the United States and implications of those approaches were discussed in this chapter.

MANAGERIAL GUIDELINES

1. Increasing demand for health care services and scarcity of health professionals will force managers to find innovative, efficient methods for service delivery.

2. Be prepared for changes in societal norms concerning consumer involvement in their health care and issues associated with access to care and quality.

3. Human resource managers should prepare the health care workforce to provide care in a manner that is culturally and linguistically appropriate for the population they serve.

4. Some strategies may exist to reduce barriers to physician acceptance of P4P, but there has been limited success in P4P programs targeted toward other health care workers.

REFERENCES

Abelson, R. (2007). Bonus pay by Medicare lifts quality. The *New York Times*. Accessed January 25, 2008 from www.nytimes.com.

Amabile, T. (1988). A model of creativity and innovation in organizations. In B.M. Staw &

L.L. Cummings (eds.), *Research in Organizational Behavior, 10*. Greenwich, CT: JAI Press.

Arbuckle, G.A. (2000). *Healthcare Ministry: Refounding the Mission in Tumultuous Times*. Collegeville, MN: Liturgical Press.

Beer, M., & Cannon, M.D. (2004). Promise and peril in implementing pay-for-performance. *Human Resource Management, 43*(1): 3–20.

Beer, M., & Katz, N. (2003). Do incentives work? The perceptions of a worldwide sample of senior executives. *Human Resources Planning, 26*(3): 30–44.

Brach, C., & Fraser, I. (2000). Can cultural competency reduce racial and ethnic health disparities? A review and conceptual model. *Medical Care Research and Review, 57,* (Supp 1): 181–217.

Brown, R., Wyn, R., Yu, H., Valenzuela, A., & Dong, L. (1998). Access to health insurance and health care for Mexican American children in immigrant families. In Marcelo M. Suarez-Orozco (ed.), *Crossings: Mexican Immigration in Interdisciplinary Perspectives* (pp. 225–247). Cambridge, Mass: Harvard University Press.

Brush, B.L., Sochalski, J., & Berger, A.M. (2004). Imported care: Recruiting foreign nurses to U.S. health care facilities. *Health Affairs, 23*(3, May/June): 78–87.

Burt, C.W., McCaig, L.F., & Rechtsteiner, E.A. (2007). Ambulatory medical care utilization estimates for 2005. *Advance Data from Vital and Health Statistics* (Number 388). Hyattsville, MD: National Center for Health Statistics.

Center for Disease Control. (2003). State-Specific Prevalence of Selected Chronic Disease Related Characteristics—Behavioral Risk Factor Surveillance System, 2001. Accessed March 18, 2009 from http://www.cdc.gov.

Chaix-Couturier, C., Durand-Zaleski, I., Jolly, D., & Durieux, P. (2000). Effects of financial incentives on medical practices: Results from a systematic review of the literature and methodological issues. *International Journal of Quality in Health Care, 12*(2): 133–142.

Chyna, J.T. (2001). Mirroring your community: A good reflection on you. *Healthcare Executive, 16*(2): 18–23.

Conrad, D.A., Sales, A.M., Chauduri, A., Liang, S., Maynard, C., Pieper, L., Weinstein, L., Gans, D., & Piland, N. (2002). The impact of financial incentives on physician productivity in medical groups. *Health Services Research, 37*(4): 885–906.

Corrigan, K., & Ryan, R.H. (2004). New reimbursement models reward clinical excellence. *Healthcare Financial Management, 58*(11): 88–92.

Daniel, P., & Chamberlain, G. (2001). Expectations and experiences of newly recruited Filipino nurses. *British Journal of Nursing, 10*(4): 254–265.

Dreachslin, J.L. (1996). *Diversity Leadership*. Chicago, IL: Health Administration Press.

Druss, B.G., Marcus, S.C., Olfson, M., & Pincus, H.A. (2002). The most expensive medical conditions in America. *Health Affairs, 21*(4): 105–111.

Editorial. (1993) How much will health care reform cost? *New England Journal of Medicine, 328*(24): 1778–1779.

Ferman, J.H. (2004a). Pay for performance gaining popularity. *Healthcare Executive, 19*(4): 50–52.

Fisher, E.S., Wennberg, D.E., Stukel, T.A., Gottlieb, D.J., Lucas, F.L., & Pinder, E.L. (2003a). The implications of regional variations in Medicare spending. Part 2: Health outcomes and satisfaction with care. *Annals of Internal Medicine, 138*(4): 273–287.

Fisher, E.S., Wennberg, D.E., Stukel, T.A., Gottlieb, D.J., Lucas, F.L., & Pinder, E.L. (2003b). The implications of regional variations in Medicare spending. Part 1: The content, quality, and accessibility of care. *Annals of Internal Medicine, 138*(4): 273–287.

Galvin, R. (2003). Purchasing health care: An opportunity for a public-private partnership. *Health Affairs, 22*(2): 191–195

Galvin, R., & Milstein, A. (2002). Large employers' new strategies in health care. *New England Journal of Medicine, 347*(12): 939–942.

Gaynor, M., & Pauly, M.V. (1990). Compensation and productive efficiency in partnerships: Evidence from medical group practice. *Journal of Political Economy, 98*(3): 544–573.

Guisinger, S. (2002). Liability of foreignness to competitive advantage. *Journal of International Management, 8*(3): 223–240.

Harvey, M., Hartnell, C., & Novicevic, M. (2004). The inpatriation of foreign health care workers: A potential remedy for the chronic shortage of professional staff. *International Journal of Intercultural Relations, 28*(2): 127–150.

Institute of Medicine. (1999). *To err is human*. Washington, DC: National Academy Press.

Institute of Medicine. (2001). *Crossing the quality chasm: A new health system for the 21st century*. Washington, DC: National Academy Press.

Institute of Medicine. (2003). *Unequal treatment: Confronting racial and ethnic disparities in health care*. Washington, DC: The National Academies Press.

Kaluzny, A.D., & Shortell, S.M. (2006). Creating and Managing the Future. In S.M. Shortell & A.D. Kaluzny (eds.), *Health Care Management: Organization Design and Behavior* (5th ed.). Clifton Park, NY: Thomson Delmar Learning.

Kohn, A. (1993). Why incentive plans cannot work. *Harvard Business Review, 71*(5): 54.

Konno, R. (2006). Support for overseas qualified nurses in adjusting to Australian nursing practice: A systematic review. *International Journal of Evidence Based Health Care, 4*: 83–100.

Meyer, H. (1975). The pay-for-performance dilemma. *Organization Dynamics, 3*: 39–50.

Mezias, J. (2002). Identifying liabilities of foreignness and strategies to minimize their effects: The case of labor lawsuit judgments in the United States. *Strategic Management Journal, 23*: 229–244.

Ohlemacher, S. (2007, September 12). Number of Immigrants Hits record 37.5 Million. *Washington Post*. Accessed March 20, 2009 from www.washingtonpost.com/wp-dyn/content/article/2007/09/12/AR2007091200071.html.

Peach, B., & Wren, D.A. (1992). Pay-for-performance from antiquity to the 1950s. *Journal of Organizational Behavior Management, 12*: 5–21.

Rollins, G. (2004). A worthy bonus. *Hospitals & Health Networks, 78*(9): 32, 35.

Robinson, J.C. (2001a). Theory and practice in the design of physician payment incentives. *The Milbank Quarterly, 79*(2): 149–177.

Robinson, J.C. (2001b). The end of managed care. *Journal of the American Medical Association, 285*: 1000–005.

Taylor, F.W. (1923). *The Principles of Scientific Management*. New York, NY: Harper and Brothers Publishers.

Troy, P.H., Wyness, L.A., & McAuliffe, E. (2007). Nurses' experiences of recruitment and migration from developing countries: A phenomenological approach. *Human Resources for Health*, 5(15).

U.S. Bureau of the Census. (2004). U.S. Interim Projections by Age, Race, and Hispanic Origin: 2000-2050. Table 2a. Projected Population of the United States, by Age and Sex: 2000 to 2050. Accessed March 20, 2009 from http://www.census.gov.

U.S. Bureau of the Census. (2008, May). U.S. Hispanic Population Surpasses 45 Million Now 15 Percent of Total. Accessed March 18, 2009 from http://www.census.gov.

Vroom, V. (1964). *Work and motivation*. New York, NY: Wiley.

Wennberg, J.E. (1984). Dealing with medical practice variations: A proposal for action. *Health Affairs*, *3*(2): 6–32.

Wennberg, J.E. (2004). PERSPECTIVE: Practice variations and health care reform: Connecting the dots. *Health Affairs*: V140–V144.

Wennberg, J.E., & Gittelsohn, A. (1982). Variations in medical care among small areas. *Scientific American*, *246*: 120–134.

Wilson-Stronks, A., & Galvez, E. (2007). *Hospitals, Language, and Culture: A snapshot of the nation*. Oak Brook Terrace, Illinois: The Joint Commission.

Wolff, J. L., Starfield, B., & Anderson, G. (2002). Prevalence, expenditures, and complications of multiple chronic conditions in the elderly. *Annals of Internal Medicine*, *162*(20): 2269–2276.

Young, G.J., & Conrad, D.A. (2007). Practical issues in the design and implementation of pay-for-quality programs. *Journal of Healthcare Management*, *52*(1): 10–19.

GLOSSARY

360-Degree Feedback Administration of a survey about a particular leader's strengths and weaknesses to his or her supervisors, peers, and subordinates. The survey results are then aggregated by a third party and returned to the leader that is the subject of the survey. This allows for a confidential, honest review of leadership ability and identifies areas to target for improvement.

Ability The mental or physical power to get something done; in other words, the quality of being able to do something.

Absolute Standards Comparative performance methods through which each individual is evaluated against written standards and several factors of performance are measured.

Accreditation A type of credentialing administered by an outside organization that shows the quality, credibility, and competency of an organization or other entity.

Action Learning A form of leadership development that occurs when groups of employees are assembled to solve a specific problem. This process is thought to promote collaborative leadership through requiring participants to apply familiar problem-solving approaches to unique or unfamiliar contexts.

Adverse Impact Adverse impact is present if the pass rate for a specific protected group is less than 80% of the pass rate for the majority group. It is unlawful to use any selection procedure that demonstrates adverse impact against a protected group, unless its use has been justified by a validation study.

Affirmative Action A policy or a program that seeks to redress past discrimination through active measures to ensure equal opportunity, as in education and employment.

Age Discrimination in Employment Act (ADEA) Prohibits discriminatory treatment of individuals 40 years of age or older for employment-related purposes, including mandatory retirement. Employment purposes include hiring, job retention, compensation, discharge, and other privileges, conditions, and terms of employment. ADEA applies to companies with over 20 employees, but certain public safety positions are exempt, such as police, fire, and uniformed military personnel.

Alternation Ranking The most common comparative performance method through which the rater repeatedly chooses the strongest then the weakest employee, each time successively choosing from the names remaining in the list. The process is continued until all employees have been placed on the ranking list, with the last two ranked in the middle.

Americans with Disabilities Act (ADA) Prohibits employers with more than 15 employees from discriminating against a qualified individual with a disability because of the disability with regard to job application procedures; hiring; job assignment, training, and advancement; employee compensation and fringe benefits; discharge of employees; and other terms, conditions, and privileges of employment.

Artifacts The first level of organizational culture. The most visible and objective aspects of the workforce culture. Artifacts are relatively easy to examine and describe, and they can include symbols; language; ceremonies and rituals; stories, myths, and legends; and heroes and heroines.

Assimilation Approach A diversity approach that expects individuals to suppress their differences and to conform to the style already dominant in an organization.

Balanced Budget Act of 1997 Reduced reimbursements to health care providers to contain government spending on health care, including caps on reimbursement for rehabilitation professionals.

Basic Underlying Assumptions The third level of organizational culture. The nonconscious system of beliefs, perceptions, and values shared by employees that work effectively and repetitively over time.

Boston Consulting Group (BCG) Business Grid A method of examining the holdings of an organization based on the market growth rate of a business and the relative market share that the business commands.

Bureau of Labor Statistics The principal fact-finding agency for the federal government in the broad field of labor economics and statistics; an independent national statistical agency that collects, processes, analyzes, and disseminates essential statistical data to the American public, the U.S. Congress, other federal agencies, state and local governments, business, and labor.

Career Sponsoring A mentoring process that focuses on enabling a protégé to pursue or assume advanced levels of responsibility and authority in an organization or in the working environment. The prime function of mentoring in this context is for the mentor to directly or indirectly influence the environment or provide counsel to a protégé so that a position, assignment, or some developmental opportunity is made available to the protégé.

Certification A type of credentialing administered by an outside organization which certifies that a professional is able to competently complete a job or task, usually by passing an examination.

Challenging Job Assignment An applied method of leadership development that involves assigning challenging jobs consisting of diverse tasks and levels of responsibility and rigor that progress with the individual as leadership is demonstrated.

Civil Rights Act of 1964 Prohibits employment treatment in hiring, dismissal, promotion, discipline, terms and conditions of employment, and job advertising that is disparate based on race, color, religion, sex, national origin, or pregnancy.

Coaching The practice of establishing a relationship between two individuals with the hope of developing one individual's career, improving his/her performance, or working through a specific challenge or issue.

Cognitive Task Analysis (CTA) The most recently developed job analysis method, created out of the recognition that when jobs involve tasks that are complex, assessing behavior alone is not sufficient. CTA focuses on the mental processes that lead to behaviors. The technique describes the cognitive processes and skills necessary to perform a job.

Comparative Methods A performance-appraisal method that compares one employee to another in order to determine performance ranking. The ranking can be a straight ranking, an alternation ranking, paired comparison, or forced distribution.

Compensation Strategy A strategy within the organization that is used to determine the forms of compensation that will be or can be offered, the workforce demographics, the business cycle, the compensation philosophy, and legal and regulatory compliance.

Compensatory Time Off (comp-time) Hours given to an employee in lieu of payment for extra time worked. Unless it is given to nonexempt employees at the rate of one and one-half times the number of hours over 40 that are worked in a week, comp-time is illegal in the private sector. Also, comp-time cannot be carried over from one pay period to another. The only major exception to these provisions is for public sector employees, such as fire and police employees, and a limited number of other workers.

Competence An underlying characteristic of a person that enables him or her to deliver superior performance in a given job, role, or situation and can be learned over time.

Competency A set of observable performance dimensions, including individual knowledge, skills, attitudes, and behaviors as well as collective team, process, and organizational capabilities that are linked to high performance and provide the organization with sustainable competitive advantage.

Competency Clusters The grouping of competencies by explicit knowledge, skills, abilities and other personal characteristics instead of detailing the specific elements required for a specific job.

Competency Code Book A book which offers organizations a menu of competencies from which they can select those which are most appropriate.

Competency Models A detailed, behaviorally specific description of the skills and traits that employees need to be effective in a job.

Competency-Based Pay Philosophy Establishing pay policies that reward employees for carrying out their tasks, duties, and responsibilities. The job requirements and responsibilities determine which employees have higher base rates. Employees receive more for doing jobs that require a greater variety of tasks, more knowledge and skills, greater physical effort, or more demanding working conditions. A number of organizations are now paying employees for the competencies they demonstrate rather than just for the specific task performed.

Competitive Analysis Identifies performance improvement that could result from changes in the competitive strategies employed in current business units of the firm.

Content Validity Indicates that the content of the assessment is relevant to the content of the job. Content validity is usually demonstrated by documenting the judgments of subject matter experts who have determined if the content of the assessment is an effective measurement of a job relevant competency.

Contingency Theory Posits that organizational strategy and design are determined by environmental conditions.

Construct Validity Encompasses both criterion-related validity and content validity, and is generally the demonstration that an assessment measures the characteristic that it purports to measure and that that characteristic is relevant to job performance.

Core Competencies Broad organizational requirements that reflect organizational goals and the strategies developed to respond to changing environments.

Cost-of-Living Adjustments (COLA) A common pay-raise practice is the use of a standard raise or cost-of-living adjustment (COLA). Giving all employees a standard percentage increase enables them to receive the same real wages in a period of economic inflation. Often, these adjustments are tied to changes in the consumer price index (CPI) or some other general economic measure.

Cost Leadership Strategy A competitive strategy in which an organization focuses on providing products or services at a lower cost than competitors through economies of scale, lean management systems, and control of resource consumption.

Cost Shifting When providers of care charge higher prices to one payer group to offset lower prices paid by other payer groups.

Counterculture A subculture that is at odds with the value structure of the overall organizational culture.

Criterion-Related Validity The statistical relationship between assessment results and actual on-the-job performance. Typically, criterion-related validity is demonstrated using a statistical correlation between the assessment score and some measure of job performance.

Critical Incident Technique This job analysis method identifies behaviors that differentiate good job performers from poor ones by interviewing incumbents and/or other job experts to compile critical behavioral incidents. Incidents are examined by determining what led to the employee's behavior, the behavior itself, and the consequences of the employee's actions. This information provides future job holders with thorough details about critical job behaviors.

Cultural Competence A set of congruent behaviors, attitudes, and policies that come together in a system, agency, or among professionals that enables effective work in cross-cultural situations.

Cyclical Workforce Shortage Temporary workforce shortages that occur over certain time periods because of circumstances that cause shifts in supply and demand and that are eventually corrected by market forces.

Degree Creep The trend of increasing degree levels in a number of health professions.

Development Activities geared toward adding new skills or experiences, usually to prepare an employee for a promotional opportunity or a different career path.

Differentiation Strategy A competitive strategy in which the organization offers products or services that are perceived by customers as unique along certain dimensions. As a result, customers are willing to pay a premium price.

Direct Compensation All tangible rewards of the working relationship. Direct compensation is the sum of base pay plus variable pay. Base pay is the basic compensation that an employee receives and is delivered as a wage or salary. The other element of direct compensation is variable pay, which is compensation linked directly to individual, team, or organizational performance. The most common types of variable pay are received as bonuses, incentives, stock options. Variable pay is often referred to as "incentive compensation" because it is used as an inducement to meet a predefined performance goal.

Disability Any physical or mental impairment that substantially limits one or more of an individual's major life activities, such as caring for him- or herself, walking, talking, hearing, or seeing. Examples of disabilities include visual or hearing impairments, mobility impairments, alcoholism, cancer, HIV/AIDS, and mental illness.

Distinct Competence An advantage that the institution holds over its competitors. The advantage may emanate from the competitive advantages of cost leadership, differentiation, and focus, or the organization may possess an asset that provides it with an advantage over competitors.

Diversity Encompasses those who are different in terms of race, age, religion, disability, marital status, ethnicity, ancestry, gender, physical abilities/qualities, sexual orientation, educational background, geographic location, income, military experience, parental status, and work experience.

Diversity Management Providing for business maximization by acknowledging people's differences, recognizing differences as valuable, preventing discrimination, and promoting inclusiveness.

Employee Attitude Surveys Surveys conducted to reveal employee needs and how those needs change over periods of time. To be effective, employee attitude surveys should be conducted often and employees should be told what the purpose is; how the data will be analyzed and used; that individual responses are confidential; and the feedback from survey findings and what changes, if any, they can expect as a result of the findings.

Employee Relations Program An organization's strategy concerning its policies regarding unions and employee relations. It is based on factors such as communication with employees, management rights, union preferences, organizational and environmental issues, and the organization's employee-relations philosophy.

Employment-At-Will Doctrine Doctrine meaning that termination of the employment relationship can occur without cause at the choice or will of either the employee or the employer, subject only to such restrictions as antidiscrimination statutes.

Enhancing subculture A subculture that is supportive of and in harmony with the principal organizational culture.

Entitlement Culture A culture that allows an automatic increase in compensation to all employees every year. Most of the employees in this type of organizational culture receive the same or nearly the same percentage increase each year. Employees and managers who subscribe to the entitlement culture believe that individuals who have worked another year are entitled to a raise in base pay. They also believe that incentives programs should always be continued and benefits should be increased regardless of changing industry or economic conditions.

Equal Employment Opportunity (EEO) Laws Make it illegal for employers to discriminate against an employee or potential employee in certain workplaces.

Equal Employment Opportunity Commission (EEOC) The federal agency, created by the Civil Rights Act of 1964, which has the responsibility to handle discrimination complaints.

Equal Pay Act of 1963 (EPA) Prohibits discrimination in pay for women and men performing substantially equal work in similar situations.

Essential Job Function A primary work activity that is necessary to perform the job. To be defined as an essential job function the activity usually must be: (1) performed by every employee holding that specific job title; (2) performed frequently, relative to other job activities; and (3) critical to accomplishing the goal of the job.

Exempt Employees Employees who hold positions classified as executive, administrative, professional, or outside sales, for which employers are not required to pay overtime. Exempt employees are paid for the job that they do, not the hours that they work.

Failure Mode Effects Analysis (FMEA) An analysis of a health care error that includes a thorough review of the actions taken and the processes involved that is focused on uncovering opportunities for training to address the mistakes in knowledge, skill, and ability. Such analyses may be used to identify the potential for errors and to provide appropriate corrective actions before they occur. FMEA is a very powerful needs assessment tool as it can highlight areas where focused training may be used to proactively prevent an error.

Fair Discrimination Making personnel decisions based on job-relevant knowledge, skills, abilities, or other competencies. The law has provided for companies to fairly discriminate between qualified and unqualified applicants in personnel decisions based on the organization's business necessity to employ individuals who can successfully perform the job.

Fair Grievance Procedure A procedure that allows employees to be able to complain about perceived problems formally without fear of subjective reprisal. If the procedures are written down and responded to promptly there should be a decreased number of complaints and employees will feel that management is concerned about their needs.

Fair Labor Standards Act (FLSA) Sets minimum wages, time-and-a half guaranteed overtime, maximum overtime pay, and prohibits employment of minors. The FLSA covers non-profit and for profit hospital employees. The Wage and Hour Division of the U.S. Department of Labor administers the FLSA, including workplace inspections and the conduct of audits.

Financial Planning The planning approach used by most organizations prior to the 1950s. It focused on budgets for a given time period, usually a year.

Focus Strategy A competitive strategy in which the organization chooses to focus on products and services that target a narrow market segment or group. This focus can be a cost focus or a differentiation focus.

Forced-Choice Method An absolute standards method through which the rater selects statements that best fit the performance characteristics of the individual employee. The rater does not know the value assigned to each characteristic, and consequently the forced-choice method can reduce bias.

Forced Distribution A comparative performance method through which the rater assigns a certain proportion of the employees to one category on each criterion. For example, 10% of employees might be in the "superior" category, 20% in the "good," 20% in the "average," with the remainder in the "poor" category.

Functional Job Analysis A job analysis method that focuses on what gets accomplished in a particular job. It uses seven scales to describe what workers do or work with: (1) Things, (2) Data, (3) People, (4) Worker Instructions, (5) Reasoning, (6) Math, and (7) Language. Each of the seven scales has several levels using behavioral statements and illustrative tasks as anchors to assist job analysts in their role.

Generic Competency Model Approach An approach to developing a competency model by defining competencies for a broad set of jobs. This approach tends to de-emphasize the technical skills and required knowledge for specific jobs, providing a more generic set of competencies.

Golden Rule Approach A diversity approach that relies on individuals to make diversity work by treating others how they would like to be treated.

Graphic Rating The most commonly used absolute-standards method for performance appraisal. The scale requires the rater to choose a value or statement along a continuum that best fits the employee for each criterion being reviewed. The advantage of a graphic scale is that it shows visually the degree to which an employee performs a job or task.

Health Insurance Portability and Accountability Act of 1996 (HIPAA) Requires the establishment of national standards for electronic health care transactions and national identifiers for providers, health insurance plans, and employers. HIPAA also addresses the security and privacy of health data.

Hierarchy-Based Rewards System A system that evaluates and rewards employees based on largely subjective criteria such as interdepartmental cooperation, interactions with consumers, interpersonal relationships, and teamwork. These rewards and evaluation criteria emphasize the importance of long-term commitment, cooperation, teamwork, and the dependence of subordinates on superiors.

Hospital-Dependent Physicians Physicians whose practice is primarily or exclusively conducted within the walls of a single hospital. This group includes the traditional hospital-based specialties (such as pathology, radiology, anesthesiology, and emergency medicine); the newer hospital-based specialists (hospitalists, intensivists, and neonatologists); and a variety of physicians who are either employed or under contract to provide medical director services to various hospital departments or units. The economic fate of all these physicians is deeply enmeshed with that of the hospital.

Hospital-Independent Physicians Physicians who spend a substantial amount of their professional time caring for hospital inpatients, but who also have extensive office-based practices. Examples might include orthopedics, cardiology, otolaryngology, gastroenterology, pulmonary medicine, and obstetrics and gynecology. This population of physicians is particularly concerned with the efficiency with which their time at the hospital is used, since much of their income depends upon their availability to see patients in their office.

Hospital-Irrelevant Physicians The third distinct population consists of those physicians who rarely if ever provide care to hospital inpatients. It includes a steadily increasing proportion of primary care physicians (internists, family physicians, and pediatricians), as well as a number of other specialties (dermatology, psychiatry, allergy, occupational medicine, etc.). Accordingly, they are relatively rarely seen at the hospital and have little or no significant involvement in medical staff governance, peer review, or quality assurance activities.

Hospitalist Hospitalist activities may include patient care, teaching, research, and leadership related to hospital care. Hospital medicine, much like emergency medicine, is a specialty associated with the site of care, rather than an organ, a disease, or the patient's age.

Indirect Compensation Pay received in the form of services and benefits is called indirect compensation. Some of the most common forms of indirect compensation are health insurance, income replacement programs (life/disability insurance), paid time off, retirement/pension plans, and educational assistance.

Industry Analysis Concerned with identifying the competitive factors that lead to success in a given product/market and determining the relative attractiveness of an industry/market for the firm.

Instructional System Design (ISD) Model Provides a framework for designing and implementing effective training programs. It suggests that training programs begin with a comprehensive training-needs assessment. Next, training objectives and strategies are developed to address identified training needs. After implementation, an explicit training evaluation is conducted. Studies have found important linkages among personal training needs, various instructional methods, and learning effectiveness.

Inter-Rater Reliability Measures statistically the amount of agreement among the various raters involved in an assessment. It can only be calculated after the assessment has been implemented because inter-rater agreement is affected not only by the quality of the assessment tools but also by the effectiveness of the raters.

Job Analysis The process by which jobs in an organization are systematically and thoroughly described by identifying and evaluating the job tasks, responsibilities, and the context or the environment associated with a particular job.

Job Applicant A person is considered a job applicant if the person makes an expression of interest in the job and follows the company's standard procedures, the organization considers the individual for a particular position, information provided indicates that the individual possesses the basic qualifications for the position, and the individual does not remove himself or herself from consideration.

Job Description A description of a job that includes job title; indirect and direct reporting relationships; committee and relating responsibilities; educational and professional certification requirements; duties and responsibilities; desired behavioral characteristics; and salary range, benefits level, and perks.

Job Specification Human attributes identified as important to the successful performance of the job, including knowledge, skills, abilities, license requirements, physical and mental demands, and experience.

Job Family Competencies Competencies that apply to broad groups of jobs.

Just Cause A principle management can use to impose discipline consistently and fairly. For management to have "just cause," the disciplinary rule must be reasonably related to efficient and safe operations, the employees must be properly warned of potential consequences of violating the rule, management must conduct a fair investigation before applying the discipline, the investigation must produce substantial evidence of guilt, the policies and procedures must be implemented consistently and without discrimination, and if a penalty results it must be related to the seriousness of the event as well as the past record of the employee.

Knowledge Familiarity with, awareness of, or understanding about a particular job requirement or competency.

KSAO Competency Components Knowledge, skills, abilities, and other personal characteristics are the varying components of a competency. Knowledge includes the information and understanding of critical rules, concepts, and work processes necessary to perform tasks. Skills are the capacity to perform mental or physical tasks to achieve desired outcomes. Abilities include the underlying cognitive or physical capabilities to fully perform a task. Other personal characteristics related to competencies might include attitudes, values, and behaviors necessary to perform effectively.

Law A body of rules of action or conduct prescribed by controlling authority and having binding legal force.

Leadership An individual's ability to not simply control day-to-day operations but also to galvanize resources and motivate employees to work collectively to further organizational goals.

Leadership Development Any activity that improves the ability of an individual to lead, including both formal and informal methods such as classroom instruction, skill-based training, challenging job assignments, team training, action learning, 360-degree feedback, and developmental relationships such as mentoring.

Level Competencies Competencies that are specific to particular jobs in a job family.

Licensing A type of credentialing administered by a government entity, usually the state, that gives professionals the legal right to practice if educational, training, and procedural requirements have been met.

Long-Range Planning The planning approach popular in the 1960s concerned with the projection of organizational goals, objectives, programs, and budgets during an extended period. This approach requires forecasting of environmental trends based on historical data.

Management By Objectives (MBO) A result-based evaluative program in which goals are mutually determined by supervisors and subordinates, and employees are rated on the degree to which these goals are accomplished. MBO stresses the value and importance of employee involvement and encourages discussion of employees' strengths and weaknesses.

Management Rights The right to prescribe certain modes of action or levels of desired productivity to justify its existence or that of the organization. May cause conflict with labor unions who question whether management should have complete power over the workforce. Organized labor attempts to shift the locus of control by seeking to obtain a voice for employees about working conditions and terms of employment.

Management Services Organization Organization established by a hospital, a physician group, or other investors to provide practice management services to individual physicians or small medical practice groups.

Market-Based Pay Philosophy Establishing specific pay policies around where an organization wishes to be positioned in the labor market. Organizations can decide whether they want to lead the market, match the market, or lag behind the market.

Medical Assistants Health care professionals who perform basic clinical procedures and administrative tasks such as drawing blood, giving shots, scheduling patients, and billing for insurance payment.

Medicare Conversion Factor The dollar amount which, when multiplied by the number of relative value units (RVUs) associated with a particular service, determines the fee paid by Medicare to the physician.

Mentoring A developmental relationship that is mutually maintained by two people for professional, social, or other benefit.

Mission Statement A statement that communicates corporate purpose, scope of operations, self-concept, and image to important stakeholders.

Monolithic Organization The first, or least effective, stage of development in managing cultural diversity. It is characterized by assimilation of diverse employees, minimal structural and informal integration of diverse others, presence of prejudice and discrimination against diverse employees, large gaps in the degree of organizational commitment of diverse versus dominant employees, and low intergroup conflict due to high homogeneity.

Motivation Theory Stipulates that individuals will gravitate toward behaviors associated with positive reinforcement and away from behaviors that produce negative reinforcement.

Multicultural Approach A diversity approach that involves increasing the consciousness and appreciation of differences associated with the heritage, characteristics, and values of many different groups, as well as respecting the uniqueness of each individual.

Multicultural Organization The final and most effective stage of development in managing cultural diversity. This organization incorporates diverse employees into its workforce by recognizing differences and valuing heterogeneity. Diverse employees are fully integrated into the organization, both structurally and informally, resulting in little intergroup conflict. Prejudice and discrimination are minimal, as are gaps in the level of employee commitment among groups.

National Labor Relations Act of 1935 (NLRA) Governs management–labor relationships of businesses engaged in interstate commerce. The NLRA defines unfair labor practices for employees and employers, authorizes the National Labor Relations Board (NLRB) to conduct secret elections for employees to determine any representation by a labor organization, and authorizes the NLRB to investigate and conduct hearings for complaints about unfair labor practices.

Needs Assessment A diagnostic process in which the organization identifies performance gaps and determines whether and how training can be used to improve performance. Training and development needs assessment occurs at the organization, department, and individual levels.

New Employee Orientation Task-related skill building that typically combines classroom instruction with on-the-job teaching. Employees learn important information about the organization and its expectations in an initial orientation, which occurs in a classroom setting.

Nonexempt Employees Employees who are paid for the hours that they work and therefore must be paid overtime under the Fair Labor Standards Act.

Nonunion Policy A formal, proactive management program that significantly reduces or eliminates the need for workers to seek union representation. It is based on the philosophy that unionization is preventable if management is doing enough of the "right things."

Occupational Safety and Health Act of 1970 (OSHA) OSHA establishes standards for occupational health and safety. OSHA has taken initiatives for the protection of health care employees from blood-borne diseases, latex allergies, needle stick injuries, tuberculosis, and waste anesthetic gases, as well as general initiatives and citations regarding employee vaccinations, ergonomics, and workplace violence.

Off-Limits Policies Relates to job-search firms. Once a candidate has entered an organization's interview process, the candidate should be considered exclusively by that organization only, and not introduced into another search until the original search is concluded. Introducing a candidate to multiple clients simultaneously is known as parallel processing. Parallel processing is not generally in the best interest of an organization as it places the search firm in the position of representing the candidate and not the organization.

Onboarding The process of helping new hires reach their optimal productivity. At minimum, onboarding usually involves some sort of orientation or initial training program.

Organizational Core Competencies Competencies based on the skills, knowledge, and attitudes and other personal characteristics of many different staff. Core competencies represent the collective learning skills within the organization and the collaborative use of different technical competencies.

Organizational Culture A pattern of beliefs, behaviors, and unspoken underlying assumptions that are conveyed to, and shared by, all members of the organization.

Organizational Learning Perspective An organizational emphasis on developing capabilities that facilitate learning through the acquisition and transfer of knowledge and insight throughout the organization.

Organizational Socialization A process by which individuals learn the values and behavioral norms of an organization through activities that facilitate social interaction and contribute to the organization's culture.

Orthogonal Subculture A subculture that partially overlaps with the principal culture by sharing some of the same values, but also simultaneously adhering to others that are different.

Paired Comparison A comparative performance method through which one employee at a time is compared to all other employees. Each time an employee is ranked higher than another employee, a tally is placed by the higher-ranking person's name. The employee with the most tallies is considered to be the most valuable, and the others are placed in order according to the number of tallies by their name.

Pay Compression Occurs when the pay differences among individuals with different levels of experience and performance becomes small. Pay compression occurs for a number of reasons, but the major one involves situations in which labor market pay levels increase more rapidly than current employees' pay adjustments.

Pay Mix The amount of emphasis that is placed on each of the elements of total compensation, including base, benefits, options, and bonuses.

Pay-for-Performance Systems These systems reward providers (beginning with hospital payments and moving to physician payments) for reporting, then performing against, certain quality performance standards.

Performance Appraisal The systematic evaluation of an employee's work behavior using valid, reliable criteria to measure important job-related activities. Appraisals are used to provide guidance for the selection of individuals for promotion, to determine increases in employee compensation, and to identify areas in which personnel need training and development.

Performance Consulting Conducted with intact work teams, performance consulting occurs in the real world environment, providing a way to observe and respond to how a team functions. By using empirical data, performance consulting effectively changes team behaviors and reinforces changes in skills and process in the work environment.

Performance Management System A system that integrates performance-appraisal systems with broader human resource systems as a means of aligning employees' work behaviors with the organizational goals to enhance employee capability and productivity. It is an ongoing, interactive process that includes performance definition, appraisal process, performance measurement, feedback, and coaching.

Performance-Based Culture A culture in which organizations do not guarantee additional or increased compensation for simply completing another year of service with the organization. Instead, pay and incentives reflect performance differences among employees. Employees who perform well receive larger compensation increases and those who do not

perform satisfactorily see little or no increase in base pay. Bonus compensation may be paid on the basis of individual, team, or organizational performance.

Performance-Based Rewards System A system that evaluates and rewards employees based on objective and measurable performance criteria. These rewards and evaluation protocols emphasize individual initiative and performance, short-term commitment, and independence from peers.

Personal Development A mentoring process associated with positively shaping a protégé's attitude about the context or environment. Focused on emphasizing values, esprit de corps, and camaraderie in the working environment so that an individual becomes more fully invested or committed to the organization and/or the mentor and associated leaders.

Personality-Based Appraisal Systems Older performance-appraisal systems through which managers are required to make personality judgments they are not qualified to make and cannot easily defend. They do not focus on how an employee performs relative to an objective standard. An evaluator can freely use personal opinions, unsupported judgments, and personal biases on evaluations.

Physician–Hospital Organization (PHO) A joint venture between one or more hospitals and a group of physicians. It acts as the single agent for managed care contracting, presenting a united front to payers. In some cases, the PHO provides selected administrative services.

Plural Organization The second stage of development in managing cultural diversity. It is still characterized by assimilation of diverse others, but has greater structural and informal integration of diverse employees, less prejudice and discrimination, smaller gaps in employee identification with the organization, and an increase of intergroup conflict due to greater heterogeneity of the workforce.

Position Analysis Questionnaire (PAQ) A 300-item questionnaire that consists of worker-oriented items focused on generalized job activities. It looks at the extent to which certain tasks are involved in the performance of the analyzed job.

Portfolio Assessment The analysis of the portfolio of SBUs operated by the firm examines the service mix of an organization to determine if the overall array of business units is appropriately balanced.

Establishes priorities and allocation of resources for the business units by comparing the anticipated future performance of all business areas.

Positioning The process of defining how an organization wishes its services to be perceived by consumers in relation to competitors providing the service.

Product Life-Cycle The progression of life stages in an organization, including development, growth, maturity, and decline of a service, business unit, or industry because of changes in demand for the service, number of competitors, profitability, cash flow, and other features of market conditions.

Protected Groups Groups that are protected by the Civil Rights Act against discrimination based on race, color, religion, sex, national origin, or pregnancy.

Public Policy Exception An exception to the employment-at-will doctrine that states that an employee has a legal claim for wrongful discharge if the employee is terminated for activity that is protected by a specific state law.

Reasonable Accommodation Any type of modification provided to enable a disabled individual to perform the job that does not cause undue hardship to the company.

Rehabilitation Act of 1973 Forbids discrimination in employment of the disabled, including advertising, recruitment, processing of applications, promotions, pay rates, fringe benefits, and work assignments.

Relative Value Units The relative value unit was established to quantify the relative work, practice expense, and malpractice costs for specific physician services to appropriately establish payment.

Reliability A measure of the extent to which a test can be expected to yield dependable and repeatable results for candidates. Reliability is measured by a reliability coefficient.

Righting-the-Wrongs Approach A diversity approach that targets groups who have suffered past discrimination and attempts to compensate for past injustices.

Rituals The habitual and customary approaches to work that convey and sustain culture, such as meetings, strategic planning, and the process of budgeting.

Role of Governance To create policies that drive strategy development and to oversee management to ensure those policies are maintained.

Role of Management To develop and execute the strategy.

Sarbanes-Oxley Act Increased the accountalty of management and governance in ensuring proper accounting, financial reporting, and internal control. Publicly owned companies have invested heavily to develop systems to increase this accountability and to obtain the assurance of external auditing firms related to these systems.

Selection Process Conducting a job analysis to determine the tasks to be performed and the qualifications required to perform them, determining the criteria for predicting employee effectiveness, deciding on a valid and reliable selection instrument, and using the instrument to select new employees.

Severance Package A continuity of salary and benefits for some specified period of time for employees terminated through no fault of their own.

Sexual Harassment Unwelcome sexual advances, requests for sexual favors, and other verbal or physical harassment. Conduct of a sexual nature when this conduct explicitly or implicitly affects an individual's employment; unreasonably interferes with an individual's work performance; or creates an intimidating, hostile, or offensive work environment. Sexual harassment includes a quid pro quo form where improved work benefits or conditions are dependent on the provision of sexual favors.

Single-Job Competency Model Approach An approach to developing a competency model that involves identifying a single critical job, collecting and analyzing data pertaining to that job, then aggregating the data into a competency model composed of an average of 8-15 competencies that include traits, knowledge, or skills, each with a definition and a list of specific behaviors.

Six Sigma Method that seeks to improve quality by identifying and eliminating defects and errors in any business process. "Sigma" is a statistical term that stands for the standard deviation from the mean in a normal distribution. Six Sigma corresponds to 3.4 million defects per million.

Skill Capacity, facility, or dexterity acquired through experience or training.

Skill-Based Training Skill based training involves initiatives targeted at the development at specific skills required for effective leadership.

Social Maintenance Activities Activities designed to meet employee needs in order to keep them from leaving or unionizing.

Straight Ranking A comparative performance method that lists employees, beginning with the strongest employee and ending with the weakest employee. This method utilizes overall job proficiency on predetermined job dimensions or characteristics.

Strategic Business Units (SBUs) The operational subunits of an organization responsible for specific sets of activities and products.

Strategic Compensation Management Linking a compensation system to the mission and strategies of the organization by assessing current compensation systems and their influence on behaviors, generating a strategy that identifies behaviors needed to meet the organization's goals, and designing and implementing a compensation system that rewards the behaviors necessary to obtain desired strategic outcomes.

Strategic Human Resource Management The management process of generating and implementing human resource policies and practices to supply the complement of employee skills, knowledge, and abilities required by an organization to attain its strategic aspirations.

Strategic Management The planning approach that is concerned with integration among administrative systems, organizational structure, and organizational culture for both strategic and operational decision making. This approach views strategic planning as one element of administrative functioning that must be blended with other management processes for an organization to function efficiently.

Strategic Planning The planning approach popular in the 1970s that defines a firm's strategy so that internal resources and skills are matched to the opportunities and risks created in the workforce environment. It involves an organization's choices of mission, objectives, strategy, policies, programs, goals, and major resources allocations. It focuses on the examination of past trends and the extrapolation of future trends based on those past trends.

Strategic Thinking Strategic thinking is a method of thinking that takes place before strategic planning and that encourages intuitive, innovative, and creative thinking at all levels of the organization.

Strong Culture A culture with a dominant and unified set of shared assumptions is adhered to consistently by the majority of members throughout the organization.

Succession Planning Leadership development activities employed by an organization that lead to the identification of a replacement for existing executives in advance of their turnover.

Supervisor-Only Based Appraisal Systems Typical performance-appraisal process involving rating of subordinates by a single supervisor, with the assumption that supervisors are objective in assessing their subordinates. Unfortunately, the performance assessment of employees by their supervisors has been found to suffer from numerous perceptual biases, such as the recency, halo, horn, similar-to-me, and leniency effects.

Talent Acquisition Function The evidence-based process of systematically using information about positions and candidates to make informed decisions about who is most likely to be successful in which roles.

Team Training Team training is a form of leadership development that occurs when members of a team interact, bringing various experiences, skills, and knowledge to the team processes.

Technical Competencies Competencies involving a particular skill or set of skills that are specific to a particular job family. Some are broadly shared across many different roles. One example in health care is the management of pain.

Three-Legged Stool This classic view of hospital activities prescribes specific roles for the board of directors, hospital administration, and the medical staff. The board establishes overall policy and provides access to community funds. Administration is responsible for day-to-day operations of the hospital. Physicians have the autonomous role of overseeing clinical services.

Time-and-Motion Studies Studies aimed at making jobs more efficient and effective. Time studies focus on the amount of time it takes to complete various job aspects, while motion studies examine the sequence of steps performed to complete a job.

Total Quality Management (TQM) A philosophy used to improve organizational processes through structured problem-solving statistical methods, the use of interdisciplinary teams, the empowerment of employees, and a focus on internal and external customers.

Training Activities geared toward improving or developing skills that an employee needs in his or her current position.

Training Motivation The direction, intensity, and persistence of learning-directed behavior in training contexts.

Undue Hardship Assessment of undue hardship may be based on unrealistic financial investment, number of employees insufficient to share job activities, inadequate safety provisions in the overall workforce, or some other significant impact on production or quality in the workplace.

Unfair Discrimination Making personnel decisions based on gender, race, ethnicity, age, or disability, which opens an organization up to potential lawsuits.

Uniform Guidelines on Employee Selection Procedures 1978 (UGESP) A set of specific requirements governing the development, implementation, and use of assessments for employee selection. UGESP was developed jointly by the U.S. Equal Employment Opportunity Commission, the Office of Personnel Management, the U.S. Department of Labor, and the U.S. Department of Justice to ensure consistency among the various Federal agencies regulating employment practices. Adherence to the detailed guidance in UGESP is absolutely critical when planning and administering talent-acquisition processes.

Validity The most important characteristic of any assessment. Validity measures how effectively an assessment measures the competency it is intended to measure. An assessment is valid if it measures a characteristic that is job relevant.

Values and Beliefs The second level of organizational culture. Values refer to the conscious outcomes that are considered desirable or meaningful to the organization. Beliefs are less of an aspiration and more of a conscious understanding of what is believed to be real and true in an organization.

Weighted Checklists Method An absolute-standards method through which the rater identifies and assigns a weight to each of the job tasks to be evaluated. The employee is then scored on each task to determine overall performance in the job.

Weak Culture A workplace culture that lacks consensus on, and commitment to, the overarching values, beliefs, and assumptions of the organization. Weak cultures emerge from the existence of splinter groups, conflicting subcultures, and a general lack of shared organization-wide values and assumptions.

Work-Oriented Methods Job-analysis methods that focus attention on tasks the worker performs, machines used, and the job context within the organization.

Worker-Oriented Methods Job analysis methods that identify what a person needs to successfully perform the job, such as the knowledge, skills, abilities, licensure requirements, and so on.

Workplace Diversity A business strategy that acknowledges diversity as a tool for success in the ever-changing environment of the future. It promotes a mix of people, skills, and cultures in the workplace that enables a range of viewpoints that challenge traditional thinking and results in a shift in people's values, attitudes, and beliefs.

Workforce Regulation Includes voluntary or self-imposed regulations by the profession, or may be governmental regulation at either the federal or state level in order to provide protection for the public against unscrupulous or unqualified individuals.

INDEX

Note: Page numbers followed by f or t refer to Figures or Tables.